Hospital Pharmacy

SECOND EDITION

Edited by
Martin Stephens   BPharm, MSc, MRPharmS, MCPP
Associate Medical Director, Clinical Effectiveness and Medicines Management
Southampton University Hospitals NHS Trust
Southampton, UK

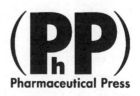

London • Chicago   **Pharmaceutical Press**

Published by Pharmaceutical Press

1 Lambeth High Street, London SE1 7JN, UK
1559 St. Paul Avenue, Gurnee, IL 60031, USA

© Royal Pharmaceutical Society of Great Britain 2011

(**P.P**) is a trade mark of Pharmaceutical Press

Pharmaceutical Press is the publishing division of the
Royal Pharmaceutical Society

First edition published 2003   ₁₀₀₆₃₆₂₉₂₉
Second edition 2011

Typeset by Thomson Digital, Noida, India
Printed in Great Britain by TJ International, Padstow, Cornwall

ISBN 978 0 85369 900 2

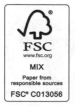

Dedication

Marjorie, thank you for your patient support.

Contents

Preface

This second edition of *Hospital Pharmacy* gathers texts on the key features of pharmaceutical services provided within and from hospital-based pharmacies in the UK. The focus falls on the National Health Service but a chapter is included on the independent sector where, within a different context, patient needs are not dissimilar. The book gives an introduction to the service, of benefit to preregistration graduates and to undergraduates. It also aims to be of benefit to recently qualified pharmacists undertaking further studies or those gaining training in rotational roles. Technicians in training or seeking broad insight into hospital pharmacy have also been considered in developing the book. As with the first edition, I trust the contents serve as a useful reference source for more experienced staff, in the UK and beyond. Indeed I hope anyone wishing to gain an understanding of pharmacy practice in UK hospitals will find the book of considerable help.

The book has been structured on functional lines; that is, there are chapters on purchasing, supply, clinical services, medicines information and so on. To some extent these boundaries are artificial and functions can be blurred; to give an example, the clinical responsibilities of a pharmacist ensuring the safe preparation and supply of total parenteral nutrition are not easily split into separate roles. However, there is a need to group in some way so a pragmatic approach has been taken.

Chapters have been included on education and training, research and development and on information technology; these make an impact on each of the other functions but they are also areas where special skills are required and indeed where specialist posts have been developed. Chapters new to the second edition include those on pharmacist prescribing, pharmacy services in mental health and consultant pharmacists.

Each chapter attempts to describe the ground to be covered, providing definitions where these assist. The historical context is set, followed by the detail of how hospital pharmacy is currently practised. Authors have also commented on any changes expected in the subject being discussed. Some key texts are suggested as further reading to support each chapter. I hope readers will gain benefit from the wide range of experience the authors have brought to the text and that the book is one which can be revisited regularly by hospital pharmacy staff and others.

Martin Stephens
December, 2010

About the editor

Martin Stephens graduated with a Bachelor of Pharmacy degree from the University of Nottingham in 1979, completing a preregistration year in South Warwickshire hospitals in 1980. He then worked in hospital pharmacy services in the West Midlands region, undertaking roles in medicines information, clinical services, community services, education and training, and dispensary management. In 1989 he became Chief Pharmacist at Wolverhampton Hospitals where he worked until 1997.

Martin was Chief Pharmacist at Southampton University Hospitals NHS trust from 1997 to 2006, where he supported the further development of clinical pharmacy, pharmacy technician roles and cross-sector collaboration on medicines management. He also held the role of clinical director for clinical support from 1998. In 2006 he became a divisional clinical director and director for clinical effectiveness. Then, in 2008, he became one of the first two national clinical directors in pharmacy at the Department of Health, whilst retaining an associate medical director role in Southampton. His masters is in health economics and management from Sheffield University. Martin is visiting principal lecturer at Portsmouth School of Pharmacy and has written *Strategic Medicines Management*, published by the Pharmaceutical Press.

Contributors

Nina Barnett   MSc, MRPharmS
Consultant Pharmacist, Care of Older People, Harrow Primary Care Trust and East and South East England Specialist Pharmacy Services, London, UK

Ian M Beaumont   BSc, MRPharmS
Director Quality Control North West, and Regional Quality Assurance Pharmacist for North West England, Stockport, UK

Trevor Beswick   BSc, MSc, MRPharmS
Director South West Medicines Information and Training, Bristol, UK

Alison Blenkinsopp   PhD, BPharm, FRPharmS, OBE
Professor of Pharmacy Practice, Keele University, Keele, UK

David Branford   PhD, MRPharmS
Chief Pharmacist, Derbyshire Mental Health Services NHS Trust, Derby, UK

Marie Brazil   BSc, DipClinPharm, MRPharmS
Consultant Pharmacist Haematology Services, Wirral University Teaching Hospitals NHS Foundation Trust, Wirral, UK

Gillian Cavell   MSc, MRPharmS
Consultant Pharmacist, Medication Safety, King's College Hospital NHS Foundation Trust, London, UK

Damian Child   BPharm, MSc, DipClinPharm, DipHospPharmMangt, MRPharmS
Chief Pharmacist, Sheffield Teaching Hospitals NHS Foundation Trust, Sheffield, UK

Jonathan Cooke   BPharm, MPharm, PhD, MRPharmS
Director of Pharmacy, University Hospital of South Manchester University NHS Foundation Trust, Manchester, UK

Phil Deady   MSc, MRPharmS
Procurement Pharmacist, Leeds Teaching Hospital NHS Trust, Leeds, UK.

Ray Fitzpatrick BSc, PhD, FRPharmS
Clinical Director of Pharmacy, The Royal Wolverhampton Hospitals NHS Trust, Wolverhampton, UK

Peter Golightly BSc, DLP(Clin Pharmacol), MRPharmS
Director Trent and West Midlands Medicines Information Services, Leicester, UK

Chris Green BSc, DipClinPharm
Director of Pharmacy and Medicines Management, Countess of Chester Hospitals NHS Foundation Trust, Chester, UK

Lyn Hanning MSc, MRPharmS
Senior Pharmacist, South West Medicines Information and Training, Bristol, UK

Karen Harrowing BPharm, BA, DpMgmt, CBiol, MSB, MRPharmS
Group Chief Pharmacist, Nuffield Health, New Malden, UK

Richard Hey BPharm, DMS, MRPharmS
Director of Pharmacy, Central Manchester University Hospitals NHS Foundation Trust, Manchester, UK

Don Hughes MSc, MRPharmS
Director of Pharmacy and Medicines Management, Central Area, Betsi Cadwaladr University Health Board, UK

Moira Kinnear BSc, MSc, MRPharmS
Head of Education, Research and Development, NHS Lothian Pharmacy Service and Lecturer in Clinical Practice, Strathclyde Institute of Pharmacy and Biomedical Science, Strathclyde, UK

Liz Mellor BPharm, MSc, MRPharmS
Clinical Governance Lead Pharmacist, Leeds Teaching Hospital NHS Trust, Leeds, UK

Christine Proudlove BPharm, MSc, DipPresSci, DipHospPharmMangt, MRPharmS
Director, North West Medicines Information Centre, Liverpool, UK

Pippa Roberts BSc, DipClinPharm, CertMangt, MSc
Clinical Director Pharmacy and Medicines Management, Wirral University Teaching Hospitals NHS Foundation Trust, Wirral, UK

Theresa Rutter   BSc, MSc, MRPharmS
Specialist Pharmacist, Community Health Services, London, UK

Graham Sewell   BPharm, PhD, MRPharmS, CBiol, MIBiol, CChem, MRSC
Head of School of Health Professions and Associate Dean (Research), University of Plymouth, Plymouth, UK

Ann Slee   BPharm, MSc, DipClinPharm, MRPharmS
Director of Pharmacy, University Hospitals Birmingham NHS Foundation Trust, Birmingham, UK

Martin Stephens   BPharm, MSc, MRPharmS, MCPP
Associate Medical Director Clinical Effectiveness and Medicines Management, Southampton University Hospitals NHS Trust, Southampton, UK

Howard Stokoe   BSc, MRPharmS MBE
Commercial Medicines Unit, Department of Health, Reading, UK

Mark Tomlin   BPharm, MSc, FRPharmS
Consultant Pharmacist, Critical Care, Southampton University Hospitals NHS Trust, Southampton, UK

Abbreviations

$5HT_2$	serotonin
ACLF	advanced and consultant-level framework
ADR	adverse drug reaction
AHP	allied health professional
AIDS	acquired immunodeficiency syndrome
AMS	antimicrobial stewardship
APC	area prescribing committee
AWMSG	All-Wales Medicines Strategy Group
BNF	*British National Formulary*
BSA	Business Services Authority
BTEC	Business and Technology Education Council
cc	complications and comorbidities
CD	controlled drug
CDAD	*Clostridium difficile*-associated diarrhoea
CHS	community health services
CIVAS	centralised intravenous additive services
CoDEG	Competency Development and Education Group
CPD	continuing professional development
CPH	collaborative procurement hub
CPOE	computerised physician order entry
CQC	Care Quality Commission
dm+d	Dictionary of Medicines and Devices
DMP	designated medical practitioner
DN	district nurse
D&T	drug and therapeutic
D&TC	drugs and therapeutics committees
DTC	Drugs and Therapeutic Centre
eMC	electronic Medicines Compendium
ePACT	electronic prescribing analysis and cost
EPR	electronic patient record
EU	European Union
FMEA	failure modes and effects analysis
GMP	good manufacturing practice
GP	general practitioner
HIV	human immunodeficiency virus
HRG	health resource group

HV	health visitor
IP	independent prescriber
IPR	intellectual property rights
IQ	intelligent quotient
IRMIS	Incident Reporting in Medicines Information System
IS ECN	Independent Sector Extended Choice Network
IS FCN	Independent Sector Free Choice Network
ISTC	independent sector treatment centre
IT	information technology
IV	intravenous
KPI	key performance indicator
LD	learning disability
LIMS	Laboratory Information Management Systems
LIN	local intelligence network
LNDG	London New Drugs Group
LSP	local service provider
MHRA	Medicines and Healthcare products Regulatory Agency
MHT	mental health trust
MI	medicines information
NDO	NewDrugsOnline
NeLM	National electronic Library for Medicines
NHS	National Health Service
NHS CFH	NHS Connecting for Health
NHSLA	National Health Service Litigation Authority
NHSTC	National Health Service treatment centre
NICE	National Institute for Health and Clinical Excellence
NPC	National Prescribing Centre
NPSA	National Patient Safety Agency
NPSG	National Pharmaceutical Supplies Group
NVQ	National Vocational Qualification
OJEC	*Official Journal of the European Community*
OTC	over-the-counter
P	pharmacy only
PACT	prescribing analysis and cost tabulation
PbR	payment by results
PCCPN	Primary and Community Care Pharmacy Network
PCT	primary care trust
PGDs	patient group directions
PIL	patient information leaflet
PL	product licence
PMSG	Pharmaceutical Market Support Group
POD	patients' own drug
POM	prescription-only medicine
PPRS	Pharmaceutical Price Regulation Scheme
PROM	patient-reported outcome measure
QA	quality assurance
QC	quality control
QIPP	quality, innovation, productivity, prevention

RAG	list red, amber, green list
RCA	root cause analysis
R&D	research and development
RPSGB	Royal Pharmaceutical Society of Great Britain
RSS	rich site summary
RWHT	Royal Wolverhampton hospitals trust
SCEP	Supply Chain Excellence Programme
SHA	strategic health authority
SLA	service level agreement
SMC	Scottish Medicines Consortium
SN	school nurse
SOP	standard operating procedure
SP	supplementary prescriber
TDM	therapeutic drug level monitoring
TPN	total parenteral nutrition
TQM	total quality management
UKAS	UK Accreditation Service
UKCPA	UK Clinical Pharmacy Association
UKMI	UK Medicines Information
UKPPG	UK Psychiatric Pharmacy Group
VAT	value-added tax
VTE	venous thromboembolism
w	with
WCPCT	Wolverhampton City primary care trust
w/o	without
WTEs	whole-time-equivalent posts

Introduction

'To begin at the beginning' would require a clear and commonly accepted definition of hospital pharmacy but that is problematic. Whilst there would be agreement on certain activities being 'pharmacy' undertaken in what is clearly a 'hospital', there has never been a definitive, universally accepted description of what hospital pharmacy comprises. Neither has there been a clear demarcation of what falls outside hospital pharmacy's remit. For example, does hospital pharmacy include dispensing for hospital outpatients? In Scotland, and in some English trusts, dispensing for hospital outpatients is not part of the service provided by the hospital pharmacy. Where such services do exist and are contracted to independent providers who deliver the service on site, perhaps that is seen as 'hospital pharmacy', but do the community pharmacies dispensing for hospital outpatients (via hospital FP10) consider themselves part of the hospital pharmacy service? And what about 'hospital at home' style of care comprising complex interventions, directed by hospital staff but delivered in the patient's home? Lack of a precise definition for hospital pharmacy is not unique to the UK. In his book on hospital pharmacy in the USA, Hassan used a 1951 American definition which describes a service under the direction of a pharmacist 'from which all medications are supplied', 'where special prescriptions are filled', where injectables 'should be prepared', where supplies are 'often stocked' – clearly room for some variation.[1]

So, a precise definition may not be available but would such a definition be helpful or desirable? Probably not – drawing very clear lines around a particular aspect of pharmacy practice may be useful for an editor deciding on the structure of a book but is of little relevance to recipients of pharmaceutical care. Indeed, in 2008 in its White Paper for pharmacy, *Pharmacy in England – Building on Strengths, Delivering the Future*, the Department of Health made the specific point that patients would be best served by a clinical pharmacy team that worked across the whole health community – doing away with the silo approach.[2] This, of course, parallels other pharmacy services that have previously delivered across organisational boundaries – medicines information, for example, answering queries for general practitioners and hospital consultants, undertaking critical appraisal of evidence for primary care organisations and for acute hospitals.

More important than a precise definition is a clear vision of the purpose of pharmacy services, services in this case provided in or from a hospital setting. Hospital pharmacy services are about providing high-quality patient care by bringing expertise on medicines to the healthcare team: in the words of the 2010 White Paper, *Equity and Excellence: Liberating the NHS*, 'optimising the use of medicines and [in] supporting better health'.[3] Hospital pharmacy is about ensuring safe use of medicines, about ensuring effective use of medicines and ensuring resources are used wisely – the cost-effective use of medicines. It encompasses preparation, procurement, provision and prescribing; it includes talking to patients about their medicines regimens, checking their understanding of how to use their medicines and involving them in the decision-making process about their medicines. Indeed, whilst the pharmacy team brings expertise about medicines it is vital that services are patient-focused, not pharmacocentric. The pharmacy team can also help provide advice to patients on broader healthy-living issues, such as diet, smoking cessation and so on.

These services are provided at individual and organisational levels, as well as anything in between. By this I mean that, as well as providing pharmaceutical care for individual patients, pharmacy services support organisational issues, be it the chief pharmacist advising on policy, the team developing a formulary or providing leadership on ensuring consistent provision of thromboprophylaxis. Nor does responsibility end at the organisation's door. Creating a community-wide clinical team has been mentioned; there is also a need to ensure patients are transferred safely between care settings. For pharmacy this includes ensuring continuity of supply of medicines and the provision of timely, accurate, explanatory information about medicines at discharge from hospital. There is also a need to work closely with primary care on the choice of medicines normally used – working with, not against local programmes for cost-effective prescribing.

In 2008, work on a generally accepted vision of pharmacy practice in a hospital setting was discussed at the International Pharmacy Federation. The consensus statements were published early in 2009.[4] The first of the overarching statements was: 'The overarching goal of hospital pharmacists is to optimise patient outcomes through judicious, safe, efficacious, appropriate, and cost-effective use of medicines'.

A further 74 statements followed, overarching and more specific, where the majority of delegates (90.4% or more) had indicated their support: not defining hospital pharmacy but certainly helping to build consensus around the key vision for pharmacy's contribution.

Though no precise definition of hospital pharmacy exists, in pursuit of the vision, a number of attempts have been made over the years in the UK to set out reasonable standards for delivering hospital pharmacy. In the 1980s the English Regional Pharmaceutical Officers developed standards for the service: the second edition (1989) contained 28 areas of practice.[5] These standards describe what is expected if a specified service is present; the standards mention purchase, supply, clinical and medicines information amongst others. Similarly, the Chief Administrative Pharmaceutical Officers in Wales drew up a standards document, which was developed into a document describing the constituents of a comprehensive pharmaceutical service and which supported audit against the standards set.[6]

In addition to these pharmacy-specific standards, there are of course elements relating to pharmacy in more general regulatory standards, such as those overseen by the Care Quality Commission, as well as more service-specific requirements such as for aseptic dispensing services. Regulatory or accreditation standards have an impact on pharmacy practice elsewhere, such as those of the Joint Commission in the USA, but a discussion of these issues goes beyond the scope of this text. However, it is worth noting that the second of the Basel statements, mentioned earlier, proposes that good hospital pharmacy practice evidence-based guidelines should be developed to help define standards and scope of hospital pharmacy practice.

The remainder of the book will explore the various elements of hospital pharmacy practice and how these services seek to deliver safe, effective and cost-effective use of medicines, including the vital specialist services such as quality assurance and provision of radiopharmaceuticals, and underpinning services such as education and training.

Progressing to 21st-century hospital pharmacy

In the first edition of this text, five key documents were set out as key shapers for hospital pharmacy practice: (1) the Noel Hall report;[7] (2) the Nuffield report;[8] (3) the *Way Forward* health circulars across Scotland, Wales and England (HC88s);[9] (4) *Pharmacy in the Future*[10] (along with *The Right Medicine: A Strategy for Pharmaceutical Care in Scotland*[11] and work from the Wales task and finish group;[12]) and (5) the Audit Commission document *A Spoonful of Sugar,* from 2001.[13] In essence, these documents supported the pioneering work that took pharmacy from 'safe suppliers of medicines' to the more complete clinical teams with which we are now familiar. Not losing our scientific underpinning, not giving up our role in safe provision, but becoming clinicians, members of the wider healthcare team.

Pharmacy in the Future focused on meeting the needs of patients, getting the most from medicines and using the pharmacist's expertise.[10] Re-engineering hospital pharmacy services to deliver the best standards was emphasised: 'one-stop dispensing' (see Chapter 4), self-administration and pharmacists working on admission wards are given as examples of good practice. Pharmacist prescribing was proposed as a way of using pharmacists' skills and giving a better service for patients, Chapter 10 of this edition sets out how that moved from proposal to practice – even if, at the time of writing, it is still relatively limited.

The Audit Commission's 2001 document *A Spoonful of Sugar*[13] recommendations included: to invest in electronic prescribing and automated dispensing; to ensure enough pharmacy staff for clinical pharmacy; to ensure all hospital staff are trained for their roles with medicines; to introduce one-stop dispensing; and to use original packs. A decade later we can see that some progress has been made, but there remains much to do.

In 2007 the Healthcare Commission reflected on the progress made in England since the 2001 report in its document *The Best Medicine*.[14] It noted: 'there has been investment in the amount of direct care provided by clinical pharmacy staff and the audit on wards demonstrated the contribution that this service makes to the safe and effective care of patients'. But the report also noted slow progress on automation and on electronic prescribing (more properly described as electronic prescribing and administration systems perhaps). The report also noted that waiting for medicines at discharge caused delay – 61% of patients experienced a delay, stating awaiting medicines was the cause. Hospital pharmacy readers may at this point be tempted to cite: 'take-home medicines are given as an excuse' or 'but it's the prescriber'. Both are probably true, but if pharmacy are the medicines experts and patient experience of care is important, then pharmacy needs to establish a system that works, with medicines ready when the patient needs them.

The Best Medicine focused on acute and specialist hospitals. Also published in 2007 was *Talking about Medicines*, the Healthcare Commission's report on the management of medicines in mental health trusts (Chapter 13 discusses these services in greater detail).[15] The specific needs of provision of medicines to mental health trusts were acknowledged. Clinical pharmacy contributions on safety were just as frequent as for acute wards, though staffing levels were seen as lower and with fewer pharmacy technicians and other supporting staff. Greater involvement of service users and of their carers in decisions about and use of medicines was stated as a key goal, along with multiprofessional working, good access to clinical pharmacy and training for staff in medicines.

Just as these documents followed up on earlier audit work, *Managing the Use of Medicines, A Follow-up Review,* published in 2009, provided a similar follow-up for Scotland.[16] Its key recommendations had parallels to those in England – e-prescribing plans to be developed, a national framework for recognising and accrediting extended roles for pharmacy technicians. In addition, the need for centrally collated and analysed data on secondary care medicines use was recognised, as well as the need for better workforce planning. The former is now being addressed in the Hospital Medicines Utilisation Database.[17]

Pharmacy in England in 2008 also addressed these themes, setting out the need for use of information technology and automation, and the need to consider training and workforce development.[2] As mentioned earlier, it also set out the important aim of developing a more integrated approach across primary and secondary care. A further issue, not yet covered, was the document's signalling of the key leadership role that chief pharmacists have in ensuring that 'safe medication practices are embedded in patient care', clearly demonstrating that pharmacy's role on medicines is not just within the department's walls but encompasses the whole organisation, providing a lead that brings along medical, nursing and other healthcare professions as well as general management.

Conclusion

This introduction has touched on a few of the documents that have helped shape hospital pharmacy's progress. There have been other developments and policy documents not covered here that have provided opportunities and challenges, for example, the development of pharmacist prescribers, the arrival of consultant pharmacists, the responsible pharmacist regulations; these issues are important and will be picked up during the course of this book.

At the time of writing, the National Health Service (NHS) faces a challenging future after a period of significant investment. In England, it also faces a major programme of organisational change. Hospital pharmacy practice will be significantly affected by these challenges. There has not been a time when the importance of delivering the right outcomes for patients and doing so safely and cost-effectively has been greater. This is pharmacy's agenda – good medicines use has a central role in reducing hospital admissions, in preventing harm and in achieving good outcomes, and pharmacy can help ensure the medicines budget is used to maximise health gains. The pharmacy team can also contribute to the health and well-being aspects of prevention. In making these contributions hospital pharmacy will also need to ensure it sets its own house in order – achieving cost-effective skill mix, providing patient-focused services, being available when needed (not just during office hours) and using technologies and improvement techniques to streamline services. The hospital pharmacy team also needs to be outward-looking – to hospital colleagues and to the primary care team. All these challenges apply irrespective of the organisational arrangements, whether these are the various models of NHS organisation across the four UK countries or whether pharmacy services are being provided in and by NHS bodies or by independent sector organisations.

Hospital pharmacy practice must respond to its changing environment and develop new ways of working as information technology moves forward. With skilled staff and leaders with vision there is no reason to doubt this can happen so that patients continue to benefit from the vital contribution the pharmacy team makes.

References

1. Hassan W. *Hospital Pharmacy*, 5th edn. Philadelphia: Lea and Febiger, 1986.
2. Department of Health. *Pharmacy in England – Building on Strengths, Delivering the Future.* London: Department of Health, 2008.
3. Department of Health. *Equity and Excellence: Liberating the NHS*. London: Department of Health, 2010.
4. The Basel statements on the future of hospital pharmacy. *Am J Health-Syst Pharm* 2009; 66: S61–S66.
5. Regional Pharmaceutical Officers' Committee. *Standards for Pharmaceutical Services in Health Authorities in England*, 2nd edn. London: Regional Pharmaceutical Officers' Committee, 1989.
6. Morgan D, Way C (eds) *Standards for Pharmaceutical Services in Health Authorities and Trusts in Wales*. Cardiff: Directors of Pharmaceutical Public Health and Chief Pharmacists' Committee (Wales), 1997.
7. Hall N, chair. *Report of the Working Party Investigating the Hospital Pharmaceutical Service*. London: HMSO, 1970.
8. Clucas K, chair. *Pharmacy: The Report of a Committee of Inquiry Appointed by the Nuffield Foundation*. London: The Nuffield Foundation, 1986.
9. Department of Health. *The Way Forward for Hospital Pharmaceutical Services*. HC88(54). London: Department of Health, 1988. Also WHC 88(66) (Wales) 1988 and 1988 (GEN) 32 in Scotland.
10. Department of Health. *Pharmacy in the Future*. London: Department of Health, 2000.
11. Scottish Executive. *The Right Medicine: A Strategy for Pharmaceutical Care in Scotland*. Edinburgh: Scottish Executive, 2002.
12. National Assembly for Wales. *Report of the Task and Finish Group on Prescribing*. Cardiff: National Assembly for Wales, 2000.
13. Audit Commission. *A Spoonful of Sugar – Medicines Management in NHS Hospitals*. London: Audit Commission, 2001.
14. Healthcare Commission, *The Best Medicine, The Management of Medicines in Acute and Specialist Trusts*. London: Healthcare Commission, 2007.
15. Healthcare Commission. *Talking about Medicines, The Management of Medicines in Trusts Providing Mental Health Services*. London: Healthcare Commission, 2007.
16. Audit Scotland. *Managing the Use of Medicines, A Follow-up Review*. Edinburgh: Audit Scotland, 2009.
17. Scottish Health Information Service, Hospital Medicines Utilisation Database website: http://www.isdscotland.org/isd/6123.html.

Further reading

Audit Scotland. *Managing the Use of Medicines, A Follow up Review*. Edinburgh: Audit Scotland, 2009.
Care Quality Commission. *Guidance about Compliance: Essential Standards of Quality and Safety. Outcome 9: Management of Medicines*. London: Care Quality Commission, 2010.

Department of Health. *Pharmacy in England – Building on Strengths, Delivering the Future.* London: Department of Health, 2008.

Healthcare Commission. *The Best Medicine, The Management of Medicines in Acute and Specialist Trusts.* London: Healthcare Commission, 2007.

The Basel statements on the future of hospital pharmacy. *Am J Health-Syst Pharm* 2009; 66: S61–S66.

1

Hospital pharmacy within the National Health Service

Martin Stephens

The National Health Service (NHS) is a large and complex organisation, responsible for the great majority of healthcare provided in the UK. Spending, at time of writing, is around £120 billion, over 8% of gross domestic product. The NHS has a workforce of over $1^1/_2$ million, including around 7500 pharmacists (this figure is for employees and excludes pharmacists delivering NHS services in community pharmacy). The responsibility for health is one devolved to the administrations in Northern Ireland, Scotland and Wales and, whilst there is much commonality in provision, there are significant structural differences across the UK. This chapter will summarise the current NHS organisational structures before describing the typical NHS acute hospital trust structure. Having established the context it will describe the range of staff and roles within hospital pharmacy and exemplify career pathways for pharmacists in the NHS.

History

The NHS became a reality in the UK on 5 July 1948. It provided general practitioner (GP) and hospital care, free at the point of delivery on the basis of need. There was optimism that good healthcare would mean a healthier nation and thus a decreasing demand for health spending. This hope of reduced demand has not been fulfilled, with demographic change, increased expectation and the ability to do more meaning an ever-increasing requirement for funding. An early response to this increase was the introduction of fees – prescription charges and dental treatments. However, the majority of care has remained free, with the NHS funded from general taxation. The 2010 White Paper, *Equity and Excellence,* reconfirmed the coalition government's commitment to a comprehensive service free at the point of use based on clinical need.[1]

Twenty-six years after its formation, the first of the major reorganisations of the NHS in England took place; the 1974 change was preceded by changes in the service in Wales and Scotland. In England, a triple-layer NHS was established above the individual hospitals. Regional health authorities (14 in all) were made responsible for area health authorities (90) which, in turn, managed district management teams (206). Within area health authorities, a parallel structure of family practitioner committees overseeing general practice was established. This change gave the opportunity to organise pharmacy services beyond individual hospitals, creating cooperation in an area pharmaceutical service along the lines of the Noel Hall report.[2]

During the 1980s and 1990s further changes occurred with area health authorities removed and general management brought in by the Griffiths report.[3] This change resulted in a reduction of the influence of senior medical and nursing staff within hospitals, with decision-making moving to general managers. A very different climate has prevailed in more recent times, retaining strong leadership but bringing clinicians in as key partners with general managers. The NHS and Community Care Act in 1990 introduced purchasers and providers of care. This split meant that responsibility for delivering healthcare (the operations, the clinics, and so on) and arranging healthcare for local populations (setting the targets for how many operations, asking for certain new services) was divided between different organisations that no longer had a direct management link. Hospitals, community health services and ambulance services became trusts. Trusts had more local control to allow them to work within the 'market' and to arrange their own finances. General practices could become fund-holding, responsible for their prescribing budget, arranging and paying for elective surgery (planned work such as hernia repairs and hip operations) and for practice staff. Though never a true 'market', there were opportunities for GPs to change the hospital to which they referred patients. This 'internal market' was criticised for creating a raft of invoicing and activity-counting.

In 1997, a Labour government was elected with a commitment to 'put right' the NHS. The internal market was abolished but with no return to line management controls from the centre. A 'third way' of partnership and collaboration was to be brought in. A White Paper *The New NHS: Modern, Dependable* set out the revised structure.[4] The purchaser–provider split was to stay, as were hospital trusts, but fund-holding was abolished, replaced by primary care groups that could evolve to primary care trusts (PCTs). In addition to these structural changes, the issues of quality of care and of health inequalities and reducing avoidable deaths were raised in *A First Class Service*.[5] and *Our Healthier Nation*.[6] The 'new NHS' saw the terminology of the market removed. Service agreements replaced contracts and purchasing was replaced by commissioning.

In 2001, further significant changes to the structure of the NHS in England were identified in the document *Shifting the Balance of Power Within the NHS: Securing Delivery*.[7] PCTs became the norm and strategic health authorities were established (28 at first, later reduced to 10). During the following years, further steps were taken to improve the NHS, though with the devolved responsibilities the changes were for England, with an increasing difference between the other UK countries.

In 2002 the Secretary of State for Health announced the plan to create foundation trusts – NHS organisations that would have greater freedoms, including the freedom from health authority performance management. The first foundation trusts came into existence in 2004, though perhaps the freedoms first envisaged were rather weaker in reality.[8]

At the same time as these structural changes, the NHS saw very significant levels of investment. Government had made a commitment to see NHS expenditure grow in real terms and to reach European average as a percentage of gross domestic product. Redesign around the needs of the patient was a recurring phrase. Many targets for change on both broad and detailed levels were set out:

- reduced waiting times; for example, no more than a 6-month wait for an operation, to be achieved by 2005, later further reduced to an 18-week maximum by the later 2000s
- maximum waiting time for accident and emergency departments – 98% of patients to be sent home or to a ward within 4 hours
- national standards to see good care everywhere
- best-practice spread, supported by the National Institute for Health and Clinical Excellence (NICE)
- more patient and user involvement in the NHS
- breaking the demarcation barriers between professions, including allowing nurses and pharmacists to prescribe
- significant investment and significant expectations.

Creating the additional capacity to reduce waiting lists also led to the creation of independent sector treatment centres – privately run facilities providing NHS care, commissioned by PCTs. By 2005 there were around 25 such centres. Chapter 2 deals with this in greater detail.

Payment by results

An important reform during this period was the introduction of a new system of paying providers for the care they provide. Historically, hospitals were paid through to block contracts, a fixed sum of money for a broadly stated service, or possibly cost and volume contracts which attempted to specify in more detail payment that related to levels of activity. However, in block contracts there was no incentive for providers to increase activity, since they received no additional funding. *The NHS Plan* set out the government's intention to link the allocation of funds to hospitals with the activity they undertake.[9] It stated that in order to get the best from extra resources there would be significant changes to the way money flows around the NHS. Hospitals would be paid for the elective activity they undertake according to a fixed tariff price (worked out as an average price, then adjusted year on year). This was announced by the Department of Health in 2002 as the payment by results (PbR) system. PbR was implemented incrementally: the system began in a small way in 2003–2004, was extended in 2004–2005, and, for the majority of trusts, included only elective care in 2005–2006. In 2006–2007 PbR was extended to include non-elective, accident and emergency, outpatient and emergency admissions for all acute trusts.

The tariff price, which of course varies between type of admission, covers all the costs of that admission. Thus for a hip replacement, the cost of surgeon, nursing care, physiotherapist, anaesthetics, antibiotics and prothesis is included in the price paid. There is also a sum included for the buildings and all other direct and indirect overheads. For each episode of care there will be a contribution for the pharmacy team, the running of the aseptic unit and so on.

For pharmacy, there is a particularly important aspect of PbR – the tariff exclusions.[10] Where medicines would make a dispropotionate element of the episode of care (admission, outpatient visit) the medicine is excluded from tariff, and the commissioning organisation pays for the medicine separately. At the time of writing, cancer chemotherapy, antitumour necrosis factor medicines, intravenous immunoglobulins, along with many others, are tariff exclusions. Significant efforts are required to ensure appropriate data are collected and recharges made; equally PCTs are keen to scrutinise the use of these medicines to ensure only appropriate payments are made.

The Next Stage Review

In 2007 the health minister, Lord Darzi, set out in an interim report the vision for the NHS for the following 10 years.[11] The vision was for an NHS that is fair, personalised, effective and safe. The point was made that there had been significant investment over the previous decade and the time had come to create a world-class service. After further work, the following year *High Quality Care for All, NHS Next Stage Review Final Report* was published – coinciding with the NHS's 60th anniversary.[12] The focus was very much on quality – quality as the guiding principle of the NHS, with a definition of quality that includes safety, effectiveness and patient experience. Table 1.1 sets out some of the key issues from the report and Table 1.2 gives more information on the three elements of quality. The document emphasised the

Table 1.1 Key issues from the *Next Stage Review*, final report[11]

Overarching theme	Detail
High-quality care for patients and the public	Focus on staying healthy • Well-being and preventive services • Bringing in private and voluntary sectors to improve health outcomes • Vascular risk assessment programme • Support for keeping healthy at work • Support GPs to help families stay healthy Give more rights and control to patients • Allow greater choice of GP practice • A constitution that gives the right of choice over where treatments are provided • Develop personalised care plans for those with long-term conditions • Explore personal health budgets • Guarantee access to NICE-approved treatments
Quality at the heart of the NHS	Getting the basics right – reducing healthcare-acquired infections NICE to set quality standards Measure and publish information on quality of care Alter payments system to support quality Increase clinical involvement in leadership Support innovation Increase uptake of innovative and cost-effective medicines Create academic centres
Work in partnership with staff	Encourage GP commissioning Improve community health services Develop clinicians as leaders No new targets Improved training opportunities

GP, general practitioner; NICE, National Institute for Health and Clinical Excellence; NHS, National Health Service.

Table 1.2 Quality defined by *Next Stage Review*[11] and used in 2010 White Paper[1]

Element	Meaning
Safety	Care provided safely, avoiding causing harm
Effectiveness	Achieving the desired outcomes, interventions that work
Patient experience	Patients involved in decision-making, given choice, treated with respect and dignity

importance of clinical leadership, pointing out that clinical staff have three key aspects to their roles: (1) providing direct care; (2) working with others and in the team; and (3) working as leaders. Pharmacists were clearly included as clinicians along with nurses and allied health professionals.

The NHS from 2010

For England, the Secretary of State for Health has responsibility for the NHS and for leading the Department of Health. In Scotland the NHS is a devolved responsibility; the Scottish parliament has legislative power and the minister for health and community care is responsible for the service. In Wales the National Assembly has responsibility for the NHS. Within the Welsh Assembly government, the Health and Social Services Secretary is lead for the service. A similar pattern applies in Northern Ireland where there is a Department of Health, Social Services and Public Safety.

England

At the time of writing, the NHS in England faces a period of very significant change. The White Paper, *Equity and Excellence – Liberating the NHS*,[1] and the supporting consultation papers, set out wide-ranging structural changes, though there is a clear intent to build upon the work of the *Next Stage Review* undertaken by Lord Darzi.[12] Strategic health authorities and PCTs will be abolished and GP consortia will be responsible for commissioning care from providers. All hospital trusts will become foundation trusts, perhaps nearer to their original design. The process-based targets, such as waiting lists, are to be replaced by outcomes measures with the Secretary of State monitoring health outcomes to see how the NHS is performing. Public health will take a more prominent role, keeping people healthy rather than simply investing to deal with illness; this is set out in the White Paper *Healthy Lives, Healthy People: our strategy for public health in England*.[13] Regulation of healthcare will be in the hands of Monitor (the economic regulator originally set up to regulate foundation trusts) and of the Care Quality Commission (CQC). CQC was established in 2009, replacing the Healthcare Commission, and regulates health and social care (for additional information see www.cqc.org.uk). Their role is to ensure 'better care is provided for everyone', which they do through a licensing system, supported by inspection and in accordance with standards. Within their guidance for health organisations, outcome 9 addresses medicines.[14]

The White Paper, *Equity and Excellence – Liberating the NHS*,[1] detailed the difficult financial challenge facing the NHS in 2010 following banking rescues and a period of recession. Whilst year-on-year investment was promised, the investment would be below that of earlier years and not at a pace that met expected new demand. The planned response was QIPP – quality, innovation, productivity, prevention.[15] In essence, increasing the quality of care to reduce costs, for example improving medicines use in asthma could prevent admissions, in all reducing the spend on care.

The White Paper also confirmed the NHS constitution, first set out in 2009, that sets out the rights and responsibilities for patients and staff using or working in the NHS.[16] The right to receive medicines approved by NICE if they are considered appropriate for the individual is enshrined in the document.

Scotland

The responsibility for NHS Scotland and for the development and implementation of health and community care policy lies with the Scottish Government Health Directorate. There are 14 NHS boards, each responsible for planning health services for its local population, with the chief executive for NHS Scotland accountable to the government for the service. Additionally, the Scottish Ambulance service and NHS 24 (the helpline for access to medical advice) is part of their responsibility. The provider–commissioner split developed in England does not play a part in NHS Scotland.

In 2010, the Scottish government published *The Healthcare Quality Strategy for NHS Scotland,* setting out the way in which high-quality care would be achieved – care that is compassionate, with clear communications, in clean environments, where there is collaboration, continuity of care and clinical excellence.[17] Specific mention is made of the need to have medicines reconciliation in place for transfers of care.

Wales

The NHS in Wales underwent a major reorganisation in 2009. The trust–health board split previously in place was removed, creating seven health boards, each responsible for organising and delivering all healthcare for its population. The stated aim was that by replacing the market-style approach, which remains in England, a better-coordinated NHS could be developed. In addition to the health boards are three trusts: (1) the Welsh Ambulance Services Trust for emergency services; (2) Velindre NHS Trust, providing specialist services in cancer care and other national support services; and (3) Public Health Wales.

Northern Ireland

There is much closer working between health and social care in Northern Ireland than in Britain. The four health and social service boards work in a similar way to health authorities in England (pre-2002) but with the addition of a social care remit. They commission services for their local population from health and social service provider organisations.

Hospital pharmacy within the NHS

Published in 2000, *Pharmacy in the Future* was the document dealing with the specific issues relating to pharmacy playing its part in the NHS for the future in

England.[18] In 2008, *Pharmacy in England, Building on Strengths, Delivering the Future* set out further plans for pharmacy's development.[19] A wide range of commitments was made, including those pertinent to hospital pharmacy. The need to ensure safe transfer of care, to develop clinical pharmacy teams across organisational boundaries and the very clear signal that chief pharmacists must focus on safe use of medicines were included. The document also announced the appointment of two National Clinical Directors, for hospital pharmacy and for primary care and community pharmacy. Aspects of this important White Paper will be recurring themes in later chapters.

NHS hospital trusts

NHS hospital trusts do not have one simple organisational pattern. Foundation trusts have specific requirements to develop memberships from which to elect a board of governors. However, the day-to-day responsibility for the trust (its finances, organisation, and so on) falls to a second board – the board of directors. Both boards are led by the trust's chair. The board of directors comprises the executives of the trust and a group of non-executives. The executives are officers of the trust, usually full-time staff with a management responsibility. The non-executives are lay members of the board with a limited time commitment to their NHS role. The non-executives have a role in ensuring that the trust meets its obligations as a public body, and in providing advice and support to the executive. The executive members of the board typically include the chief executive, the medical director, the nursing director and the finance director. Other executives can be a general manager (deputy chief executive, for example) or a human resources lead for the trust. A director of planning and, increasingly, of modernisation may also be included.

The trust will then have a group that oversees its strategic and operational management. This would be the executives joined by other senior managers in the trust. Size and membership of this group will vary between trusts; often there will be clinical representation beyond the nursing and medical directors. *A Spoonful of Sugar*[20] recommended that the chief pharmacist should have influence at this level; chief pharmacists are more likely to be included if they head a directorate or division, perhaps representing other non-medical groups.

The trust will then be organised into a number of manageable groups, typically divisions or directorates or care groups. Divisions group together a range of services led by a management team or general manager. An example of a division would be surgical specialties, which could include general surgery, orthopaedics, ophthalmology and gynaecology. In larger trusts a division may include over 1000 staff and have a budget of tens of millions, with a drug spend of several millions. A directorate or care group structure would be along similar lines but, as the name suggests, a larger number of smaller

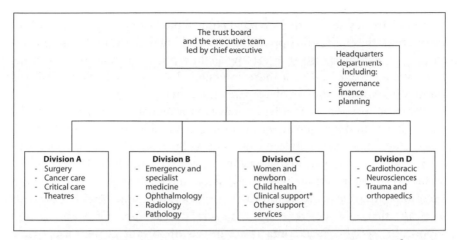

Figure 1.1 Southampton University Hospitals National Health Service trust structure. *, Includes pharmacy.

groupings. Orthopaedics, child health and general medicine could each form its own directorate. Figure 1.1 shows the divisional structure for Southampton University Hospitals NHS trust in 2010.

The management groupings of the organisation (directorate or division) would typically have a mixture of general, financial and clinical management input. Usually a senior nurse as well as a doctor would be part of the management team. Information officers, planners and governance leads would also support the business of the directorate or division.

Pharmacy's place in a trust

The move to involve doctors in management of trusts in the 1990s often left pharmacy as a loose end. No single structure has emerged as the way in which pharmacy should fit into a hospital's organisation. In a directorate structure a large pharmacy service could stand alone, headed by the chief pharmacist, although the size of budget, even in larger departments (£5–10 million, excluding drugs), would be small for a typical directorate. Combination with other non-medically led services such as physiotherapy or dietetics has been a path followed in a number of trusts. Chief pharmacists may act as clinical lead or general manager for these groupings. Another model is where a general manager, possibly at executive level, has responsibility for a range of services that includes pharmacy. Grouping pharmacy with other non-bed-holding specialties such as pathology, theatres and radiology in clinical support divisions is also possible. Whatever the structure, it is important that the chief pharmacist has responsibility for the service and the way in which medicines are used in the trust, having access to the executive team when necessary and contributing to the governance group for the trust.

The development of clinical pharmacy has led to staff specialising in various clinical areas. There are examples of pharmacists moving from a central pharmacy service to individual clinical directorates or divisions. This can increase the ability and opportunity of working with the multidisciplinary team and for specialists to feel ownership for their pharmacy service. However, it could lead to a more fragmented service or leave an isolated rump service of the non-devolved part of pharmacy.

Pharmacy needs to be involved not just in the management structure of the trust but also in the wide variety of committees and groups within the trust. Once again, these vary between trusts but will include groups that deal with clinical governance, risk management, patient liaison, clinical effectiveness audit, control of infection, health and safety, and medicines. Pharmacy managers and staff need to create informal networks and contacts within the trust to ensure that, as issues relating to medicines arise, appropriate advice and support are sought. Such contacts are just as important as the formal trust structures.

Pharmacy staff

Hospital pharmacy has developed a range of support staff roles. The introduction to this book mentioned several documents that encouraged the development of the technician roles. Ensuring other support staff underpin and allow good use of resources is also important for pharmacy. Pay modernisation was part of revising the NHS: *Agenda for Change* introduced changes in

Table 1.3 Pharmacy staffing groups

Job title	Qualifications
Pharmacists	Registered with the General Pharmaceutical Council (Great Britain) or the Pharmaceutical Society of Northern Ireland Having obtained a pharmacy degree and successfully undertaken a 1-year preregistration programme.
Pharmacy technicians	Registered with the General Pharmaceutical Council (from 2011) Qualified staff, having BTEC or NVQ (level 3) or an earlier equivalent in pharmaceutical science
Assistants	Not formally qualified in pharmaceutical science but usually undergoing relevant competency or in-house training to undertake practical tasks in pharmacy or NVQ (level 2)
Clerical and administrative staff	Undertaking personal assistant, administrative roles at senior level or in supportive capacity May have considerable experience and relevant qualifications or be undertaking training
Other staff	Graduates from science or other backgrounds may take on roles within the service, for example, in quality control laboratories. Roles in store-keeping or purchasing or information technology may also bring in experienced or non-pharmaceutically qualified staff

BTEC, Business and Technology Education Council; NVQ, National Vocational Qualification.

pay structures and had an impact on career structures.[21] It is possible that there will be greater variation across the NHS as foundation trusts develop local pay structures. The roles and job titles seen in pharmacy at the time of writing are shown in Tables 1.3–1.5.

Table 1.4 *Agenda for Change* pharmacist posts

Agenda for Change band	Typical role
5	Preregistration graduate
6	Pharmacist, contributing to service but also having undertaken general training or in early year of more focused training
7	Described as 'pharmacist specialist' in job profile. Probably specialising in a particular aspect of service, still developing specialised skills. May have specific management responsibility
8 a–b	Described as 'pharmacist advanced' in job profile. More experienced pharmacist; may be leading a section or providing specialist services, possibly a clinical lead for service to a directorate or division
8 b–c	Described as 'pharmacist team manager' – similar to above but leading a section with defined management role
8 b–d	Consultant pharmacist – see Chapter 18 for details
8 c–d or 9	Chief pharmacist – described as 'professional manager pharmaceutical services'

Note: at January 2011, without allowances, band 6 salary was £25–£34k, band 9 maximum £97k.

Table 1.5 *Agenda for Change* technician posts

Agenda for Change	Typical role
Trainee, paid percentage of band 4	Student pharmacy technician
4	Pharmacy technician – dispensing, aseptic services, may have some ward roles
5	Pharmacy technician with additional responsibilities, probably providing final checks in dispensing, may be ward-based, may have a supervisory role
6	Pharmacy technician with a management or coordinating role, may be responsible for a section. May provide training
7	Described as 'pharmacy technician team manager' – managing provision of a technical pharmacy service, possibly a large section
8	No specific pharmacy technician profiles exist but, where a service is managed by a technician with significant personnel or financial responsibility, an alternative Agenda for Change profile may be used

Note: At January 2011, without enhancements, salary range was £18k at bottom of band 4 to £40k at top of band 7.

Table 1.6 Some career pathways for hospital pharmacists	
Case A	Hospital pharmacy preregistration training Junior hospital pharmacist post Independent sector – project relating to secondary care Senior IT pharmacist in hospital Senior pharmacist for dispensary services Chief pharmacist teaching trust Head of pharmacy and therapy services in multisite teaching trust
Case B	Hospital–industry preregistration training Junior pharmacist – clinical diploma Resident pharmacist Clinical pharmacist in various specialties Medicines information pharmacist Senior medicines information pharmacist Critical appraisal pharmacist in medicines information centre Principal pharmacist for medicines information centre
Case C	Hospital–industry preregistration training Resident pharmacist PhD studies in pharmacology Pharmacy industry – pharmacovigilance Specialist hospital pharmacist Consultant pharmacist (in same specialist area as above)

Progression through the current grades follows a variety of routes. Aspirations and career pathways do not follow a simple pattern; however, Table 1.6 gives a few examples of career histories based on current senior pharmacists. The Modernising Pharmacy Careers programme will also bring significant changes to the development and career structure for pharmacy staff.

The future

The new structure of the NHS in England will take shape, as it has done previously, and is doing in Wales at the time of writing. Organisational structures and committee arrangements will also change as new challenges are faced. Throughout this, pharmacy will need to ensure there are suitable arrangements to provide advice on the safe, clinical and cost-effective use of medicines if patients are to be protected and good outcomes achieved. Pharmacy leaders at a local level must build good working relationships with medical, nursing and general management colleagues to achieve this.

References

1. Department of Health. *Equity and Excellence: Liberating the NHS*. London: Department of Health, 2010.
2. Hall N, chair. *Report of the Working Party Investigating the Hospital Pharmaceutical Service*. London: HMSO, 1970.

3. Griffiths report. *NHS Management Enquiry*. London: HMSO, 1983.
4. Department of Health. *The New NHS: Modern, Dependable*. London: The Stationery Office, 1997.
5. Department of Health. *A First Class Service, Quality in the New NHS*. London: The Stationery Office, 1998.
6. Department of Health. *Our Healthier Nation*. London: The Stationery Office, 1999.
7. Department of Health. *Shifting the Balance of Power Within the NHS: Securing Delivery*. London: The Stationery Office, 2001.
8. Department of Health. *A Short Guide to NHS Foundation Trusts*. London: Department of Health, 2005.
9. Department of Health. *The NHS Plan*. London: The Stationery Office, 2000.
10. Department of Health guidance on high cost medicines excluded from PbR. Available online at: http://www.dh.gov.uk/en/Managingyourorganisation/NHSFinancialReforms/DH_114339 (accessed 17 August 2010).
11. Department of Health. *Our NHS, Our Future, NHS Next Stage Review, Interim Report*. London: Department of Health, 2007.
12. Department of Health. *High Quality Care for All, NHS Next Stage Review, Final Report*. London: Department of Health, 2008.
13. Department of Health. *Healthy Lives, Healthy People: Our strategy for public health in England*. London: Department of Health, 2010.
14. Care Quality Commission. *Guidance About Compliance: Essential Standards of Quality and Safety*. Outcome 9: management of medicines. London: Care Quality Commission, 2010.
15. Department of Health. *The NHS Quality, Innovation, Productivity, Prevention Challenge, An Introduction for Clinicians*. London: Department of Health, 2010.
16. Department of Health. *The NHS Constitution*. London: Department of Health, 2009.
17. Scottish Government. *The Healthcare Quality Strategy for NHS Scotland*. Edinburgh: Scottish Government, 2010.
18. Department of Health. *Pharmacy in the Future*. London: Department of Health, 2000.
19. Department of Health. *Pharmacy in England, Building on Strengths, Delivering the Future*. London: Department of Health, 2008.
20. Audit Commission. *A Spoonful of Sugar – Medicines Management in NHS Hospitals*. London: Audit Commission, 2001.
21. Department of Health. *Agenda for Change, Modernising the NHS Pay System*. London: The Stationery Office, 1999.

Further reading

Department of Health website: http://www.dh.gov.uk.
Foundation trusts: http://www.dh.gov.uk/en/Publicationsandstatistics/Publications/Publications PolicyAndGuidance/DH_4126013.
National Health Service Constitution: http://www.dh.gov.uk/prod_consum_dh/groups/ dh_digitalassets/@dh/@en/@ps/documents/digitalasset/dh_113645.pdf.
National Health Service website: http://www.nhs.uk.

2

Pharmacy in the acute independent sector

Karen Harrowing

Introduction

Independent providers have been at the centre of pharmacy service provision for some considerable time. For example, Boot and Company Limited was founded in 1883 with their first pharmacist appointed in 1884 and, by 1933, there were 1000 Boots stores open. Independent hospitals also have a long history and some, such as King Edward VII's Hospital: Sister Agnes (founded in 1899) in London, continue to operate as independent charitable hospitals today.

Since the National Health Service (NHS) was formed in 1948 there have always been independent contractors providing NHS service delivery, the most obvious examples being general practitioner services. This situation has been accepted as the norm for over 60 years, whereas the position of independent sector hospitals has not been as well integrated into the NHS over much of that period. However, there have been significant changes in the past 10 years, including greater cooperation between the NHS and independent sector to maximise capacity. There have also been changes in the regulation of hospital services during 2010 that mean both NHS and independent sector hospitals are regulated under the same legislation, namely *The Health and Social Care Act 2008*[1] with the Care Quality Commission (CQC) as regulator, as discussed in Chapter 1.

In this chapter these significant changes will be reviewed under the following headings:

- independent sector background and large hospital groups
- independent sector and the NHS – from concordat to free choice
- *The NHS Plan*[2] and the independent sector
- treatment centres – NHS and independent sector

- plurality of provision and patient choice
- regulation of the acute independent sector – from homes to acute services
- medicines management – delivering consistency of outcome to all service users
- independent sector background and hospital groups.

The independent sector supports a wide range of healthcare needs, including diagnostic services, surgery, physiotherapy, assisted conception services, maternity services, oncology and palliation, as well as treatments not provided by the NHS, such as cosmetic surgery.

Patients decide to use the independent sector for a variety of reasons, including ability to choose consultant or hospital, and the availability of treatments. Historically, length of waiting time was a significant issue and, whilst this has reduced, the greater flexibility to choose when to come to hospital remains attractive. Where fees are required for services these are often covered by private medical insurance, which may be through a personal policy or as a benefit of a patient's employment. Other patients choose to pay fees directly: the proportion varies according to the market. Independent sector hospitals also provide NHS-funded treatment: this is where those commissioning care for local populations have contracted with the independent sector to provide care. In these situations patients may choose the independent sector via the NHS patient choice scheme – no fees are paid by these NHS patients.

Independent healthcare providers are extremely diverse, ranging from single charitable hospitals to large groups of hospitals. However, all are regulated and monitored by the CQC. The larger hospital groups operating in the UK cover a wide geographical area and a wide range of procedures and treatments. The larger hospital groups include:

- BMI Healthcare, which is the largest independent provider of healthcare in the UK and has 60 hospitals. It is a division of General Healthcare Group, managed by a consortium led by the South African company Network Healthcare Holdings Limited (Netcare)
- Spire Healthcare, which has 36 hospitals in the UK and is owned by Cinven; it is a European company with large acquisitions in France, the Netherlands, Spain and the UK
- Nuffield Health, which is the UK's leading health charity, and has 30 hospitals and, in addition, provides a network of other services, including a nationwide physiotherapy service
- Ramsey Health Care, which is an Australian healthcare group, is the fourth largest operator of private hospitals with 22 acute hospitals across the UK.

There is a focus of independent sector hospitals in and around London, and some groups, such as HCA International and Aspen Healthcare, have fewer but larger hospitals in a smaller geographical area. These hospitals may also specialise; for example, the Portland Hospital (HCA) for women and children, and the Parkside Oncology Clinic (Aspen). Further information on independent health, community care and childcare can be obtained from Laing and Buisson (http://www.laingbuisson.co.uk/).

Pharmacy service models vary in the independent sector depending on the size and specialities of the facility. Since hospitals are often much smaller than NHS trusts, the pharmacy team works more closely with the hospital senior management team, which may include a general manager and/or matron. The role of accountable officer for controlled drugs (see Chapter 5) is usually held by either the manager, who is often the registered person for the facility, or the matron.

Independent sector and the NHS – from concordat to free choice

The NHS Plan and the independent sector

As mentioned in Chapter 1, *The NHS Plan* was published in July 2000 and it created the platform for significant reform both within the NHS and between the NHS and the independent sector.[2] The document set out challenging targets to reduce NHS waiting times. As part of the plan to meet those targets the document proposed that there was a need to engage more constructively with the independent sector in order to use extra capacity to benefit NHS patients. This approach has been termed the 'plurality' of service provision.

Before *The NHS Plan* the NHS had procured services on a local basis in an ad hoc manner, using a range of independent providers including hospitals, nursing homes and hospices. In 2000 the consistency, quality and value for money of service delivery by the independent sector were not monitored nationally. Reform was required to ensure that the £1 billion of public money being spent in the independent sector at that time was being used effectively and patient safety could be assured.

The NHS Plan described the creation of a concordat between the NHS and independent providers that would make better use of facilities, so long as value for money and standards of patient care could be demonstrated. Therefore the independent sector was required to comply with NHS standards in addition to compliance with the *National Minimum Standards* published in 2002.[3] Furthermore, from 2002 the independent sector was required to move to a single approach to pricing procedures based on the national NHS tariff, published and revised annually by the Department of Health.[4]

Fundamental to the new partnerships was that the core principle of the NHS would not be compromised, namely, that healthcare should be available on the basis of need and not ability to pay. In addition to the quality and safety principles another key requirement of the independent sector was that they should augment the clinical staff pool rather than rely on those same clinicians who deliver services in the NHS. It was recognised that full utilisation of existing and new capacity in the independent sector could not be realised if the procedures were delivered by the same NHS consultants; thus 'additionality' clauses were added before contracts for services were awarded.

Treatment centres – NHS and independent sector

The imperative to reduce waiting times in the NHS provided the impetus for the development of new treatment centres run by the NHS (NHSTC) or the independent sector (ISTC) for treatment of NHS patients. Treatment centres were designed to offer choice to patients and to provide streamlined, safe and effective surgery and diagnostics tests for prebooked patients.[5] Treatment centres were often, although not exclusively, designed to manage procedures from one specialty, for example orthopaedics or ophthalmology, where waiting lists had traditionally been long.

In 2003 central contracts, which included national key performance indicators (KPIs) to support clinical and financial governance, began to be awarded to international independent healthcare companies who were able to offer 'additional' staff. New ISTC capacity initially became available towards the end of 2004. NHS patients treated by the independent sector are not private patients but remain NHS patients and they have access to all NHS services. To ensure patients are not confused, the ISTCs are required to comply with NHS branding requirements.

Two supplementary contracts were also established with the independent sector in 2004 to ensure that there was a timely reduction of waiting lists while further treatment centre contracts were agreed and building projects established. These contracts made use of existing spare capacity in independent hospitals already established in the UK, for example Nuffield Hospitals (now Nuffield Health) and Capio (now Ramsey Health Care).

The ISTC programme was designed to allow the independent sector to work in partnership with local healthcare economies to provide solutions that met local requirements. Another aim was to stimulate innovative models of service delivery and drive up productivity.[6] The ISTCs provide care for elective surgical patients, not unplanned emergency care. This results in a streamlined process for patient care informed by preassessment and following defined pathways of care, including the discharge process. Many of the ISTCs are day-case facilities and therefore patients with low risk and fewer or no comorbidities are selected.

Use of ISTCs has not been without criticism, both in the press and from politicians, with claims of higher costs for cases in ISTCs and limited contribution to waiting-list reductions.[7, 8] However, from the evidence that outsourcing to the independent sector was already significant it seems that more capacity was essential and these possible inefficiencies are inevitable when a significant growth over a very short timescale was sought, with the very clear goal of greatly reduced waiting times. Furthermore, it was potentially difficult for providers to voice criticism of purchasers when in tendering situations. However, there was a general concern in the independent sector that the cumbersome contractual processes developed by the Department of Health did not support the initial intentions and innovative approaches that could be gained from working with private business.

Pharmacy service provision to ISTC will vary depending on the model of care and the procedures undertaken. There may be an on-site pharmacy providing products and services in a similar manner to any acute hospital pharmacy service. In should be noted that the base pharmacy department may be remote from the ISTC and may be provided by a subcontractor – hospital- or community-based. The innovation and productivity aims of the ISTC programme mean that pharmacy providers have also had to come up with ways for effectively supporting the programme, for example protocols for medicines from admission to discharge.

Plurality of provision and patient choice

The treatment centre programme has supported the drive to reduce waiting lists. However, there is a longer-term aim to have a more integrated model for patients to move between the NHS and the independent sector as part of the 'choice' agenda. There is a right for patients to make choices about their NHS care and to have information to support these choices, as defined in the NHS constitution.[9]

The Independent Sector Extended Choice Network (IS ECN) and Independent Sector Free Choice Network (IS FCN) are frameworks for independent sector providers, who demonstrate that they meet NHS standards and costs, to offer 'choice' and reduce waiting times to NHS patients. As part of the membership requirements for IS ECN and IS FCN the independent sector location must be registered with the CQC for the activities to be delivered. In addition the independent sector providers are required to demonstrate compliance with certain NHS standards, for example the *NHS Litigation Authority (NHSLA) Risk Management Standards*.[10] The NHSLA standard for managing risks associated with medicines requires processes to be in place to monitor accurate, safe and effective prescribing, administration and self-administration, and the disposal of medicines. This requirement is similar to that required by the CQC and therefore NHS and independent sector organisations can use similar evidence to demonstrate compliance.

Formed in 2005, the NHS Partners Network is an alliance of independent (commercial and not-for-profit) healthcare providers involved in all aspects of NHS care. Its aim is to increase integration of independent healthcare in order to continue to improve patient choice and value for money for patients and taxpayers. In June 2007 NHS Partners Network was incorporated into the NHS Confederation. NHS organisations are supported, through networks, briefings and publications, by the NHS Confederation, which seeks to ensure we have a national health system that delivers first-class services and improved health for all.

Regulation of the acute independent sector – from homes to acute services

Until 2002 the *Registered Homes Act 1984* provided the legislative framework for independent hospitals (as well as independent care homes, nursing homes and mental nursing homes).[11] Part II of the Act covered a wide spectrum of activities under the definition of 'nursing homes', including nursing homes through to clinics, acute hospitals and psychiatric hospitals. NHS hospitals were exempt from the 1984 Act.

The *Care Standards Act 2000* provided for the establishment of the National Care Standards Commission in England.[12] (There were and remain differences in the way other home countries deal with these issues.) The Secretary of State was given powers to make relevant regulations and to issue national minimum standards applicable to all the relevant services.[3] The registration authorities and providers were required to demonstrate compliance with regulation and national minimum standards through a process of self-assessment and inspection.

The 2000 Act also defined the meaning of an 'independent hospital', previously not well defined. An independent hospital is 'any establishment which has, as its main purpose, the provision of psychiatric or medical treatment for illness (including palliative care) or mental disorder (including detention under the *Mental Health Act 1983*[13]) or which provides one or more of the specific "listed services" (for example hyperbaric oxygen therapy)' and which is not a health service hospital.

This definition of an independent hospital also includes private and voluntary hospitals previously not regulated, for example those run by bodies established under Royal Charter or by special Act of Parliament. Furthermore the 2000 Act defined the meaning of an 'independent clinic' as 'an establishment (other than a hospital) where medical practitioners provide services' thereby bringing private primary care services into the regulatory framework for the first time. Registration under the *Care Standards Act 2000*[12] continued in the independent sector until 30 September 2010; NHS services were excluded from the 2000 Act.

In April 2002 *The Private and Voluntary Health Care (England) Regulations 2001*[14] came into force and set out the regulations by which the independent sector in England would be monitored. Organisations falling within the regulations were required to appoint a registered manager for each establishment and provide the names and date of appointment to the Commission. The fitness of the registered manager is defined within the 2001 regulations and later a formal process of 'fit person' interviews was introduced.

The registered manager/person is required to define the 'statement of purpose' for the establishment and can then only provide services in accordance with that statement. In addition the registered manager/person is responsible for ensuring that services meet the needs of the individual service users and are in accordance with research evidence and other good practice. For medicines management the quality of service provision regulation 15 (5) states that:

> The registered person shall make suitable arrangements for the ordering, recording, handling, safe keeping, safe administration and disposal of medicines used in or for the purposes of the establishment, or for the purposes of the agency.[14]

From 1 April 2010 the *Care Quality Commission (Registration) Regulations 2009*[15] came into force and provide for the registration of persons carrying on a regulated activity. On 1 October 2010 the regulations came into force for adult social care and independent healthcare providers. All health and adult social care providers (whether NHS or independent sector) who provide regulated activities will be required by law to be registered with the CQC. For the first time acute care has been brought under the same definition, namely acute services, and includes:

- acute NHS hospitals
- acute independent hospitals
- NHS community hospitals
- ISTCs
- cosmetic surgery clinics.

The *Health and Social Care Act 2008* also provides regulations that include the quality and safety of the service provision, for example, the management of medicines.[1] Regulation 13 states:

> The registered person must protect service users against the risks associated with the unsafe use and management of medicines, by means of the making of appropriate arrangements for the obtaining, recording, handling, using, safe keeping, dispensing, safe administration and disposal of medicines used for the purposes of the regulated activity.

The CQC will also monitor providers against a set of outcomes defined within the *Essential Standards of Quality and Safety*.[16] The management of medicines outcome 9 states that:

People who use services:

- will have their medicines at the times they need them, and in a safe way. Wherever possible will have information about the medicine being prescribed made available to them or others acting on their behalf.

This is because providers who comply with the regulations will:

- handle medicines safely, securely and appropriately
- ensure that medicines are prescribed and given by people safely
- follow published guidance about how to use medicines safely.

The outcome is associated with a series of prompts that support providers in how to demonstrate compliance with the outcome.

Although the regulatory framework has become aligned across the acute NHS and independent sector providers, there has been an area of medicines management practice in the independent sector that has fallen outside both CQC and General Pharmaceutical Council regulation, namely injectable cosmetic treatments. However, from 2010 the provision of injectable cosmetic treatments, including dermal fillers and botulinum toxin, will be controlled for the first time under a shared regulation scheme operated by the Independent Healthcare Advisory Service and monitored by Caspe Healthcare Knowledge Systems. The registration, certification and inspection scheme has been developed by the injectable cosmetics industry to promote compliance with medicines management and training standards to improve the safety of patients.

Medicines management – delivering consistency of outcome to all service users

Medicines are the most common treatment intervention and the majority of care pathways in hospitals involve medicines. The independent sector and NHS treatment pathways for patients have become more integrated as the 'plurality of provision' objective continues to become embedded in healthcare delivery models and regulation by the CQC becomes consistent across all acute hospital provision.

The way pharmacy services are provided has changed and the models of provision are increasingly varied, for example community pharmacy providing the service, NHS acute provision to independent sector, as well as independent sector acute provision to the NHS. There is also a potential for mixed provision across individual service lines; for example, a service may comprise ward pharmacy and medicines information from NHS acute provider, outpatient dispensing from community pharmacy and stock supplies direct by wholesaler.

These changes in service delivery options to a more 'virtual' pharmacy platform require improved communication channels, service level agreements and KPIs. These avoid assumptions being made by any party. The important point is that the outcomes of essential standards are met by all providers and 'people who use services will have their medicines at the times they need them, in a safe way with the relevant information'.[16] This is the objective of the *Medicines in Commissioning Toolkit*, that is, to 'get medicine use right', and is intended to support both commissioners and providers of medicine-related services.[17] The toolkit covers various areas and these are identified in Text box 2.1.

Box 2.1 Medicines in Commissioning Toolkit [14]

Assess needs and provision review

There must be clarity of strategic position, definitions and delivery outcomes between commissioners and providers. Information and data requirements must be clearly defined and assumptions used within a sector avoided, for example quality measurement and criteria may differ between National Health Service and independent sector.

Deciding priorities and investments

The position on priorities must be explicit, for example with reference to any economic requirements to adhere to National Institute for Health and Clinical Excellence guidance that may not be an existing requirement in the independent sector.

Patient safety and governance

Commissioners should ensure policy and procedure documents are based on relevant standards for the service being delivered.

Legal aspects

Commissioning pharmacy or medicines management for acute services from community pharmacy providers will require explicit reference to acute standards since community practice will be regulated and monitored under the standards of the General Pharmaceutical Council rather than the Care Quality Commission.

Service delivery

Service delivery requirements must be explicitly defined within agreements and monitored.

Staff training and competency

The standards and rules of the General Pharmaceutical Council, as well as the compulsory registration of pharmacy technicians, will help to reduce ambiguity in the roles and competency of registered pharmacy personnel delivering service across different sectors. However, there may be other personnel issues to consider, for example the presence and level of Criminal Records Bureau checks and safeguarding training that may be required in certain establishments where services are delivered, particularly those involving children and vulnerable adults.

Patient experience

The experience of the patient should be able to be compared across sectors. Local service delivery models need to ensure that patient experiences metrics are fully defined and monitored.

Funding aspects

The toolkit provides many examples of funding issues to be considered, including the provision of FP10 prescriptions for NHS patients being treated in the independent sector. Primary and secondary NHS care providers have greater clarity of the responsibilities for medicine supply, including shared-care protocols. The acute independent sector supplies the majority of medicines in accordance with the medical insurance company contracts for NHS patients arrangements would need to be explicit in contracts, including management of shared care.

With respect to governance arrangements, these will become more aligned between independent sector and NHS. However, policy and procedure development has been based on difference standards, namely the *National Minimum Standards* in the independent sector[3] and the *Standards for Better Health* in the NHS.[18] Commissioners should ensure this is addressed.

An area that continues to differ between the acute providers in the NHS and independent sector is in relation to consultant staff. In the NHS they are employed whereas in the independent sector the majority of consultants operate privately under a licensing system called practising privileges. This is a robust framework used across the independent sector; however, the indemnity arrangements for any prescribing as part of local contracts would need to be clarified explicitly.

The patient safety agenda is a key focus for all pharmacy and medicines management providers. It is important to note that there are differences in how National Patient Safety Agency (NPSA) and other alerts are disseminated and managed. For example, community providers may not receive direct communications whereas many acute independent sector providers are part of the NHS Central Alerting System. At the time of writing only NHS providers have access to the feedback process that demonstrates compliance with NPSA alerts. Therefore a mechanism for reporting compliance to NPSA and other medication safety alerts may need to be incorporated into service level agreements and KPIs.

Regarding legal issues, when the service delivery model is dependent on the use of patient group directions the differences in the NHS and independent sector must be understood, for example requirement for CQC registration and sign-off by the registered manager in the independent sector.

Historically, there have been issues in monitoring service delivery between the independent sector and the NHS. In July 2007 the Healthcare Commission published a review of the quality of care in independent sector treatment centres and made a number of recommendations, including improving the quality of data, the need for common data sets and improving the partnership relationship between independent sector treatment centres and the NHS.[19] Whilst many of the recommendations have been addressed in central contracting processes, commissioners and providers of local service delivery models need to ensure any differences are fully defined and monitored.

Patient experience

The experience of the patient should be able to be compared accurately across sectors; however, this was not found in the Healthcare Commission's review of quality of care in independent sector treatment centres.[19] Local service delivery models need to ensure that patient experience metrics are fully defined and monitored.

In conclusion, the safe and effective use of medicines delivered by pharmacy services should be of a consistent standard irrespective of the provider and whether that provider is NHS or independent sector. This is the principle behind the management of medicines requirements in the *Essential Standards of Quality and Safety*.[16]

References

1. *The Health and Social Care Act 2008*. London: The Stationery Office, 2008.
2. Department of Health. *The NHS Plan*. London: The Stationery Office, 2000.
3. Department of Health. *National Minimum Standards for Independent Healthcare*. London: Department of Health, 2002.
4. Department of Health. *Reforming NHS Financial Flows, Introducing Payment by Results*. London: Department of Health, 2002.
5. Department of Health. *Treatment Centres: Delivering Faster, Quality Care and Choice for NHS Patients*. London: Department of Health, 2005.
6. Department of Health. *Commercial Directorate – ISTC Manual*. London: Department of Health, 2005.
7. Public Finance report – MPs call for more scrutiny of Department of Health contracts. Available online at: http://www.publicfinance.co.uk/news/2006/mps-call-for-more-scrutiny-of-doh-contracts/ (accessed 31 May 2010).
8. House of Commons Health Committee. *Independent Sector Treatment Centres. Fourth Report of Session 2005-6*, vol. 1, together with formal minutes. HC934-I. London: The Stationery Office, 2006.
9. Department of Health. *The Handbook to the NHS Constitution*. London: Department of Health, 2010.
10. NHS Litigation Authority. *NHSLA Risk Management Standards for Acute Trusts, Primary Care Trusts and Independent Sector Providers of NHS Care*. London: The Stationery Office, 2010.
11. *Registered Homes Act 1984*. London: The Stationery Office, 1984.
12. *Care Standards Act 2000*. London: The Stationery Office, 2000.
13. *Mental Health Act 1983*. London: The Stationery Office, 1983.
14. *The Private and Voluntary Health Care (England) Regulations 2001*. SI 2001 no. 3968. London: The Stationery Office, 2001.
15. *Care Quality Commission (Registration) Regulations 2009*. London: The Stationery Office, 2009.
16. Care Quality Commission. *Guidance About Compliance: Essential Standards of Quality and Safety*. London: Care Quality Commission, 2010.
17. East and South East England Specialist Pharmacy Services. *Medicines in Commissioning Toolkit – A Toolkit to Help Ensure Safe and Accessible Services for Patients*, version 2. East of England, London, South Central and South East Coast. London: NHS, 2009.
18. Department of Health. *Standards for Better Health*. London: Department of Health, 2006.
19. Commission for Healthcare Audit and Inspection. *Independent Sector Treatment Centres – A Review of the Quality of Care*. London: The Stationery Office, 2007.

Further reading

Care Quality Commission. *Guidance About Compliance: Essential Standards of Quality and Safety*. London: Care Quality Commission, 2010.

3

Purchasing medicines

Howard Stokoe and Phil Deady

This chapter describes how National Health Service (NHS) hospitals contract for the supply of medicines and explains typical local arrangements for obtaining medicines, invoicing and stock management. The focus is on England and, whilst approaches are reasonably consistent across the whole of the UK, readers should note that the home countries organise themselves in different ways and that systems vary across the whole of Europe.

Background

Expenditure

The pharmaceutical market in the UK forms the context for hospital purchasing. The UK represents around 3% of the global market for medicines. NHS hospital expenditure, at just over £3.6 billion, represents about a third of the NHS total for prescription medicines, with the balance being spent in primary care (Table 3.1). This sum excludes value-added tax (VAT: a purchase tax), but it should be noted that hospitals do pay VAT on medicines (where applicable – some items do not incur VAT) and this element is included in the expenditure figures – figures for general practitioner prescribing costs do not include VAT. Overall expenditure on medicines at over £11 billion forms around 12% of NHS expenditure.

The Pharmaceutical Price Regulation Scheme (PPRS)

The PPRS is a UK government scheme that controls the prices of branded prescription medicines supplied to the NHS by regulating the profits that pharmaceutical companies can make on their sales to the NHS.[1, 2] At the same time, the scheme supports an industry that will continue to offer innovative medicines and is competitive internationally. Indeed, the UK

Table 3.1 Expenditure on medicines in the National Health Service (NHS) in England (2008–2009)						
Primary care		Hospital sector		Total drug spend		As % of total NHS spend
Gross		Gross		Gross		Gross
Outturn (£m)	Year-on-year growth (%)	Outturn (£m)	Year-on-year growth (%)	Outturn (£m)	Year-on-year growth (%)	(%)
7749	1.1	3647	11.4	11 397	4.2	11.9

Sources:

1. Primary care figures are from the Prescription Pricing Division of the NHS Business Services Authority and primary care trusts (PCTs) audited summarisation schedules

2. Hospital and community health services figures are from NHS trusts and PCTs finance returns and foundation trusts consolidated accounts.

3. The figures exclude value-added tax (VAT), but it should be noted that hospitals do pay VAT at the standard rate on medicines and the NHS is funded to take account of this non-recoverable VAT. Medicines in primary care are zero-rated for VAT.

pharmaceutical industry is seen as a significant asset; *The NHS Plan* made this clear and also stated there needs to be opportunity for companies to undertake research with reasonable haste.[3]

Under the PPRS suppliers are allowed to introduce major new medicines (new active substances) to the NHS at prices that they determine but can only increase prices with the Department of Health's agreement. The PPRS distinguishes the UK market from all others in the European Union (EU), though at the time of writing a value-based pricing approach is being considered.

Generic substitution

Unlike the current system in primary care, NHS hospital pharmacies have dispensed medicines generically, irrespective of how they are prescribed, for some time. Thus, a brand name may be used by the doctor but a generic version issued. Exceptions are made if the branded product has unique characteristics that could result in a clinically important effect if substituted (modified release, for example).

Aims of the service

Obtaining medicines from manufacturers, wholesalers and short-line stores is an essential part of the pharmacy service. Medicine purchasing needs to be carried out with probity and to be undertaken efficiently. There are conflicting demands on the service: to avoid failing to meet a patient's need but also avoiding excessive stock within the pharmacy. Too large a stock holding means that trust money is tied up in an asset; high stock levels may also lead to waste and will require more space than would a reasonable stock level; there is also a risk that a change in clinical practice could lead to wastage. The average stock holding for a hospital pharmacy has been estimated at approximately 1 month's supply, a stock turnover of about 12 times per year. Although there may be pressure on hospital pharmacies to decrease stock holding and thus increase turnover, the decrease in value of asset needs to be balanced against increased costs to place orders and clear invoices, as well as the risk of 'stock outs'.[4]

How the service has developed

The first hospital contracts

Regional pharmaceutical officers and supplies managers introduced some of the first hospital contracts for medicines during the 1970s in the days of the regional health authorities. At that time purchasing was organised on a regional basis. As branded medicines came off patent, and generic versions were introduced, these contracts were awarded to reflect a fall in price, as well as the additional benefits that came from competition between generic suppliers. Given that hospital pharmacists were able to dispense generically, the contracts delivered immediate cash savings that were then available to support the funding of newer, relatively more expensive and innovative medicines.

The impact of broader government policy and NHS reorganisations

The established contracting model has survived numerous NHS reorganisations that have otherwise fundamentally reshaped the procurement environment. NHS trusts continue to support collaborative procurement through their pharmacy purchasing groups that are, in England, now aligned to current strategic health authority boundaries. For the most part these groups use a national procurement organisation, the NHS Commercial Medicines Unit (CMU), as their contracting authority.[5]

Perhaps the greatest impact has come as a result of a wider government initiative. The Gershon report, *Releasing Resources to the Front Line*, was published in 2004 with the aim of driving greater efficiencies across the whole of the public sector.[6] Within the NHS this resulted, amongst other things, in the Supply Chain Excellence Programme (SCEP). SCEP, without changing the established pharmacy contracting model, forced through a more structured approach and enabled the development of new information systems that are described below. SCEP also introduced collaborative procurement hubs (CPHs). These CPHs, and equivalent organisations, are now able to offer the pharmacy purchasing groups additional local support, thus enabling them to extend the scope of their activities. To avoid confusion around their roles and involvement, and to avoid duplication of effort, a list of products and services allocated to CPHs for tender is maintained.[7]

Hospital procurement and the application of EU legislation

Background and requirements

Overlaid on this background and history has been the impact of EU legislation. The UK is a member state of the EU and an aim of the EU is to create a single European market devoid of all trading restrictions and barriers – a marketplace in which all businesses have an equal opportunity to compete. The EU regulates and monitors all large-scale public sector procurement through EU directives covering the supply of goods, services and works.[8] In the UK the directives apply to all NHS contracting authorities and NHS trusts.[9]

As a result of EU membership, hospital procurement is subject to the directive within the Treaty of Rome, including Article 12 (prohibition of discrimination on grounds of nationality), Article 28 (free movement of goods within the EU) and Article 81 (prohibition of agreements that prevent, restrict or distort competition).

The main requirements are:

* the advertisement of large public contracts to a standard format in the supplement to the *Official Journal of the European Community* (OJEC) so that suitable suppliers from all EU and government procurement agreement countries have the opportunity to declare their interest. Prescribed minimum periods for responses
* the use of technical specifications which are non-discriminatory and which refer to EU or other recognised international standards wherever possible
* the use of objective criteria for selecting participants and awarding contracts.

The directives only apply where the value of the procurement exceeds a given threshold. This is quoted in euros but, as a rule of thumb, means any contract with a value of £100 000 is included. It should be noted that the figure is for the contract's lifetime, not an annual figure; thus, a contract for £30 000 per year for 3 years must go through this process.

Types of procedure

The regulations recognise three contracting procedures – open, restricted and negotiated. These have slightly different requirements and advantages, and are summarised in Text box 3.1.

> *Box 3.1 Types of contracting procedure*
>
> ## Open procedure
>
> Available in all circumstances and involves only a single stage. All offers received must be considered, provided that candidates have passed any minimum short-listing criteria. The open procedure can be conducted more quickly than the restricted procedure but there is no possibility of limiting the number of bids received.
>
> ## Restricted procedure
>
> Available in all circumstances but involves a two-stage procedure. From amongst the candidates expressing interest (the first stage) it is possible to shortlist a limited number from whom to invite offers (the second stage).
>
> ## Negotiated procedure
>
> The most flexible but the least transparent of the three procedures. It is used only in very limited circumstances (for example, where goods are needed urgently due to reasons that were unforeseeable by, and not attributable to, the buyer).

Offer evaluation

The directives require that any contract must be awarded to the candidate who submits the lowest-priced tender or the tender that is the most economically advantageous (buyers almost invariably select the latter because it gives greater flexibility). The factors that may be used to determine economic advantage include price, quality of service and running costs: the chosen factors must be stated in the OJEC notice or the contract documents.

Negotiation within the process

Where the open or restricted procedures are being used, the rules forbid buyers to engage in post-tender negotiations with candidates. These are defined as negotiations with candidates on fundamental aspects of their bids, for example, price. Discussions aimed as clarifying or supplementing the content of the bids are, on the other hand, permitted, provided all candidates are treated equally. Pre-tender discussions with potential suppliers, conducted on an equitable basis, are critical to designing contracts that will perform and deliver.

Types of contract

There are two types of contract: the commitment contract and the framework contract. The commitment contract commits a legal entity (such as an NHS trust) to purchase a defined quantity of product at a defined price; the framework contract does not guarantee to deliver commitment. Rather, based on estimated volumes it provides (for example, on behalf of a group of hospitals represented as a purchasing group) a framework against which purchase orders will be placed by hospitals covered by the agreement. The framework agreement sets the terms and conditions of the purchase by the hospital, including price/pricing schedules, with the trust contract being formed when individual hospitals place their purchase order.

Framework contracts are normally used on behalf of purchasing groups in recognition that an agent (such as the NHS CMU) or a hospital within the purchasing group cannot deliver absolute commitment to volume on behalf of the group.

The strengths of the contracting process

It may appear sometimes that the contracting process is cumbersome and bureaucratic. However, recognition must be paid to its inherent strengths. These are that the process is auditable, is legal (so minimising the risk of challenge, particularly when the lowest bid is not accepted), provides a framework for equal treatment for all bidders, establishes a clear trading basis between the NHS and its suppliers (through standard terms and conditions) and provides a fair test of value for money on behalf of the NHS.

The organisation of hospital contracts

Hospitals have contracts at various levels: purchasing group, trust contracts, national. The principles of purchasing group contracts are straightforward. Hospitals aggregate their purchasing power through their pharmacy purchasing groups and the NHS CMU then competitively tenders, awards and manages the resulting contracts, as an agent, on behalf of the groups. Each trust must nominate an individual to represent the interests of its hospital managers, clinicians and budget-holders (as well as its local relationships with primary care trusts) on its purchasing group. The nominee's roles include sharing information, adjudicating contracts and participating in collective dialogue with the NHS CMU buyer dedicated to work with the group.

The nominees use their knowledge and experience that originate in managing medicines on a day-to-day basis (particularly through formulary management systems that are linked to drugs and therapeutic committees, and input into the prescribing process) to direct the management of the contracts.

In England there are six main purchasing groups operating on a geographical basis with some, varying by main group, being divided into smaller groups. Each main group 'owns' contracts of between 1500 and 2000 lines, representing upward of 200 suppliers. Whilst the contracts on behalf of these groups are framework contracts that do not guarantee commitment, the ownership of the contracts (through the participation of their member trusts) ensures that these contracts are highly effective.

The framework contracts on behalf of each purchasing group can vary in length. However, typically they last for a maximum period of 2 years and include options to extend for an additional 2 years.

Following SCEP the NHS now supports a nationally coordinated programme to contract for the supply of its generic medicines. This is organised to reflect the characteristics of the generics that are involved and is summarised in Table 3.2.

Alongside the generic contracting programme there are tenders for branded medicines in the same way but by local agreement with NHS CMU, making awards to reflect volume discounts. This enables the NHS to benefit from competition between therapeutically similar medicines where this exists. Some product ranges can be separated out from the model to reflect the strategic development of their procurement; these are shown in Table 3.3.

Table 3.2 Characteristics of generic medicines as the basis for the design of National Health Servcice (NHS) contracting programme

Type of generic	Characteristic	Objective
Transitional product	Loss of patent of brand and generic competition emerging	Agreements in place as quickly as possible to maximise benefits to NHS as generic versions become available
Injectable products	NHS is the market for these products. There are risks to patient care if supply is compromised. This risk increases if there is a loss of supply capacity	NHS business is tendered on behalf of two purchasing groups at 8-month intervals, with the aim of keeping at least two suppliers in the market wherever possible
Oral preparations	The NHS does not represent the market as predominant use is in primary care	NHS business is tendered with the recognition that business will most often be awarded to one supplier with limited risk of damaging supply capacity

Table 3.3 Specific contracting activities for certain product type

Product range	Contract
Infection control products	By National Health Service supply chain to enable direct-to-ward supply
Clotting factors	On behalf of haemophilia centres through a direct relationship
Immunoglobulins	Through a single national tender; to match supply against commitment by purchasing group
Vaccines	Through commitment contracts on behalf of the Department of Health to support the delivery of its national vaccination programmes

Pharmacy purchasing groups – branded medicines and other activities

Contracts at purchasing group level are more important when decisions around the clinical choice of medicines can be influenced at a local level. Product ranges contracted for at this level include: branded medicines; bulk fluids; therapeutic tenders (where branded medicines have the same therapeutic outcome); service contracts (for example home care, aseptic compounding and over-labelling services).

Trust contracts

Some medicines will still be contracted for at trust level, though the driver is to move as much contracting to purchasing group and national level as possible, where aggregation of usage improves purchasing power.

Systems and processes

Pharmacy specialists and working relationships with procurement

The technical and procurement specialists within pharmacy strengthen the contracting arrangements, especially where they are employed by a trust to support and work with a purchasing group. Pharmacy quality control (QC) arrangements are involved in assessing product quality as part of the tendering process, as well as on a day-to-day basis (see Chapter 7 for further details on QC services).

Specialist involvement, combined with day-to-day working relationships between trusts and their buyer, minimises duplication of effort through shared access to central contract management and associated procurement expertise.

NHS CMU management systems

NHS CMU manages the contracting process using a system called Phacter. Phacter maintains a database of all suppliers and product lines. It generates invitations to tender (through an electronic format that suppliers access through an electronic portal Bravo) and produces comparative evaluations to support contract adjudication before finally generating award notices to suppliers and contract details to trusts through a web-accessed catalogue.

NHS CMU also collects, at each month end, in electronic format, hospital pharmacy purchasing information through a system known as Pharmex. Pharmex data are used to scope NHS secondary care business for tender. They also provide individual trusts and NHS CMU with measures reporting the performance of the contracting arrangements.

Through a third system, PharmaQC, NHS CMU collects and stores product images and supply chain information from suppliers. The QC pharmacists access this system to record their product assessments. Available at adjudication, via the system, this information ensures that QC product quality and risk assessments are reflected when contracts are awarded.

Meeting structures

The totality of the contracting arrangements is underpinned through meeting arrangements and communication structures. The pharmacy purchasing groups, elected chairs and their buyers meet regularly to share information, adjudicate contracts and monitor performance. At the national level the Pharmaceutical Market Support Group (PMSG), consisting primarily of the specialist procurement pharmacists and NHS CMU specialists, brings pharmaceutical expertise around a focus of contract management, making sure that security of supply is placed above savings. PMSG is supported by various working groups dedicated to specific workstreams. It reports to the National Pharmaceutical Supply Group (NPSG). NPSG membership consists of NHS trust chief pharmacists and PCT advisors. Its role is to provide advice to NHS CMU to ensure that it manages and develops its service in line with NHS requirements. Lastly, the chairs of both NPSG and PMSG attend regular meetings with the Department of Health chief pharmacist, the NHS CMU general manager, amongst others, to ensure that there is an exchange of information with Department of Health colleagues working at policy level.

Recent changes

All of the following changes will have long-term impact.

Home care

The growth in the supply of medicines to patients at home, either as components of packages of care or just simply as a route of supply, has been dramatic. Home care now represents a major part of NHS business. The NHS focus lies with the National Homecare Committee.[10]

Other service contracts

Stimulated by policy, by National Patient Safety Agency guidance and increasing demands on its finite capacity, the NHS is increasingly outsourcing other services such as outpatient dispensing, the provision of aseptically prepared products and 'specials' in addition to home care. Over time these changes will have an impact on contracting and procurement.

Payment by results and NICE

As described in Chapter 1, for England, payment by results has started to change the dynamics within the market for those high-cost medicines that are not included in the payment by results tariff (and particularly those approved by the National Institute for Health and Clinical Excellence (NICE): see Chapter 11). *The PPRS 2009*[1] allows pharmaceutical companies to propose patient schemes to improve the cost-effectiveness (cost per quality-adjusted life-year) of medicines. If NICE approves or partially recommends the medicine, these schemes become operational in order to achieve the cost-effectiveness approved by NICE. Types of scheme include free stock, rebates, straight discounts (applied to invoices at order point) and dose caps. Whilst providing access via the NHS to a wider range of medicines at cost-effective rates, these schemes have added a not inconsiderable burden to NHS medicines purchasing teams.

Security of supply

Globalisation within the pharmaceutical industry, associated with company mergers, rationalisation of manufacturing capacity, product discontinuations, extended supply chains, strengthened regulation and shifts in the sourcing of active pharmaceutical ingredients from China, are all contributing to increasing stresses within the supply chain, increasing risks to supply. The risks associated with the supply of counterfeit medicines are also increasing. The Department of Health (supported by the Medicines and Healthcare products Regulatory Agency), the PMSG, NHS CMU and the trade associations all work together to minimise these risks.

Product coding

The establishment of the Dictionary of Medicines and Devices, its acceptance and increasing application mean that the NHS has, for the first time ever, access to nationally recognised coding and product descriptions. Linked to bar coding (GS1), which is currently underutilised within hospital pharmacy, this will create unprecedented opportunities to improve hospital pharmacy supply management.

Local arrangements

The majority of pharmacy departments now use information technology systems for ordering, goods receipt and invoice processing. These systems are configured so that the audit requirement for segregation of these tasks between different staff members is delivered. Procedures must be consistent with the trust's standing financial instructions. Manual systems are occasionally used but these will be phased out and will not be covered here.

Ordering

Items which need to be ordered will be identified by the computer system or by pharmacy staff. Computer systems maintain live stock levels and, as these fall to the reorder level, the item is flagged for reorder. The reorder level is either fixed or can be calculated by the system based on an algorithm of average daily usage, time it takes to be delivered (lead time) and a preset safety factor. Infrequently used items may be flagged so that they are only placed on order by authorised staff.

The system will allocate these items to a preferred supplier that will be one of the following:

- the contract holder
- the manufacturer offering an NHS price
- a short-line store
- a wholesaler

These lists of items will be reviewed and amended by an authorised member of staff and orders generated. The supplier may be charged if the lead time is not appropriate for patient needs or the preferred supplier is out of stock. The orders will be sent to the supplier by one of the following methods:

- verbally by phone – this method is useful if the item is urgent or patient-specific. If used routinely, verbal ordering is labour-intensive and subject to transcription errors
- faxing: this reduces transcription errors but requires re-entering of data by the supplier and is dependent on the quality of the faxed copy
- electronic data interchange: this is exchange of electronic order data. It is the objective of all NHS ordering. The accuracy is dependent on the upkeep of product codes and so on, but it has the potential for rapid, accurate transfer, with minimal time commitment for staff. Examples include use of the Pharmacy Messenger system and Medecator
- post: this route is now rarely used due to time delay and cost.

Goods receipt

On receipt, goods will be checked visually for damage and expiry date. They will then be checked against the delivery note and against either a hard copy or computer copy of an order. The aim is to ensure that quantities and products are correct and that there are no obvious defects. Any discrepancies will be notified to the supplier immediately. Many trusts collect data on errors and timeliness of deliveries since supplier performance is a key consideration at contract adjudication. Once checks are complete, items will be entered into the computer system and stock levels updated.

Batch number details are recorded in some trusts, although the benefit of this is reduced by the inability to track batches to the end-user. There is a requirement to do this with blood products and medicines used in reproductive health services.

When controlled drugs are ordered and receipted, the requirements of the *Misuse of Drugs Regulations* must be followed.[11] Records of receipt are made in a register and the balance of stock received updated (see Chapter 5 for a more detailed discussion of controlled drugs)

Invoicing

Practice varies between trusts: this function is carried out by pharmacy staff in approximately 80% of trusts and by finance staff in the remainder. Wherever it is carried out, the system requires input of invoice data into the computer system and checking of price invoiced against price expected on the original order. Most trusts require exact matching of contract line prices and agreed tolerances with non-contract prices but use last purchase price on the orders.

Historically, invoices have been received in hard copy with details manually entered into the computer system. The receipt of electronic invoice files and subsequent matching of items is developing rapidly and is used to some extent in 20% of trusts. These systems automatically process items with complete matching of data and allow trust staff to focus on price or delivery discrepancies.

Acceptance of invoice details will update the unit cost of the item(s) on the computer system and also authorise payment to the supplier.

Looking forward

In the future we can expect a continuation of recently established trends, particularly the outsourcing of pharmacy-related services. With increasing demand on NHS resources the supply chain will come under ongoing scrutiny to improve its performance. The long-anticipated introduction of integrated electronic patient records systems across the NHS and the development of web-based e-commerce packages will radically change the procurement of pharmaceuticals and change will begin to occur at an accelerating rate. The increasing and disproportionate growth in high-cost medicines will force the relationships between clinical pharmacists and their procurement colleagues to strengthen to make sure that these medicines are sourced and managed with maximum efficiency. Similarly, the need to purchase with safety in mind requires close collaboration between the pharmacy purchasing team and frontline staff.

This will change the role of pharmacy staff from being process-focused to a more strategic role supporting the clinical objectives of the trust. The Audit Commission has indicated the need for trusts to make best use of supplies expertise and contract purchasing.[12] The demand to achieve effective and efficient purchasing for hospital medicines will continue. The procurement role will continue to form a building block for effective pharmacy services.

References

1. Department of Health. *The PPRS 2009*. Available online at: http://www.dh.gov.uk/en/ Publicationsandstatistics/Publications/PublicationsPolicyAndGuidance/DH_091825.
2. Pharmaceutical Price Regulation Scheme. Findings of OFT study (2005). Available online at: http://www.oft.gov.uk/OFTwork/markets-work/completed/pprs.
3. Department of Health. *The NHS Plan*. London: The Stationery Office, 2000.
4. Karr A. Procuring medicines – key issues for all pharmacy staff. *Hosp Pharm* 2006; 13: 391–393.
5. National Health Service Commercial Medicines Unit website: http://www.cmu.nhs.uk.
6. Department of Health. Gershon efficiency programme 2004–2008. Efficiency technical note. Available online at: http://www.dh.gov.uk/en/Publicationsandstatistics/Publications/ PublicationsPolicyAndGuidance/DH_081430.
7. Pharmaceutical Market Support Group products and services list. Available online at: http:// www.cmu.nhs.uk/Medicines/Pharmaceuticalproductsandservices/Pages/LandingPage.aspx.
8. Procurement policy and application of EU rules and regulations. Available online at: http:// www.ogc.gov.uk/procurement_policy_and_application_of_eu_rules_uk_regulations_.asp.
9. Procurement policy and application of EU rules and guidance. Available online at: http:// www.ogc.gov.uk/procurement_policy_and_application_of_eu_rules_guidance_on_the_UK_ regulations.asp.
10. National Homecare Committee website: http://www.cmu.nhs.uk/homecare/Pages/NHMC. aspx.
11. *The Misuse of Drugs Regulations 2001*. London: The Stationery Office, 2001.
12. Audit Commission. Procurement and supply, 2002. Available online at: http://www.audit-commission.gov.uk/nationalstudies/health/other/Pages/procurementandsupply.aspx.

Further reading

Brown S, Lamming R, Bassat J *et al. Strategic Operations Management*. London: Butterworth-Heinemann, 2005.
Department of Health. *Necessity not Nicety*. London: Department of Health, 2009.
Guild of Healthcare Pharmacists Procurement and Distribution Special Interest Group website: http://www.pdig.org.uk.
Karr A. Specialising in procurement. *Hosp Pharm* 2004; 11: 379–382.
Samways D, Wind K, Page J. Towards 'intelligent' purchasing. *Hosp Pharm* 2001; 8: 144–146.
Wind K, Aubrey P. Hospital drug procurement – more a can of worms than a can of beans. *Hosp Pharm* 2005; 12: 242.

4

Medicines supply and automation

Chris Green and Don Hughes

Supply of medicines is part of a multidisciplinary process, triggered by the writing of a prescription and ending with the administration of a medicine to a patient. As nearly every patient admitted to hospital will receive a medicine in one form or other, the safe and secure handling of medicines is an essential part of a hospital's medicines management system and is subject to the standards set out in the requirements for trusts to register with their regulator, for example the Care Quality Commission in England.[1] Medicines management therefore needs to be undertaken within a framework of policies, procedures, staff training and quality assurance measures.

Most National Health Service (NHS) hospital organisations define responsibilities for each component of medicines management in their medicines policy. Whilst the chief executive has the overall statutory responsibility for every activity within the hospital, the chief pharmacist is responsible for ensuring that systems are in place to address appropriately all aspects of the safe and secure handling of medicines, accountable directly to the chief executive for this purpose across the whole of the organisation. This re-emphasises the role of the 'senior pharmacist' described in the revised Duthie report, which also gives guidance on the responsibilities of other professionals in the handling of medicines.[2]

History

A key milestone in the adoption of security measures into medicines supply occurred with the publication of the Aitken report in 1958, which recommended practices that are still followed today.[3] However, the key driver in the development of systems has been the desire to improve medication safety. This was recognised as a major cause for concern during the 1960s and resulted in the introduction of new prescribing and administration recording systems, which form the basis for those in use, even today. Many hospital organisations are using prescription forms which have changed little in 20 years (an example is given in Chapter 9).

Most hospitals operated a 'stock' and 'non-stock' system for medicines on their wards, though few still operate this system. Stock medicines were those that were in routine use on that particular ward and specialty. 'Non-stock items' were supplied individually for those medicines that were not routinely used on that particular ward. This also applied to medicines that the hospital wanted to restrict or monitor. More recently, with the advent of payment by results, as mentioned in Chapter 1, English trusts may wish to issue medicines which are excluded from the regular tariff payment scheme to individual patients, so that dispensing data can be interrogated to ascertain which patients have received which medicines and, in some cases, for what purpose. It may be used to promote return to pharmacy of unused, less common medicines when the patient is discharged.

Current systems

In recognising that many processes had changed little since the 1970s and 1980s, a number of factors have influenced the systems and processes for the supply of medicines in UK hospitals over the past decade. Hospitals have a much higher occupancy rate, with reduced lengths of stay. There has been an increased emphasis on clinical governance and growing awareness of medication errors. Patients have more chronic illnesses and complex medication regimens. The *European Community Directive 92/27* was incorporated into UK law on 1 January 1999.[4] It required, amongst other things, that all medicines supplied to patients should include a patient information leaflet (PIL) and be labelled with the product batch number and expiry date. The directive was one of the key drivers behind the introduction of original pack dispensing into hospital practice. Traditional practice of limiting discharge supplies and splitting packs risked non-compliance with the law and possible prosecution.

Along with individual patient dispensing and the more recent models of supply, the use of patient bedside medicine cabinets is now widely adopted as an established practice across the NHS. The benefits of the cabinets are that individual patients' medicines are kept at their bedside, reducing the risk of selection errors and errors of omission and, in addition, the traditional nursing drug trolley, which was traditionally crammed with a huge array of medicines, is now a much more streamlined operation which also has the benefit of reducing selection error.

It is perhaps helpful to mention the arrangements under which hospital pharmacies operate at this point. Unlike community pharmacies, hospital pharmacy departments do not require premises registration with the

General Pharmaceutical Council to provide services to their wards and out-patients. Whilst at the time of writing the Medicines Act is under review, the current exemption is based on section 10 of the Act and relates to a 'hospital's normal business'. Hospital pharmacies do have quality systems and detailed standard operating procedures for dispensing and supply just as required for registered pharmacies. However, many hospital pharmacies do register: this became common when Crown immunity was removed over 20 years ago. This permits them to undertake other activities – not 'normal business of a hospital' – and where this is the case the responsible pharmacist requirements apply. A detailed discussion of this is beyond the remit of this chapter. Details about responsible pharmacist can be found on the General Pharmaceutical Council website at http://www.pharmacyregulation.org/regulatingpharmacy/thephar-macyregister/responsiblepharmacist/index.aspx.

Non-stock dispensing

The choice of inpatient supply system for a hospital lies anywhere on a spectrum between total stock and almost complete individual dispensing. Whilst the former was the traditional Scottish system and the latter is favoured in private hospitals because it facilitates charging, the choice in NHS hospitals throughout the UK should now be based on a careful risk appraisal of the options and resources (principally staff) available.

'One-stop dispensing'

Original pack dispensing has now been widely adopted across most hospitals in the UK and is referred to as 'one-stop dispensing' or 'dispensing for discharge'. The concept is to combine inpatient and discharge dispensing into a single supply, labelled with directions for use. In this system, patients' medicines are supplied as soon as they are needed, and labelled for discharge so that only one supply is made during the patient's stay. Manufacturers' original packs are usually dispensed and the patient is discharged with what remains after use in hospital. If this is less than a minimum quantity agreed with local general practitioners (GPs), usually 2 weeks' supply, an additional pack is issued. Large numbers of individually dispensed items cannot be handled in a conventional medicines trolley, so each patient normally has a bedside medicines cabinet, which can also be used for the patient's own drugs (PODs: see later in chapter) or in a self-administration scheme. To operate efficiently, a judgement needs to be made about which medicines can be relabelled for discharge early in the patient's admission, and which cannot. For example, aspirin 75 mg tablets for cardiovascular disease are almost universally prescribed and taken by patients as a once-daily dose and, similarly, statins are also taken once at night. Therefore it would be reasonably safe to make the assumption that, provided the patient continues to take the medicine after discharge, the directions will probably not change. However, in the case of warfarin, corticosteroids or antibiotics, for example, it is likely that doses or duration of treatment will change before or at the point of discharge, such that labelling them before this point is somewhat risky. These also reduce the risk of medication error by limiting the choices for selection at administration times and allow nurses to give more individualised patient care. There is a need to keep the contents of cabinets up to date with prescription changes and, at discharge, to check that the pack quantity and label are still appropriate and that the cabinet is empty, all of which may be undertaken by a pharmacist or technician.

Patients benefit by having PILs provided and by avoiding the wait for discharge medicines to be dispensed, provided that the prescription is written in good time, and also by having more time before ordering repeat prescriptions. The hospital can meet its legal obligation on PILs and also benefits from speedier discharges.

The Royal Pharmaceutical Society's Hospital Pharmacists Group has produced useful guidance on the introduction of one-stop dispensing, use of PODs and self-administration schemes.[5] Using patient packs at the time of discharge, a possible intermediate step to one-stop dispensing, has also been successful.[6]

The review of medicines management in NHS hospitals undertaken by the Audit Commission in 2001 and the recommendations made have had a profound impact on the modernisation of the dispensing process.[7] Many NHS hospitals have installed automated dispensing systems in the past decade as a consequence of the recommendations. A number of commercial systems are now available that accurately pick original patient packs to support the one-stop dispensing process and support re-engineering of services. Figure 4.1 provides

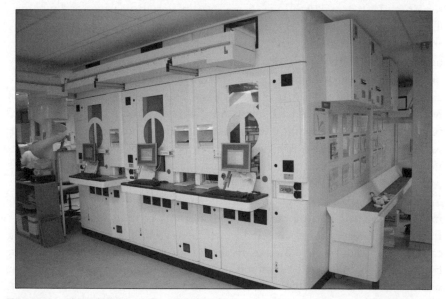

Figure 4.1   The ARX Rowa commercial system.

an example of such a system – the ARX Rowa from the Countess of Chester NHS Foundation Trust.

Scanning of bar codes is also used in loading such machines, enabling the robot to identify different products, strengths or pack sizes. Products can be packed very compactly because any gaps can be filled without regard to any human need for selection, as positions are memorised by the system's computer. The machines can also occupy less floor space than an equivalent amount of conventional shelving. A number of studies have shown the beneficial impact on dispensing errors, reduced dispensary turnaround times, simplified ordering systems, improved reliability of service and more efficient use of staff.[8–10]

Patients' own drugs

Patients admitted to hospital are usually asked to bring their medicines with them to facilitate the recording of their drug history and some trusts run publicity campaigns on bus adverts and in GP practices to promote this. Traditionally, PODs were routinely returned to pharmacy for destruction once a hospital supply was obtained. However, the move to dispensing of prescriptions in primary care using manufacturers' original packs has given much greater confidence in their continued usefulness, but only for the patient to whom they were originally supplied. Before use their suitability must be assessed, with this being variously undertaken by pharmacists, technicians, doctors or nurses at different hospitals. Most hospitals will have a policy or set of procedures covering this. Reuse of patients' own medicines has a number of benefits, including the reduced risk of medication errors, since PODs can be used a reference to patients' medicines consumption prior to admission.

When the directions are inappropriate, relabelling by pharmacy staff may be permissible. As with one-stop dispensing, further checks on directions and quantities are required on discharge. The importance of these, including the check that the locker has been emptied, has been shown by reported errors, which also highlight the need for thorough training of those involved.[11] Guidance on implementation includes the need for publicity to encourage patients to bring in their medicines.[5]

Unit dose systems

Unit dose systems have been adopted quite widely in North America and many European countries but have only been tried to a limited extent in the UK. The concept is that pharmacy provides medicines to wards in single-unit packages, either just prior to the time of administration or on a daily or (for long-stay) weekly basis, placing them in the patient's individually labelled drawer in a medicine cabinet, trolley or cassette. Because of the labour-intensive nature of this work, and the advent of original pack dispensing, it has not been widely adopted in the UK.

Storage arrangements

Responsibilities

Each hospital's medicines policy will set out the roles and responsibilities for the safe and secure storage of medicines on wards. For the most part, the appointed registered nurse in charge of the ward or clinical area (usually the ward manager or theatre manager) or other professionally qualified person (possibly an operating department practitioner or radiographer) must ensure that systems for the safe use and security of medicines are followed and that stocks are safeguarded.[2] He or she may delegate some of the duties, such as access, to another nurse or to a member of the pharmacy staff, but the responsibility always remains with him or her. In almost all instances, medicines will be stored in locked cupboards or another secure receptacle, such as patients' medicines cabinets, described above. The pharmaceutical service may assume responsibility for replenishment of these stocks, advise on the type and location of cupboards, regularly inspect and audit them and assure the quality of the product at the time of use. However, pharmacy staff are rarely in a position to do more than this as they do not administer or use the items stored. What is clear is that this arrangement does present some risks if the wrong patient's medicines, stock items or medicines that are no longer needed are left in the patient's locker and not managed appropriately.

Keys

The keys to medicines stock cupboards, drug trolleys and patients' medicines cabinets should be labelled, kept separate and carried on the person of a nurse (or other qualified person in charge). Controlled drug (CD) cupboard keys should be kept on a separate ring that can be readily identified and carried by the assigned nurse in charge, that is, the senior registered nurse on duty for the ward or clinical area, identified as nurse in charge for that shift. This all has the effect of minimising unnecessary access to medicines. For self-administration schemes patients may hold the key for their own medicines locker; the appointed nurse in charge as described above should keep a master key.

Cupboards and trolleys

Separate lockable cupboards should be available for internal and external medicines (constructed to the British Standard specification) and CDs.[2] In small units, if space does not permit a separate cupboard for external medicines, they must be kept on a separate shelf, below those for internal use. A separate lockable medicine refrigerator must be available in all areas where medicines may require it, with a maximum minimum thermometer to enable regular checks that temperatures are maintained in the range 2–8°C. A number of hospitals are now using automated systems to monitor the fridges used to store medicines: these fridges are linked to alarm systems in the event of fridge failure.

Medicines in current use on wards are either kept in a lockable trolley or in individual patient medicine cabinets or drawers, usually at the bedside; none of these must be used for permanent storage. The trolley must be immobilised when not in use, locked either in a cupboard or to a wall; it is not normally used for CDs. Patient medicine cabinets or drawers must be lockable and not readily portable. In some hospitals, patients' medicines lockers are attached or an integrated part of their bedside locker, tend to be on wheels and are therefore portable to some extent. However, in practice this is seen as acceptable in many British hospitals.

Security

There are no published data to quantify the volume or cost of medicines that are misappropriated by hospital staff. Although the concept of diversion is rarely discussed, there are a number of anecdotal examples that suggest it is more common that most people would assume. Unpublished studies have suggested that as much as 20% of the medicines supplied to a ward will be unaccounted for.

Procedures and documentation need to minimise opportunities for misappropriation and some departments ask nursing staff to sign for deliveries to ensure there is an audit trail from the point of ordering to the point of delivery to wards.

A minimum requirement to give an audit trail in a manual system is that the requisition has the signature of the ordering nurse, that pharmacy can verify, the issuer's and checker's signature is entered and a receipt is obtained. Serial numbering and book-fast copies (kept for a minimum of 2 years) minimise the opportunity for destruction of records to go undetected. Where requisition books are used there should be only one in each ward or department, kept locked away, with new ones treated as controlled stationery, stocked only in pharmacy.

Exceptions

In some cases, organisations may decide that some medicines should be left in more readily accessible locations. Although this may not be ideal, a risk assessment may identify that this is an appropriate course of action.

Examples might include:

- medicines in emergency kits or on emergency drug trolleys, in clearly labelled boxes with a tamper-evident seal, kept readily accessible
- intravenous fluids, antiseptic and irrigation solutions
- medicines considered appropriate for some patients to administer under the supervision of a registered nurse, unless there is a hazard to other patients.

The last situation is distinct from participation in a formally recognised self-administration scheme, which allows greater independence of action for patients and no limit on the range of medicines covered. There must be a valid prescription for the medicine. The prescriber may specify that the patient should have ready access to the preparation but generally this is not specifically required in medicines policies. The registered nurse may decide (and this should be documented) on whether to have the medicine on the patient's bedside locker. The patient must be capable of administering the medicine correctly and willing and able to tell the nurse when a dose has been taken so that this can be recorded on the prescription sheet. Clearly, where a patient is using a medicine on a when-required or regular basis, a lack of awareness that the patient is doing so, that is, a lack of documentation on the drug administration record or prescription sheet, may mask a clinical issue that the team caring for the patient may wish to address. Examples include an increased use of glyceryl trinitrate spray, reliever inhalers or increased use of insulin devices. The medicine is likely to be in one of the following categories:

- inhalers
- glyceryl trinitrate sublingual tablets or spray
- oral contraceptives and hormone replacement therapy products – ointments or creams
- insulin preparations.

Ordering ward stock

Nurse requisitioning

Safety and security are key issues here. Ward staff tend to accept that what is supplied by pharmacy is correct, even though the supply may be based on an ambiguous or poorly written requisition, without sight of the prescription. On occasion, nursing staff may even identify an error made in the pharmacy department, but assume that because it has come from pharmacy, it is the correct product.

Traditionally, pharmacy would make a supply to patients on the strength of a requisition alone. One of the drivers for the development of clinical pharmacy was to encourage the review of prescriptions by a pharmacist in order to keep prescription and administration charts on wards, where they are in constant clinical use. An additional incentive was that it was easier to address problems with prescriptions at ward level in conjunction with the patient and the nursing and medical staff than it is in isolation in a pharmacy dispensary. More recently, most hospitals will not dispense an item without sight of the prescription chart and a check by a clinical pharmacist at ward level or in the dispensary. CDs are discussed in Chapter 5.

Topping up

Responsibility for routine ordering of ward stock is transferred, under this system, from nursing staff to pharmacy technicians or assistants, who check and replenish this to predetermined levels, usually weekly or twice weekly depending on the storage capacity and turnover of the wards concerned. The requirements are entered on either a computer-printed copy of the ward stock list or one stored on a hand-held computer, for example a personal digital assistant or bar code-scanning device. The stock list should be based on usage and agreed between the appointed nurse and a designated member of pharmacy staff, usually a technician, while clinical input from a pharmacist is also essential. The content of a ward stock list should be a balance between having readily available supplies of commonly used medicines and trying to cover every eventuality, which means stock lists which are greater than ward storage capacity allows and will probably result in stock items unnecessarily going out of date. Supplies are usually dispatched to the ward, in locked boxes, for nursing staff to put away and store. A delivery note recording what has been supplied should be sent to the ward with the products requested, and a copy should be retained in pharmacy once it has been signed by the nursing staff on the ward to confirm receipt. The top-up system is useful because it allows planning of workload, and reduces the need for nursing staff to spend significant amounts of time ordering medicines and the likelihood of commonly used medicines not being available to patients who need them.

Supply to outpatients

A number of options are available to allow patients access to medicines following an outpatient consultation in a hospital. The reason that these options exist arises from perverse arrangements for funding outpatient prescribing, and the application of value-added tax (VAT) to hospital-dispensed medicines, but not to those dispensed in the community.

Community dispensed route

The advantage to the hospital is that it does not pay VAT on medicines prescribed via this route; patients can be seen in clinic and then leave the hospital and go to their own community pharmacy, or at least one of their own choosing. This route also allows hospital pharmacy resources to be focused on the needs of inpatients and timely discharge processes. The disadvantages are that it is difficult to police what prescribers are writing on the forms in terms of formulary compliance and quantity, and the information arising from this has a lag time of approximately 3 months while the data are processed and collated by the prescription pricing authority. Another disadvantage is that prescriptions dispensed via this route do not attract contracted NHS discount prices and, in some cases, this cost differential may exceed that of VAT. In terms of public funding, the VAT reduction for the organisation using this route is matched by a reduction in revenues to the treasury. (Forms used by hospitals for dispensing in the community are known as FP10 in England, WP10 in Wales and GP10 in Scotland; the term has also been suffixed with (HP) to distinguish from GP forms.)

Hospital pharmacy dispensing

Similarly, prescriptions dispensed for outpatients from the hospital pharmacy may be more convenient for patients to collect while in the hospital, and may provide some reassurance to them. Hospitals pay VAT on medicines, whereas dispensing by community pharmacists is zero-rated and advantageous prices obtained through hospital contracts may be insufficient to counterbalance this difference. A major disadvantage to the hospital is that outpatient dispensing deflects pharmacists and technicians from a clinical role on the wards. In 1988 the Department of Health, in a health circular requiring health authorities to plan for implementation of clinical pharmacy, suggested that 'subject to a satisfactory local option-appraisal exercise', FP10(HP) forms could be used, 'thereby releasing hospital staff for other duties'.[12] Outpatient dispensing by hospitals is further challenged in the Audit Commission report, which in paragraph 64 suggests that 'the practice should be questioned'.[7]

Prepacked medicines

Suitably labelled prepacked medicines for standard treatments may be issued to departments (such as accident and emergency or outpatient clinics) for medical or nursing staff to add the patient's name and minor alterations to directions. Predictable requirements for day-case patients following surgery may be able to be dispensed in advance and issued after the pharmacy has closed. The advantage of this is that a limited list of products is supplied and is available to patients immediately following a consultation. This means that patients are accessing medicines without having to use resources in the hospital pharmacy, possibly bought at contract prices, and they do not have to wait.

GP referral forms

These forms are a benefit to the hospital in that prescribing costs are not picked up by the hospital, but they are inconvenient to patients since, in order to collect their medicines, they need to visit the GP, hand in the form, wait for 24–48 hours while the form is processed, collect the prescription from the GP and then go to the community pharmacy. This is hardly an efficient use of resources or helping the patient experience. The option of referring patients back to their GP for prescribing is dependent on the acceptability of transfer of clinical responsibility.[13] In Scotland the GP always retains this: the out-patient is referred to the hospital only for a consultation, so prescription on GP10 forms is the norm. In England and Wales such transfer of prescribing was often seen as 'cost-shifting' of expensive treatments from hospital budgets to primary care. This was unpopular with GPs, when they had insufficient information to manage the patient safely, since ultimate liability lies with the doctor who signs the prescription.[13] These problems can be overcome with shared-care agreements between the consultant and the GP on continuing care, once the patient's condition is stable, under a protocol normally provided by the hospital.[14] For some patients the GP may prefer to initiate long-term treatment with a drug from the practice formulary.

'RAG lists'

Many areas have a 'RAG list' (red, amber, green list) that is a list of medicines suitable for prescribing either in hospitals, or by GPs, or both. For example, most cytotoxic preparations or retinoids would always be 'red' and hospital-only prescriptions, whereas antibiotics or antihypertensives would always be 'green'. There may be exceptions to this general rule, where a new class of drug is introduced or the drug is for a niche indication. 'Amber' drugs tend to be medicines that might be initiated by the hospital, and then once the patient is reasonably stable, care would be taken over by the GP via a shared-care protocol, for example, methotrexate.

Home care

Since the late 1990s, the use of home care has expanded enormously. Hospitals enter an arrangement with a home care company, of which there are several, to supply medicines to their patients. The consultant seeing the patient completes a bespoke prescription form that goes to the home care company. The company then supplies the medicines directly to the patient, either by post or by courier, and in some instances will also provide nursing support, including either administering the drug or training patients to do it themselves. Such arrangements should have suitable financial and clinical governance arrangements.

Community pharmacy partnerships

A more recent development is the introduction of independent pharmacies to hospital sites. The model is such that the community pharmacy dispenses outpatient prescriptions from the hospital. The medicines used in the supply to patients are purchased at contract prices which would routinely be available to that hospital, and also dispensed at zero VAT, resulting in potentially significant cost savings to the trust. In this way, hospitals will be able to take advantage of zero-rated VAT and, in addition, receive a double saving via contracted discounts.

Overall, it may be that a number of routes are appropriate for a hospital to make the most of cost-efficient prescribing strategies. For example, when providing antitumour necrosis factor-alpha therapies such as etanercept, where there is no contract price, and VAT is significant, the home care route is attractive. Similarly, the prescription of urgently needed antibiotics or analgesics might best be provided via the FP10 route while supply of anti-retrovirals might be suited to a partnership with a community pharmacy on the hospital site. For extemporaneous preparations, the hospital pharmacy is an appropriate route because of the costs associated with prescription via FP10 and supply via specials manufacturers. However, the complexity of this section highlights the inefficiencies and lack of a seamless approach to the supply of medicines to outpatients.

Clinical trials

A clinical trial is an investigation by a doctor or dentist involving administration of a medicinal product to a patient to assess the product's safety and efficacy (a Medicines and Healthcare products Regulatory Agency definition).[15] The pharmacist has a key role in the organisation and management of clinical trials, which is much wider than the supply function; this is reflected in good clinical practice. A definition from EU Directive 2001/20/EC, article 1, clause 2 states that 'Good clinical practice is a set of internationally recognised ethical and scientific quality requirements which must be observed for designing, conducting, recording and reporting clinical trials that involve the participation of human subjects'.[16]

All medicines, or constituent ingredients, for clinical trials should be ordered, stored and dispensed by the hospital pharmacy. Separate stocks should not be kept elsewhere in the hospital. Accurate records must be maintained of receipt, dispensing, issue, administration and disposal and 'regularly audited by pharmacy staff, with reconciliation, where necessary'.[16] All staff involved in dispensing clinical trials must have been trained to do so, and record of this training kept in each trial folder. Disposal of unused products in a company-sponsored trial must be according to the company's instructions.

New and emerging technologies

With increasing use of electronic prescribing, the opportunity arises for the seamless transfer of an order, generated from the electronic prescription, and in many cases, linked to the use of bar codes. This means that orders can be generated and transmitted to pharmacy in real time, unlike paper that needs to be delivered, and this order does not hold the risk of transcription error. Indeed, by routing these orders directly from the electronic prescribing system to an integrated or via an interface to a separate dispensing system, any human intervention can be removed, significantly reducing the risk of error.[17] Some hospitals will have a prescribing system separate to that of their dispensing system such that the prescribing system generates a paper order which is then transferred to the dispensing system by pharmacy staff. Although this generates the opportunity for human error, there are usually issues around the functionality of the prescribing system to act as a dispensing system that make this an issue, and one that needs to be considered during procurement exercises.

Medicines management systems and processes should be chosen to minimise the potential for medication errors wherever possible. Techniques such as failure modes and effects analysis can be used to break down processes into steps and determine the steps in the process that may result in an error, and identify opportunities to make the process safer and more efficient.[18] In addition, security measures should minimise the risk of misappropriation of medicines by staff, to protect them and the wider community.

Pneumatic conveying (air tube) systems are being increasingly used for rapid delivery of ward stock and discharge medicines within a hospital. Until electronic prescribing is more widely available, time and effort are saved by sending prescriptions to pharmacy this way. They can help to support pharmacy staff who are working in a decentralised, clinically based system. The only problem may be if the system fails, if delivery is not then necessarily to the intended destination.

Ward automation of medicine supplies

In line with other industries, hospitals are introducing new technologies to manage stocks of supplies and medicines automatically in clinical areas. A number of manufacturers are producing purpose-built advanced vending machines suitable for storage of medicines and other consumable products.

Most share a number of common features, which offer significant advantages over existing storage facilities and processes. In principle, the systems consist of a number of frames containing a number of drawers and storage cupboards that come in a range of shapes and sizes. Access is computer-controlled and, most commonly, restricted via use of a pin number, swipe card, fingerprint scan or combination of the three. Product selection and identification are usually supported by a fixed location within the system, restrictions on how much drawers can open, directional light technology and a visual display, possibly of a photograph of the product, on the system's computer monitor. Bar code technology is frequently used to control the stock in the system, which is intended to minimise the likelihood of selection and replenishment errors.[19, 20] Medicines administration can also be supported by the on-screen option to view or print guidelines and protocols while accessing the product. Most have a refrigerator attached which is controlled by a magnetic lock, and some have external storage options, that is, shelves or cupboards, and stock movement is monitored using bar code scanners. Similar facilities in hospital wards and departments in the USA have shown a number of key benefits. These include significant reductions in time spent on nurse and pharmacy medication-related activities, high user acceptability and significant reductions in medication errors.[21–25] It is anticipated that these types of systems will become the recommended storage facilities for medicines in UK hospitals in the next few years.

Clearly the opportunity to link electronic prescribing, ward automation and the 'bar-coded patient' allows the development of a closed-loop system in which patient safety is supported by the use of bar codes.[21] This approach has the potential to be the future of medicines management at ward level.

References

1. Care Quality Commission website: http://www.cqc.org.uk/ (accessed 19 August 2010).
2. Royal Pharmaceutical Society of Great Britain. *The Safe and Secure Handling of Medicines: A Team Approach. A Revision of the Duthie Report (1988) led by the Hospital Pharmacist's Group of the Royal Pharmaceutical Society.* London: RPSGB, 2005.
3. Department of Health and Social Security. *Report on Control of Dangerous Drugs and Poisons in Hospital – The Aitken Report.* London: HMSO, 1958.
4. *European Community Directive 92/27.* Brussels: Council of European Communities, 1992.
5. The Hospital Pharmacists Group. One-stop dispensing, use of patients' own drugs and self-administration schemes. *Hosp Pharm* 2002; 9: 81–86.
6. Jeffery L. 28 day patient pack discharge medication. *Pharm Manage* 2001; 17: 24–25.
7. Audit Commission. *A Spoonful of Sugar – Medicines Management in NHS Hospitals.* London: Audit Commission, 2001.
8. Farrar K, Slee A, Hughes D. Implementing an automated dispensing system. *Pharm J* 2002; 268: 22–23.
9. Fitzpatrick R, Cooke P, Southall C *et al.* Evaluation of an automated dispensing system in a hospital pharmacy dispensary. *Pharm J* 2005; 274: 763–765.
10. Dean Franklin B, O'Grady K, Voncina L *et al.* An evaluation of two automated dispensing machines in UK hospital pharmacy. *Int J Pharm Prescribing* 2008; 16: 47–53.

11. Cousins DH, Upton DR. Take care when using PODs. *Pharm Pract* 1998; 8: 26–32.
12. Department of Health. *The Way Forward for Hospital Pharmaceutical Services.* HC(88)54. London: The Stationery Office, 1988.
13. NHS Executive. *Responsibility for Prescribing Between GPs and Hospitals.* EL(91)127. London: The Stationery Office, 1991.
14. Stephens M. Shared care arrangements. In: *Strategic Medicines Management.* London: Pharmaceutical Press, 2005, p. 149.
15. Medicines and Healthcare products Regulatory Agency standards on regulation. Available online at: http://www.mhra.gov.uk/Howweregulate/Medicines/Inspectionandstandards/GoodClinicalPractice/index.htm.
16. Good clinical practice. Available online at: http://www.eortc.be/Services/Doc/clinical-EU-directive-04-April-01.pdf.
17. Dean-Franklin B, Jacklin A, Barber N. The impact of an electronic prescribing and administration system on the safety and quality of medication administration. *Int J Pharm Pract* 2008; 16: 375–379.
18. Williamson S, Wake N, Donovan G. FMEA: a new approach to manage high risk medicines. *Br J Clin Pharm* 2009; 1: 329–332.
19. Arden-Jones J, Hughes DK, Rowe PH *et al.* Attitudes and opinions of nursing and medical staff regarding the supply and storage of medicinal products before and after the installation of a drawer-based automated stock control system. *Int J Pharm Pract* 2009; 17: 95–99.
20. Arden-Jones J, Hughes DK, Rowe PH *et al.* The impact of a ward-based automated vending unit on nursing tasks and time in the emergency department. *Int J Pharm Pract* 2009; 17: 1–5.
21. Dean Franklin B, O'Grady K, Donyai P *et al.* The impact of a closed loop electronic prescribing and administration system on prescribing errors, administration and staff time: a before and after study. *Qual Safe Health Care* 2007; 16: 279–284.
22. Guerrero RM, Nickman NA, Jorgenson JA. Work activities before and after implementation of an automated dispensing system. *Am J Health-System Pharm* 1996; 53: 548–554.
23. Schwarz H, Brodowy B. Implementation and evaluation of an automated dispensing system. *Am J Health-System Pharm* 1995; 52: 823–882.
24. Kimble C, Chandra A. Automation of pharmacy systems: experiences and strategies of a rural healthcare system. *Hosp Topics* 2001; 79: 27–32.
25. Borel J, Rascati K. Effect of an automated, nursing unit-based drug dispensing device on medication errors. *Am J Health-System Pharm* 1995; 52: 1875–1879.

Further reading

Care Quality Commission website: http://www.cqc.org.uk/, in particular the management of medicines guidance (accessed 19 August 2010).
Royal Pharmaceutical Society of Great Britain. *The Safe and Secure Handling of Medicines: A Team Approach. A Revision of the Duthie Report (1988) led by the Hospital Pharmacist's Group of the Royal Pharmaceutical Society.* London: RPSGB, 2005.
Responsible pharmacist and hospital practice:
http://www.rpsgb.org.uk/pdfs/rprequirementshospstat.pdf (when to register).
http://www.rpsgb.org/pdfs/rprequirementshospguid.pdf (detailed discussion of implications).

5

Controlled drugs in hospital pharmacy

Liz Mellor

Background: legislative framework

The management of controlled drugs (CDs) in hospitals, although a multidisciplinary responsibility, is a key element of medicines management governance. It is helpful, when considering CD issues, to understand the basic legislative framework, and a little of why and how it has developed over the past decade. Most CD legislation is consistent across the UK, though there are slightly different arrangements that underpin the delivery of these requirements across the four regions of the UK. This chapter refers predominantly to the legislation in England.

The conviction of Dr Harold Shipman for the murder of 15 of his patients using CDs and the subsequent findings of the independent public inquiry, led by Dame Janet Smith, laid much of the foundation for the Department of Health's *Safer Management of Controlled Drugs* programme.[1] The inquiry's *Fourth Report* focused on the methods used by Shipman to divert large quantities of CDs for his own purposes, and considered how he was able to do this for so long without detection.[2] It concluded that there were serious shortcomings in the systems for regulating CDs and, in response, the government proposed a series of measures which involved amendments to existing, as well as new, legislation.

The Department of Health is responsible for *The Health Act 2006*, which applies across the UK and with its associated regulations provides the basis for the new legislation strengthening the governance and monitoring arrangements for CDs.[3] Whilst continuing to encourage good practice, it introduced and strengthened systems aimed at detecting unusual or poor practice, criminal activity or risk to patients. It is this Act that introduced the requirement for healthcare organisations to appoint a CD accountable officer.

No one agency holds complete responsibility for CDs or for CD legislation and it is important to remember that the overall legislative framework which applies to all medicines is the *Medicines Act 1968*,[4] and subsequent regulations, which are managed by the Medicines and Healthcare products Regulatory Agency (MHRA).

CDs are simply a group of substances, some of which are used as medicines, that have the potential for abuse. For this reason the Home Office has placed additional controls on these substances through the *Misuse of Drugs Act 1971*.[5] The *Misuse of Drugs Act* imposes a complete ban on the possession, supply, manufacture, import and export of CDs, except in situations allowed by regulations or by licence. In the Act substances are divided into three classes, A, B and C; this categorisation is linked to the maximum penalties that may be imposed in criminal law on a person convicted of an offence under the Act. The Act also introduced the Advisory Council on the Misuse of Drugs, a body that keeps under review substances that are likely to be misused or constitute a social problem in the UK and provides advice on measures to prevent misuse.

It is the *Misuse of Drugs Regulations 2001* which permit the clinical use of CDs as medicines, many of which are extremely valuable to patient care.[6] *The Misuse of Drugs Regulations (Northern Ireland) 2002* are broadly similar to the *Misuse of Drugs Regulations 2001*.[6, 7] The 2001 regulations categorise CDs into five schedules according to the level of control they need: schedule 1 CDs are subject to the highest level of control and schedule 5 CDs are subject to the lowest level of control. Few substances in schedule 1 are used therapeutically and so it is schedule 2 substances used in medicinal products that are the focus of the most stringent procedures in hospitals. Detailed information relating to each schedule can be found using the further reading and reference resources provided at the end of this chapter.

The controls placed on each drug in a specific schedule relate to all aspects of medicines management, including medicine production and supply, possession, prescription, record-keeping, preservation of records and supervision of destruction; the controls reflect a judgement balancing the therapeutic benefit against potential harm if the substance were to be misused. Hospital pharmacy staff play a crucial role in ensuring CDs are available for use in patient care when clinically indicated. Strengthened controls, implemented through local procedures, should support healthcare professionals and encourage good practice whilst providing monitoring tools that can help to indicate when potential misuse or misdirection might be a concern. Misuse of CDs can occur in any aspect of their management.

The accountable officer

The Health Act 2006 requires all healthcare organisations, which are described as 'controlled drug designated bodies', to appoint an accountable officer.[3] This includes NHS organisations, including primary care trusts and foundation trusts, as well as independent hospitals that are registered with the Care Quality Commission under relevant service user categories.

Accountable officers must be senior executives in the organisation with professional credibility and sufficient seniority to enable them to take action regardless of how a concern about CDs is raised.[8] They should not be personally involved in the routine prescribing, supply, administration or disposal of CDs. Hospital accountable officers are most frequently a chief pharmacist, chief nurse or medical director.

The accountable officer in each healthcare and social care organisation must ensure the safe management of CDs at a local level.[9] There are a number of specific aspects they have to oversee in order to do this:

Standard operating procedures

Accountable officers must ensure adequate and up-to-date standard operating procedures (SOPs) are in place within their organisation;[10] these should support strong governance arrangements and must be compliant with the relevant current legal framework.

SOPs must cover the following as a minimum:

- who has access to CDs
- where and how CDs are stored
- how CDs are transported within the organisation
- how CDs are destroyed and disposed of
- who is alerted if complications or concerns arise or incidents occur
- what records need to be maintained, including relevant CD register requirements
- how records of schedule 2 drugs that have been returned by patients are kept and managed

The accountable officer should make sure that additional SOPs are available within the organisation, where required, to ensure all aspects of CD management and accountability are clearly defined and agreed. Most hospitals will have similar core SOPs but their content and detail may vary, as they should be specifically tailored to the healthcare setting and reflect the roles and responsibilities agreed within the organisation.[10]

Hospital pharmacists are in an ideal position to observe day-to-day practice with CDs in clinical areas and can help to identify when local SOPs may need review or where additional training may be required.

Routine monitoring and auditing

The accountable officer must ensure that the use of CDs is monitored through routine processes such as data analysis, audit and clinical governance, all of which should form an integral part of the organisation's normal governance systems.[9]

Hospital pharmacists are key members of the multidisciplinary team supporting accountable officers in their monitoring role. Different models and approaches to routine monitoring and auditing exist across hospitals but it is generally recommended that the security of CDs is checked, by pharmacy staff, at least every 3 months.[11, 12]

The process of monitoring should include aspects of both audit and reconciliation, and should occur in all locations where CDs are stored. This independent assessment of local CD management supported by knowledge and data can help assess and detect discrepancies between amounts supplied and amounts prescribed and used. Even simple acts such as roughly correlating supply and prescription can act as indictors to trigger more in-depth investigations and help eliminate error, misuse or misdirection. E-prescribing, electronic data collection and automated data analysis tools have been developed within some organisations to provide reports which can be used to support the audit and reconciliation processes.

The same principles of having an independent approach to the monitoring of CD stock held within hospital pharmacies should be considered best practice. It is recommended that organisations arrange for periodic checks of pharmacy-held CDs by appropriate personnel who do not routinely work in the particular pharmacy service.[12]

The focus of clinical area – including pharmacy – checks is often solely on schedule 2 CDs for which a register or record book is required. However, it should be remembered that all drugs classified in the misuse of drugs legislation are known to have the potential for misuse.[13] Therefore, hospital pharmacies should develop systems to assess periodically the local management and use of other medicines with the potential for misuse, including medicines in schedules 3 to 5.

Currently, primary care trust accountable officers are required to monitor all prescriptions for CDs dispensed in the community through the Electronic Prescribing Analysis and Costs (ePACT) data analysis tools available from the Prescription Pricing Division of the NHS Business Services Authority. Hospitals who issue FP10 (HNC) prescriptions, which are dispensed in the community, should ensure that their hospital CD ePACT reports form part of their local CD prescription monitoring processes.

Systems were introduced in 2006 to control and collect data on all private prescriptions for schedule 2 and 3 CDs dispensed by community pharmacies.[14] Non-NHS prescribing of schedule 2 and 3 CDs, which are to be dispensed by a community pharmacist, must be on a dedicated prescription form (FP10PCD) and each prescriber must be allocated a unique six-digit private CD prescriber's code. Private prescriptions issued and dispensed within the same hospital are not currently subject to the same requirements; this is one area where the hospital accountable officer may require additional specific and comprehensive monitoring arrangements if such a service is provided.

The Care Quality Commission (CQC) is required to produce an annual report on the safer management of CDs. This provides data and an overview against which certain aspects of hospital prescribing and medicines use can be further analysed.

Inspection, self-assessment and declaration to the relevant authority

All healthcare organisations providing clinical services and relevant social care organisations must complete a periodic declaration on whether or not their organisation keeps stocks of CDs and whether there are any special circumstances that might explain any unusual patterns of prescribing or supply.

NHS trusts are required to register with the CQC in relation to their compliance with the essential standards of quality and safety. The CQC registration framework incorporates CD management within the medicines management outcome.[15] The CQC has developed a CD self-assessment tool to support acute NHS trusts and primary care organisations in considering the comprehensiveness of their own local practices and procedures. The tool also forms a helpful educational resource.[16]

Collaboration and local intelligence networks

Accountable officers must establish and operate arrangements for sharing information. Currently, primary care trust accountable officers have additional responsibilities, as they are required to establish and operate a local intelligence network (LIN).[8, 9] With the revised structures emerging for the NHS in England, similar arrangements will be put in place once PCTs are abolished.

A LIN must involve all accountable officers from local hospitals: NHS, including foundation trusts, independent sector, hospices, ambulance trusts and local care providers along with representatives from any relevant local and national agencies who may be involved in any aspect of CD management or inspection, such as professional regulatory bodies, the CQC and police forces. Although the *Health Act* placed a legal duty of collaboration on responsible bodies, the precise make-up of a LIN is decided locally.

LINs often have their own local information-sharing codes and procedures; they provide an excellent forum to share learning from CD incidents or investigations and can also act to encourage good practice developments.

The LIN enables concerns to be raised and encourages intelligence and information-sharing, which may include situations involving individuals who give cause for concern. Each accountable officer in the LIN must present quarterly occurrence reports to the primary care trust accountable officer who leads the network. Each occurrence report will describe details of any concerns the organisation has regarding the management of CDs, or confirmation that they have none.

All hospital pharmacy staff should be clear how they report concerns about CD issues, either through their management arrangements or in some instances directly to their organisation's accountable officer.

The CQC is responsible for making sure that healthcare providers and regulators are creating a safer environment for the management of CDs. Designated bodies must notify the CQC of the appointment of their accountable officer and of any subsequent changes; the CQC is required to publish a list of accountable officers in England and this list can be found on the CQC website (http://www.cqc.org.uk/).

Medicines management

All aspects of CD medicines management and governance should be detailed in local CD SOPs; these should reflect relevant aspects of CD legislation as well as NHS guidance and any additional local requirements specified in the trust's medicine policies. The following paragraphs are intended to provide an overview of some areas where the law and guidance meet and suggest further best-practice considerations. More detailed guidance can be found in the further reading provided at the end of this chapter.

Storage

It is the *Misuse of Drugs (Safe Custody) Regulations 1973* that impose controls on the storage of CDs, requiring safe custody, in certain types of premises.[17] Retail dealers (pharmacies), including any registered pharmacy premises in hospitals, private hospitals and care homes, must store their CDs in a CD cabinet or safe which complies with the specifications in the regulations or obtain a police certificate to confirm an adequate degree of security.[18]

NHS hospitals are required to keep CDs in a 'locked receptacle' which can only be opened by a person who can lawfully be in possession of CDs, for example a pharmacist or a senior registered nurse in charge of a hospital ward or department. It is generally considered good practice to ensure that wards store CDs in a specific cupboard that conforms, as a minimum, to an appropriate British Standard (for example, BS2881).

Additional security measures may be considered necessary for areas where staff are not present for 24 hours in a day or closure occurs at weekends. CD cupboards should not be used to store anything else, including patient valuables, to minimise the occasions when access is required.[12]

Some organisations apply CD secure storage and recording procedures to CD medicines which are not subject to the legal safe storage requirements, for example, midazolam, or where these procedures are used as a means of reducing the risk of inadvertent selection or administration, for example, concentrated potassium-containing products.[19] Local SOPs should make these situations clear to staff and they should form part of induction and training activities.

Ordering and transport

All stationery which is used to order, return or distribute CDs must be stored securely and access to it should be restricted. Stock of CDs for wards, operating theatres and departments is obtained from a hospital pharmacy by an authorised practitioner using duplicate requisitions, most frequently in the standard NHS CD supplies order book. It is good practice to verify that the person placing the order is authorised to do so through a system such as having a list of authorised signatories available at the point of dispensing, ideally validated and authorised through appropriate management routes. Registered operating department practitioners and senior registered nurses or acting senior registered nurses are authorised to order, possess and supply CDs.[12]

It is considered good practice to have systems and SOPs that ensure at each point where a CD moves from the authorised possession of one person to another, a retrievable record is made which contributes to the maintenance of a full audit trail for each product.

Administration

A record of the administration of schedule 2 CDs should be made in patient-specific documentation or medical record systems and in a CD stock record book, following local organisational procedures. The Nursing and Midwifery Council recommends that the record of administration of CDs within secondary care, or similar healthcare setting, requires a second signatory.[20]

Controlled drug record-keeping requirements

A record should be kept of all schedule 2 CDs that are received or issued, throughout the hospital. The Nursing and Midwifery Council recommends that all entries must be signed by two registrants and that the stock balance of an individual preparation must be confirmed to be correct after every administration when the balance is recorded in the CD record book.

It is good practice to require that the stock balance of all medicines entered in the CD record book should be checked and reconciled with the amounts in the cupboard with sufficient frequency to ensure that discrepancies can be identified and investigated in a timely way. If long periods lapse between stock checks it becomes far more difficult to identify the cause of any discrepancy and, indeed, those staff who may be linked to the event.

Before 2007 the legally required CD register was of a prescribed layout. This was replaced with the requirement that a CD register must contain specific headings.[21] A standard NHS register for hospital pharmacy receipts and issues and a generic ward CD record book are still the predominant documentation used to maintain a complete audit trail of all CDs received into, supplied and used across hospital services. Additional purpose-specific record books are now also being developed and used in some hospitals, for example, theatre CD record book and patients' own medicines CD record book.

The amended regulations also included a new requirement to add specific information to the legally required CD register, to record information about the identity of the person collecting schedule 2 CDs.[21]

This requires that a record is made of the person collecting the schedule 2 CD, be this the patient, patient's representative or healthcare professional, and if the person who collected the drug was a healthcare professional acting on behalf of the patient, that person's name and address.

A 'yes/no' is recorded against two questions:

1   Was proof of identity requested of patient/patient's representative?
2   Was proof of identity of person collecting provided?

In hospitals the recording of schedule 2 CD medicines supplied to a patient to take home at discharge should be subject to clear local procedures which may also encompass recording some of these additional elements of information, as diversion can occur at any point in the supply and transport processes, particularly when multiple steps are involved.

Controlled drug prescribing

In hospital practice, inpatient medicine charts are used to provide written directions for the administration of medicines. If a supply on an individual-patient basis is made the prescription must meet the requirements of the *Misuse of Drugs Regulations 2001*.[6] This applies in outpatient settings and for discharge. The usual approach for inpatients is to supply on a ward stock basis.

Doctors and dentists may prescribe all CDs. Nurse independent prescribers can prescribe from a specific list of products for specific medical conditions. Further amendments to the *Misuse of Drugs Regulations 2001* are planned to allow nurse and pharmacist independent prescribers additional authority in relation to CDs. Registered supplementary prescribers can prescribe a CD as long as it is within the clinical management plan specific to that patient and is agreed between the independent prescriber (doctor or dentist), supplementary prescriber and patient.

A limited number of specified CDs can be included in patient group directions.[22]

Controlled drug destruction

Schedule 1 and 2 CD stock ('stock' is defined as product not supplied to or dispensed for an individual patient) can only be destroyed in the presence of a person authorised under the *Misuse of Drugs Regulations 2001* who acts as witness for the destruction. Accountable officers can nominate personnel within their organisation to witness the destruction of CDs. Accountable officers for CDs cannot undertake the role of witness to destruction themselves. This authority allows accountable officers to ensure that out-of-date or surplus CD stocks are appropriately destroyed in a timely manner so they cannot be diverted or misused.[23] Hospital pharmacists should also consider how unwanted medicines classified in other CD schedules are safely disposed, minimising the risk of misuse.

The method of disposal should ensure that the CD is rendered unrecoverable prior to onward safe disposal. Guidance on suitable approaches is provided by the Royal Pharmaceutical Society[24] and in the Department of Health *Safer Management of Controlled Drugs: A Guide to Good Practice in Secondary Care (England or Northern Ireland).*[12]

In some hospital clinical areas the use of CD products is routine, for example in palliative care services, intensive care units and operating department theatres. Destruction procedures should not only direct the management of unwanted or out-of-date stock medicines but should also set out the expected management of CD product excess to patient care needs. Healthcare practitioners should not forget that there is a potential to misuse or misdirect any CD product, including unused product issued for patient care, and it is important that procedures require that all CD product is accounted for in appropriate documentation or recording processes, and actions such as destruction of unwanted product are always witnessed.

Patients' own CD medicines, prescribed through a hospital or in the community, that are no longer wanted or required may be returned or left in the hospital. Hospital SOPs should include procedures detailing how records of schedule 2 drugs returned by patients are stored, managed and disposed.[8]

Mixing medicines prior to administration in clinical practice

The MHRA recently put in place changes to medicines regulations to enable the mixing of medicines prior to administration in clinical practice.[25] The

MHRA has also approached the Home Office and the Advisory Council for the Misuse of Drugs with the Commission on Human Medicine's recommendation that corresponding amendments for CDs are made to the *Misuse of Drugs Regulations*. Meanwhile, existing good-practice arrangements should continue on mixing, which may include a CD, before administration.

Nurse and pharmacist independent prescribers

In March 2007 a public consultation to consider options that might support the independent prescribing of a broader range of CDs by both nurse and pharmacist independent prescribers was initiated.[26] The Department of Health, the Home Office and the Commission on Human Medicines supported the consultation and we now await the required amendments to the *Medicines Act* and the *Misuse of Drugs Act*. On a related matter, legislative changes which could affect patient group directions and the supply and/or administration of certain CDs in specific circumstances are being considered at the time of writing.

Conclusion

The pharmacy team has an important role in ensuring medicines covered by CD legislation are handled appropriately. As well as ensuring pharmacy processes are fit for purpose, pharmacy has a responsibility for providing support and advice throughout the organisation.

References

1. Department of Health and Home Office. *Safer Management of Controlled Drugs, the Government's response to the Fourth report of the Shipman Inquiry*, 2004. Available online at: http://www.dh.gov.uk/en/Publicationsandstatistics/Publications/PublicationsPolicyAndGuidance/DH_4097904 (accessed 31 May 2010).
2. The Shipman Inquiry. *Safer Management of Controlled Drugs in the Community, The Fourth Report of the Shipman Inquiry*, 2004. Available online at: http://www.the-shipman-inquiry.org.uk/images/fourthreport/SHIP04_COMPLETE_NO_APPS.pdf (accessed 31 May 2010).
3. Department of Health. *The Health Act 2006*, Chapter 2. London: The Stationery Office, 2006.
4. *Medicines Act 1968*. Available online at: http://www.legislation.gov.uk/ukpga/1968/67/contents.
5. *Misuse of Drugs Act 1971*. Available online at: http://www.statutelaw.gov.uk/legResults.aspx?LegType=All+Legislation&title=The+Misuse+of+Drugs+Act+1971&searchEnacted=0&extentMatchOnly=0&confersPower=0&blanketAmendment=0&TYPE=QS&NavFrom=0&activeTextDocId=1367412&PageNumber=1&SortAlpha=0.
6. *The Misuse of Drugs Regulations 2001*. London: The Stationery Office, 2001.
7. *The Misuse of Drugs Regulations (Northern Ireland) 2002*. Statutory Rules of Northern Ireland 2002 no. 1. London: The Stationery Office, 2002.
8. *The Controlled Drugs (Supervision of Management and Use) Regulations 2006*. Statutory Instrument 2006 no. 3148. London: The Stationery Office, 2006.

9. Department of Health. Safer management of controlled drugs: (1) Guidance on strengthened governance arrangements. Gateway 7553. Available online at: http://www.dh.gov.uk Northern Ireland: Safer management of controlled drugs: a guide to strengthened governance arrangements in Northern Ireland. Available online at: http://www.dhsspsni.gov.uk.

10. Department of Health. Safer management of controlled drugs: Guidance on standard operating procedures for controlled drugs. Gateway 7585. Available online at: http://www.dh.gov.uk. Northern Ireland: Safer management of controlled drug guidance on standard operating procedures for Northern Ireland. Available online at: http://www.dhsspsni.gov.uk.

11. Department of Health. The safe and secure handling of medicines: a team approach (the revised Duthie report) 2005. Available online at: http://www.rpharms.com/support-pdfs/safsechandmeds.pdf.

12. Department of Health. Safer management of controlled drugs: a guide to good practice in secondary care (England). Gateway 8913. Available online at: http://www.dh.gov.uk/en/Publicationsandstatistics/Publications/PublicationsPolicyAndGuidance/DH_079618. Northern Ireland: Northern Ireland government. Safer management of controlled drugs guidance – a guide to good practice in secondary care. Available online at: http://www.dhsspsni.gov.uk.

13. Drugs classified under the misuse of drugs legislation. Available online at: http://www.home-office.gov.uk/drugs/drug-law/.

14. Department of Health. *Safer Management of Controlled Drugs: Private CD Prescriptions and Other Changes to the Prescribing and Dispensing of Controlled Drugs: Guidance for Implementation.* Gateway 6820. London: Department of Health, 2006.

15. Care Quality Commission. Guidance about compliance. Essential standards of quality and safety. Available online at: http://www.cqc.org.uk/publications.cfm?fde_id=13512.

16. Care Quality Commission. CQC self-assessment tool. Available online at: http://www.cqc.org.uk/guidanceforprofessionals/healthcare/allhealthcarestaff/managingrisk/controlled-drugs/self-assessmenttool.cfm.

17. *The Misuse of Drugs (Safe Custody) Regulations 1973.* Statutory instrument no. 798. London: HMSO, 1973.

18. *The Misuse of Drugs and The Misuse of Drugs (Safe Custody) (Amendment) Regulations 2007.* Statutory instrument no. 2154 (see Home Office circular 027/2007 for explanation). London: The Stationery Office, 2007. Northern Ireland: *The Misuse of Drugs (Safe Custody) (Northern Ireland) Regulations 1973.* Available online at: http://www.dhsspsni.gov.uk/index/pas-lie/pas-medreg-legislation.htm.

19. National Patient Safety Agency (NPSA) *Patient Safety Alert. Potassium Solutions: Risk to Patients from Errors Occurring During Intravenous Administration.* NPSA reference number 1051. London: NPSA, 2002.

20. Nursing and Midwifery Council. *Standards for Medicines Management.* London: Nursing and Midwifery Council, 2008.

21. Department of Health. Safer management of controlled drugs: changes to record keeping requirements. Guidance for implementation (England). Gateway reference 8712, 2008. Available online at: http://www.dh.gov.uk/en/Publicationsandstatistics/Publications/PublicationsPolicyAndGuidance/DH_079574.

22. National Prescribing Centre (NPC). *A Guide to Good Practice in the Management of Controlled Drugs in Primary Care (England).* Liverpool: NPC, 2009.

23. Department of Health. *Safer Management of Controlled Drugs: Guidance of the Destruction of Controlled Drugs – New Role for Accountable Officers.* Gateway reference 8700. London: Department of Health, 2007.

24. Royal Pharmaceutical Society of Great Britain. Controlled drug guides. Guidance on changes in the management of controlled drugs. Available online at http://www.rpsgb.org.

25. Department of Health. *Changes to Medicines Legislation to Enable Mixing of Medicines Prior to Administration in Clinical Practice.* Gateway reference 13337. London: Department of Health, 2010.

26. Home Office Public Consultation (MLX 338). Independent prescribing of controlled drugs by nurse and pharmacist independent prescribers. March 2007. Available online at: http://www.mhra.gov.uk/Publications/Consultations/Medicinesconsultations/MLXs/CON2030628.

Further reading

When considering controlled drug issues it is important to ensure you are always using the most
up-to-date legislation or and guidance. Development of additional controlled drug legislation
and guidance is still ongoing.

Refer to the Office of Public Sector Information website: http://www.opsi.gov.uk.

Or one of the regularly updated summary reference sources, such as:

The health departments' websites across the UK (controlled drug sections):

http://www.dh.gov.uk

http://www.dhsspsni.gov.uk

http://www.scotland.gov.uk

http://www.wales.nhs.uk.

General Medical Council website: http://www.gmc-uk.org/.

General Pharmaceutical Council website: http://www.pharmacyregulation.org/index.aspx.

National Prescribing Centre website: http://www.npci.org.uk/cd/public/home_page.php.

Nursing and Midwifery Council website: http://www.nmc-uk.org/.

Royal Pharmaceutical Society website: http://www.rpharms.com.

Department of Health. *Safer Management of Controlled Drugs: a guide to good practice in secondary care (England)*. London: Department of Health, 2007. Gateway reference 8913 provides an overview of controlled drug issues for the hospital pharmacist. Available online at: http://www.dh.gov.uk/en/Publicationsandstatistics/Publications/PublicationsPolicyAndGuidance/DH_079618

6

Technical services

Graham Sewell

The term 'technical services' usually refers to the elements of hospital pharmacy organisational structure related to pharmaceutical production, manufacturing and associated quality assurance (QA) functions. The definition has been modified to suit local situations and changes in emphasis within hospital pharmacy production and preparation. For the purposes of this chapter, 'technical services' will include:

- pharmaceutical repackaging
- non-sterile manufacturing
- sterile manufacturing (terminal sterilisation)
- aseptic preparation, including:
  - parenteral infusions
  - cytotoxic infusions
  - total parenteral nutrition (TPN) solutions
  - radiopharmaceuticals.

In some centres, the different aspects of aseptic preparation are grouped under the heading centralised intravenous additive services (CIVAS). However, this does not adequately describe aseptic preparations requiring more complex manipulations than simple addition or the preparation of parenteral products for non-intravenous administration. For this reason the term 'compounding' is increasingly used to describe aseptic preparation services. Chapter 7 deals with QA.

This chapter will outline the development of technical services and then describe current practice across the range of services listed above. The responsiveness of technical services to clinical need and changes in practice is illustrated with selected examples of development and progress. These also serve to emphasise the interdependence of hospital pharmacy clinical, procurement and technical services. Finally, the new challenges facing technical services will be explored in the context of future trends in healthcare services.

History

The focus of production and repackaging activities in hospital pharmacies has changed dramatically over the past 40 years. In the early 1970s, it was common practice for even small district general hospitals to engage in a wide range of production activities. Non-sterile production would have typically included a range of oral liquids and mixtures (often preserved with chloroform water), antiseptic skin-staining solutions for use in theatre, suppositories, creams, ointments and powders. Many of the formulae for these products were obtained from official literature such as the *British Pharmaceutical Codex*, although a number of formulations were 'developed' in house.[1]

Many hospitals had also realised the benefits of preparing stocks of commonly used solid-dosage forms as prepacks on a small-batch scale. These become known as 'ward packs' and were prepared using manual (for example, the tablet triangle) or semiautomatic tablet- and capsule-counting systems. Labels were often preprinted and batch-specific details were either hand-written or typed.

With few exceptions, non-sterile manufacturing and prepacking occurred on an ad hoc, small-scale basis, with little central coordination. Batch records, procedures and production facilities were all extremely variable and little thought was given to process validation, shelf-life assignment, QA and control.

The manufacture of terminally sterilised products was also more widespread in the 1970s than is currently the case. The presence of small autoclaves, dry-heat sterilisers and steam baths was common in district general hospital pharmacies, and many hospitals were self-sufficient in their provision of most sterile products, buying only the bulk intravenous (IV) infusions from industry (for example, 0.9% sodium chloride and 5% glucose). The product range typically included bladder irrigation solutions, multidose eye drops, antiseptic solutions and oily preparations for sterile wound dressings. In some centres, specialist injectables for IV, intramuscular and intrathecal administration were also produced. In most cases, bulk solutions were prepared in uncontrolled or perhaps 'socially clean' areas and were invariably filled into glass containers which were sealed with a rubber stopper and screw cap arrangement. A basic filtration procedure was usually incorporated for parenteral products and eye drops; some of the more specialised units had ampoule sealing equipment which was, at best, only semiautomatic. Sterilisation processes were poorly controlled and rarely validated, particularly in the case of steam baths (for heating with a bactericide) and dry-heat sterilisers. Quality control (QC) was usually rudimentary, with only an inspection of the product for visible particulates and an examination of sterilisation cycle temperature–time charts prior to batch release.

As the 1970s progressed, sterile production became more organised with the emergence across the UK of specialist sterile product units on a coordinated, regional basis. Many of these units concentrated on the production of sterile large-volume irrigation solutions that were normally presented in semirigid plastic containers (for example, Schubert containers). These units benefited from considerable investment to fund automatic filling lines, hermetic sealing technology and large double-ended autoclaves. A few UK centres were equipped to fill flexible-film polyvinyl chloride containers for the manufacture of large-volume IV infusions and small blow-moulded containers for eye drops. By comparison with sterile and non-sterile manufacturing, aseptic preparation was a relatively minor component of hospital pharmacy work in the mid-1970s.

In 1976 the Breckenridge report was published, recognising the hazards associated with infusion preparation on hospital wards.[2] This prompted the development of embryonic CIVAS in a few of the larger teaching hospitals, which prepared TPN and other infusions considered of insufficient stability to withstand terminal sterilisation processes. As with other types of hospital production of that era, facilities, controls and documentation were often neglected. The preparation of radiopharmaceuticals at the time was largely confined to nuclear medicine departments, where medical physics staff under the supervision of medical staff carried out the work.

An attempt to rationalise hospital technical services activities through the introduction of rigorous costing policies was made in 1984 with the issue of health circular HC(84)3 by the Department of Health.[3] This circular recommended that hospitals should not produce pharmaceuticals that were commercially available and that the economic viability of in-house manufacture should be assessed. This included taking into account the full cost of staff, facilities, equipment, maintenance, heating, lighting and depreciation when calculating the cost of products. At the time, this health circular was not well received by technical services pharmacists and, apart from encouraging further rationalisation through regional production units, its impact was limited.

Of greater significance was the loss from National Health Service (NHS) hospitals of Crown immunity in 1990. Under new guidelines, manufacturing activities above specified levels were required to be licensed by the Medicines Control Agency,[4] now known as the Medicines and Healthcare products Regulatory Agency (MHRA). For many smaller production units, the cost of upgrading facilities to the standards required to obtain a Medicines Control Agency specials manufacturing licence was prohibitive. The loss of Crown immunity coincided with the introduction of trust status for many NHS hospitals. The combination of new, higher standards and a more cost-conscious environment in the NHS significantly changed the emphasis of technical services activities. More recently, the issue of guidance note 14 and enforcement by the MHRA have, in effect, eliminated products made under a manufacturing specials licence where a licensed equivalent is available.[5] Although seeking to raise the standards of preparation of medicines, this has led to concerns about intellectual property rights (IPR) of hospital-developed formulations which can be copied by industry and sold back to the NHS at high cost in a protected market. This guidance may also prevent hospital manufacturing units responding to supply problems, now more prevalent in the pharmaceutical industry.

Licensing issues

With the exception of a limited number of lines produced by specialist hospital manufacturing units, medicines produced by hospital technical services departments are unlicensed and have no product licence (PL) or marketing authorisation. If the production of an unlicensed medicine is conducted under the supervision of a pharmacist, and the batch size and frequency of preparation are within MHRA-defined limits, section 10 of the 1968 *Medicines Act* provides exemption from the requirement to hold a manufacturer's licence.[4] (At the time of writing, the *Medicines Act* is under review.) In addition to the above restrictions, manufacture under section 10 exemption does not permit the supply of the product outside the NHS trust in which it was made and imposes limits on the maximum shelf-life which may be assigned to certain product types.

For the production of larger batches, and in the case of medicines sold outside the production unit's trust, a manufacturer's specials licence is required. The specials licence is regulated by the MHRA and permits the manufacture of products that are not subject to a PL. The licence specifies the type of manufacture permitted (that is, non-sterile, aseptic manufacture, and so on) and the product categories to which the licence applies (large-volume IVs, antibiotics, cytotoxics, biologicals). Hospitals holding a specials licence are subjected to regular audits by the MHRA, including an inspection of facilities and a full audit of good pharmaceutical manufacturing practice, QA and QC systems. Advertising of products manufactured under a specials licence is not permitted, although it is permissible to advertise a specials manufacturing service.

Repackaging (prepacking, assembly)

Scope

Repackaging is a process in which liquid or solid-dose formulations are packed from bulk into smaller, ready-to-use containers (prepacks). The presentation of prepacks, in terms of the number of tablets or capsules or volume of liquid, the label details and the container type, are designed to meet a specific clinical need. Until the mid-1990s, the most common prepackaging activity undertaken by hospital pharmacy departments was the production of ward packs. Bulk packs of tablets and capsules (typically 500–5000 dose units) and large containers of liquid medicines (up to 2 litres) were economic to purchase, particularly from manufacturers of generics. However, it was neither economical nor safe to place such large containers on hospital wards as stock medicines. Therefore ward packs were produced by repacking bulk medicines into pack sizes of typically 25–50 solid-dose units per pack or 50–200 ml of liquid medicines per bottle. Repackaging also provided an opportunity to improve the clarity of labelling. The proprietary or trade name of the medicine was often prominent on bulk packs but the prepacks could be labelled with the approved name of the medicine to reduce the risk of drug administration errors on the ward.

In recent years the increased availability of commercially produced ward packs which carry full UK marketing authorisation has reduced the need for in-house production of ward packs. Also the introduction of patient packs containing strips of blister-packed tablets and capsules has provided another presentation that can be adapted for ward use by simply overlabelling the outer carton. Although there will be a continued demand for a limited range of ward packs which are not commercially available, the emphasis of hospital repackaging activities is now directed towards more patient-specific packs which are not commercially viable. These include prepacks for hospital discharge medication and packs designed to meet the requirements of specific treatment protocols or patient group directives in primary, secondary and tertiary care settings. The objective in both cases is to produce a presentation that exactly meets specific clinical and patient requirements while minimising repetitive, labour-intensive dispensing work. Providing the exact number of doses needed by the patient also reduces drug wastage. The MHRA provides guidance on the requirement for a special assembly licence for repackaging, depending on the batch size and the frequency with which batches are produced.[4] Increasingly, hospital repackaging has become more centralised in specialist units with automated packing lines. Although repackaging whole strips of blister-packed medicines into different containers is acceptable, the removal of tablets or capsules from blisters for repackaging is not advisable since stability cannot be guaranteed. However, any repackaging needs to be considered in terms of whether value is truly added and standardisation to a limited range is advisable.

Facilities and equipment

In its simplest form, repackaging is a manual operation in which counting of tablets, capsules and measuring of liquids are achieved with tablet triangles, capsule trays and glass measures. Containers are also capped and labelled by hand, although all labels are either preprinted or produced on a computer labelling system. Repackaging activities require a clean, uncluttered, designated area. Walls, floors and work surfaces should be of a smooth, impervious finish and should be readily accessible for easy cleaning. Although most tablets are now coated, dust containing active drug can be generated during repackaging and a localised dust extraction system should be fitted.

The degree of automation of repackaging processes ranges from semi-automatic tablet and capsule-counting machines to fully automated packing lines. In the case of the latter, empty containers are sorted, oriented and then transported to the filling zone by a conveyor track. Tablets or capsules are fed from a hopper over a chip-sieve to counting heads, which fill the correct number of dose units into each container. The containers progress to an automated capping system before preprinted labels are applied automatically.

Alternatively, automatic packing lines can pack solid doses into preformed blisters or foil pouches to produce blister and foil packs.

Many packing lines are fitted with localised dust extraction in critical areas and also electronic check-weight systems to assure correct counting and filling processes. An example of a fully automatic packing line is shown in Figure 6.1. This type of equipment must be easily dismantled and re-assembled to permit cleaning and inspection between batch runs.

Process

Whilst repackaging processes are simple, errors can occur. To avoid transposition of medicines or labels it is essential that only one batch is repackaged at a time in a designated area and that the work area is cleared of all labels, containers and medicines from the previous batch. With solid-dose forms, it is good practice to organise the repackaging schedule so that medicines differ from the previous batch repackaged in colour, shape, size or appearance. This makes it easier to detect the odd rogue tablet or capsule transposed to another batch of a different product in error.

It is also important that cleaning procedures for equipment are carefully validated, particularly if sensitising antibiotics such as penicillins are repackaged, to ensure that medicines are not contaminated with dust from previous batches.

When repackaging liquids (particularly suspensions) it is essential to shake the bulk container thoroughly before distributing the liquid to the prepack containers. This ensures that the concentration of drug in all

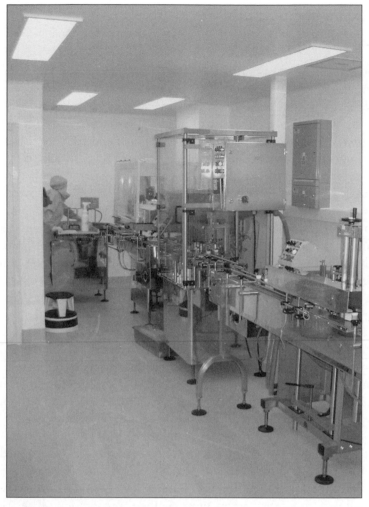

Figure 6.1   Automated solid-dose repackaging line at Royal Devon and Exeter Hospital.

prepacked containers is homogeneous. In practice, these processes are mainly controlled through standard operating procedures, batch documentation, staff training and competency assessment. In the case of liquid suspensions, routine sampling and QC testing during a batch run are introduced to ensure the homogeneous content is maintained. The reconciliation of the number of dose units used, the number of packs produced and the number of labels issued and used all require particular consideration. These controls should be part of a comprehensive QA system, which will also include QC, self-inspection, error reporting and feedback from 'customers'.

Non-sterile manufacture

Scope

The manufacture of traditional non-sterile oral liquids and topical preparations, usually in accordance with *British Pharmaceutical Codex* formulae, has declined in the hospital sector over recent years.[1] This is largely due to the commercial availability of licensed products and also the growth of non-sterile specials manufacturing services operated commercially. However, a non-sterile production service is still required to support several clinical specialties, particularly dermatology and paediatric. Many dermatologists have their own variants of standard preparations, often differing only in the type of diluents or base used or in the concentration of active components. Although there is little scientific evidence to support the use of these non-standard preparations, custom, practice and clinical experience have, until recently, provided a continuing demand. Attempts are being made to reduce the range of products used to allow standardisation and simplification. The British Association of Dermatologists' preferred list was issued in 2008 to support this approach.[6]

Conversely, the clinical justification for using medicines outside their licensed indications for adults in the paediatric setting is well accepted. The unit dose of commercially available preparations of medicines designed for adult use is usually too large for paediatrics. Also, some of the larger tablets and capsules would be difficult for children to swallow. Safe and reproducible paediatric dosing therefore requires preparations of lower dose, usually in the form of oral liquids, suspensions or powders.

Department of Health information reported in 2002 suggested that dermatology preparations (coal tar, salicylic acid and dithranol) were the most frequently prepared non-sterile products by hospital pharmacy departments, although in recent years most of these preparations have become commercially available.[7] Some hospitals have developed commercial non-sterile manufacturing units to supply other hospitals and community pharmacies. This type of activity helps to offset the costs of maintaining facilities of a high standard and meeting the regulatory requirements of MHRA specials licences.

In some hospitals, dispensary services have been reorganised and extemporaneous dispensing work has been transferred to the technical services section. A wide range of non-commercially available extemporaneous preparations is required for individual patients, including oral liquids, creams, ointments, powders, suppositories and pessaries. This approach provides variety and clinical interest for manufacturing staff and ensures that extemporaneous products are produced in accordance with the principles of good manufacturing practice.

Facilities and equipment

Typically, non-sterile manufacture is carried out in a European Union (EU) grade D environment with a single stage change.[8] Although some units require production staff to wear sterilised coverall gowns, most centres rely on clean two-piece gowns of low-lint-shedding material, over-shoes, hats and gloves. To reduce the microbiological bioburden, drains and potable water supplies are excluded from production areas and all surfaces should have a smooth impervious finish to facilitate effective cleaning. Weighing areas should be separate from the main production area (linked to it with a pass-through hatch) and should be fitted with localised dust extraction. Although containers for non-sterile products are not reused, a facility for washing and drying containers before use may be required. Separate areas should be provided for labelling and reinspection of products.

The *Rules and Guidance for Good Pharmaceutical Manufacture and Distribution* strongly recommend the use of stainless-steel measures and mixing vessels to avoid the risk of contaminating product with spicules from glass equipment.[8] Large-scale manufacture will require the use of industrial mixers and homogenisers. Automated liquid filling lines may be deployed for large-scale liquid handling and some units with a significant output of creams and ointments have also invested in tube-filling and sealing equipment. Figure 6.2 illustrates small-scale non-sterile manufacturing facilities.

Process

All raw materials, containers and labels used in the production process must be approved by the person responsible for QC. To reduce the microbiological bioburden, limits are placed on the level of microbiological contamination of raw materials and only sterile water (usually water for irrigation BP) or freshly distilled water is used for manufacture. All product formulae, storage conditions and shelf-life assignments require prior QC approval.

The manufacturing process is controlled through the use of approved standard operating procedures and batch documents. Particular care is required to ensure that mixing processes produce a homogeneous product for distribution into the individual containers that constitute the batch. This process must be validated for each product type to ensure uniformity of content in the finished batch. The avoidance of cross-contamination between different products is also essential. Only one batch may be prepared in a designated work area at any one time and the cleaning of equipment and work surfaces must be carefully validated and monitored.

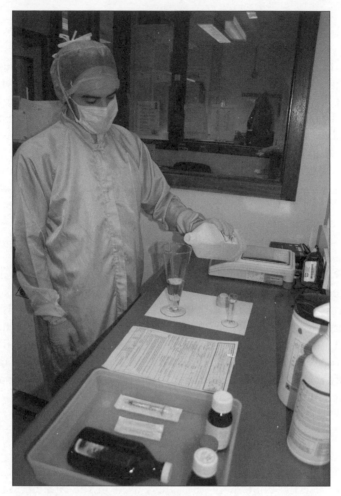

Figure 6.2   Small-scale non-sterile manufacturing facilities.

Filled containers should be visually inspected for product homogeneity and the absence of any extraneous matter. The security of container closures should be checked and the quality and accuracy of labels determined against a master label for the product. It is essential that the batch documentation includes reconciliation between the amounts of raw materials, number of containers and number of labels used in the process and the yield of finished product. All variations must be recorded and investigated.

Although some regulators have attempted to discourage non-sterile manufacturing in hospital pharmacies, there are compelling reasons why sufficient capacity in this activity is retained. The ongoing need for paediatric doses of both new and existing medicines that are commercially available in adult doses must be recognised. There is also a requirement to formulate medicines for patients with particular clinical needs, such as patients with dysphagia. It is preferable for these medicines to be produced by trained pharmacy staff in appropriate facilities, using fully documented procedures, than to have undocumented manipulation taking place in clinical areas by nursing staff.

Sterile manufacture

Scope

All terminally sterilised medicines produced in hospitals are made under a manufacturer's specials licence, except in a few cases where PLs have been obtained. The range of products made generally reflects gaps in the portfolio of licensed products available from the pharmaceutical industry. The limited number of specialist sterile manufacturing units remaining in the NHS provides an essential service in making available sterile parenteral and topical products that are not commercially viable for industry to produce. Such products include non-standard concentrations and presentations of injections and eye drops, specialist injectables for paediatrics, anaesthetics and palliative care, and various sterile topical products.

In some cases, NHS hospital sterile product units have developed products to support pharmacy CIVAS units. These include electrolytes for addition to TPN feeds such as concentrated sodium chloride injection, potassium phosphate injection and zinc sulphate injection. A range of sterile bulk solutions for filling into syringes and other devices is also produced. These include bupivacaine injection, morphine sulphate injection and fentanyl injection. Sterile manufacture also supports research, and small runs of experimental drugs in parenteral formulations are prepared for clinical trial use.

The container and filling technologies employed in hospital units encompass glass vials, glass ampoules, glass bottles and polyvinyl chloride infusion bags for parenteral products, and a variety of glass and rigid plastic containers for topical solutions. No lyophilised presentations are available since freeze-drying technology is beyond the scope of hospital sterile product units.

Facilities and equipment

In general, the weighing and solution preparation areas required would be similar to those described previously for non-sterile manufacture. However, the filling, sealing and capping stages must be accomplished in a higher-quality environment, usually EU grade A, to minimise particulate contamination and reduce the microbiological load prior to sterilisation. This is usually achieved by local laminar flow of high-efficiency particulate air-filtered air at the filling zone. After filling and sealing, containers and their contents are sterilised by steam in an autoclave (aqueous solutions) or by dry heat in a hot-air oven (non-aqueous liquids, powders). The sterilisers and associated monitoring equipment can be located in a lower-grade environment and are normally sited so that maintenance staff can access them without the need to enter critical production areas.

Dedicated space for reinspection of the finished product, labelling, packing and quarantine is also required. Regulatory requirements for sterile production facilities and sterilising equipment are strictly defined and require extensive validation.[8] The design and construction of sterile manufacturing units should only be undertaken by specialist contractors. The increasing use of automated systems, particularly for filling, sealing and reinspecting ampoules, and the sophistication of modern steriliser technology have contributed to the rapid rise in capital and maintenance costs associated with sterile manufacturing units. National coordination and strategic planning of new units are essential to maximise the cost-effectiveness of these expensive but important resources.

Process

In addition to the processes outlined under non-sterile manufacture, above, sterile production normally includes a filtration process (for liquids) and sterilisation of the product. These processes are critical to product quality and require rigorous validation and control. The microbiological bioburden must be minimised, particularly in the case of injectables, to reduce the release of bacterial pyrogens into the product, because these will not be destroyed by sterilisation. This is achieved by limiting the number of viable microorganisms in starting materials and by minimising the time between preparations of the bulk product, filling and sterilisation.

The sterilisation cycle for each batch is clearly monitored to ensure that all containers in the batch have received the pharmacopoeial-approved temperature and time combinations.[9] Printouts of the load temperature, usually taken at the coolest location of the autoclave or dry-heat oven, are recorded throughout the cycle and are scrutinised as part of the release process. Additional measures are taken to ensure that products sterilised by autoclave or hot-air oven are not at risk from microbial contamination of cooling water or non-sterile air, respectively, which could enter through closures during the cooling phase of the cycle. Figure 6.3 shows an autoclave and its control systems in a large sterile production unit.

The QC of sterile products includes analysis of active components, sterility testing, subvisual particulate measurement and tests for the absence of bacterial pyrogens. This means that batches must be quarantined for at least 14 days (the time taken for sterility test incubation) before release. Production

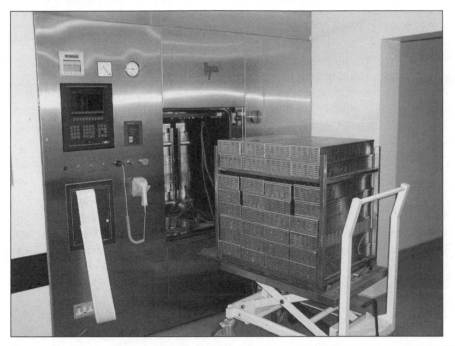

Figure 6.3 Autoclave at Pharmacy Manufacturing Unit, Torbay Hospital.

managers and users of sterile products need to consider this when drawing up production schedules and managing stocks.

Aseptic preparation

Scope

Most aseptic preparation work undertaken in the hospital setting is described by the following categories:

- IV additions
- TPN
- cytotoxic infusions/syringes
- radiopharmaceuticals.

Stability issues frequently preclude the provision of 'ready-to-use' parenteral medicines by the pharmaceutical industry. Many drugs, including antibiotics, opioid analgesics and cytotoxics, are degraded by hydrolysis. In order to assign a reasonable shelf-life to these medicines, parenteral formulations are presented as vials containing lyophilised powders, which require reconstitution (in some cases dilution) before administration to the patient. Aseptic manipulation is also necessary for clinical reasons, in which doses or formulations need to be tailored for individual patients, requiring the preparation of 'bespoke' infusions.

The same principles of aseptic preparation apply to all four categories (above), although there are subtle differences in the processes and equipment used for each product type. Many hospitals group the first three activities under the heading CIVAS, although others consider TPN and cytotoxic work to be separate.

Aseptic preparation work is a high-risk activity; the risk of calculation or compounding errors and the risk of microbiological contamination must be controlled to ensure the safety and efficacy of aseptic preparations. The UK CIVAS group conducted a national study on failure rates in media-fill simulations of aseptic processes and found this to be approximately 1 in 500.[10] However, these risks need to be placed in the context of the alternative to hospital pharmacy-based aseptic services. Although evidence is limited, intuitively it is clear that the risk of calculation and compounding errors and the incidence of microbiological contamination will be considerably higher if aseptic manipulations are carried out by untrained nursing and medical staff in clinical areas. Certainly the Audit Commission supported the use of CIVAS in its *A Spoonful of Sugar*: 'making up aseptic preparations in hospital wards should be stopped'.[11] With the ongoing problem of hospital-acquired infections associated with clinical areas, this would seem sensible advice. The need to move from ward preparation to pharmacy provision was also included in the 2008 pharmacy White Paper.[12]

Since the unfortunate deaths of children from contaminated parenteral nutrition solutions, the regulation of aseptic preparation has been strictly enforced by the UK Health Departments.

Hospitals preparing aseptic products under a specials manufacturing licence are subject to rigorous inspection by the MHRA. Unlicensed units (those working under *Medicines Act* section 10 exemption) must follow the guidance set out in *Aseptic Dispensing for NHS Patients*.[13] The authority for enforcing compliance with this document has been delegated to regional QA pharmacists by the Department of Health. The document also restricts the shelf-life assigned to products produced in unlicensed facilities to a maximum of 7 days, irrespective of whether stability data would support a longer shelf-life.

Intravenous additives

Many medicines for parenteral administration are provided as concentrates or lyophilised powders. These require reconstitution and/or dilution followed by transfer to a device (such as a syringe or infusion bag) for administration to the patient. The need for pharmacy-based IV additive services was recognised in the Breckenridge report of 1976.[2] However, studies in the north-west of England have shown that only 35% of medicines requiring aseptic manipulation are prepared by the hospital pharmacy department.[14] Most CIVAS departments target high-risk areas for their services. These include the provision of various doses for paediatric patients, analgesics and antibiotics and also anaesthetic analgesic combinations for epidural infusion. Many hospitals also provide subcutaneous infusions of drug combinations used in palliative care, as well as prefilled syringes to support patient-controlled analgesia. They also provide antibiotic infusions in disposable infusion devices for domiciliary patients with cystic fibrosis or osteomyelitis. A Department of Health survey placed infusions of morphine, bupivacaine, desferrioxamine and three antibiotics into the top 10 aseptic products produced by hospitals.[7]

Total parenteral nutrition

Fewer hospitals are now preparing TPN solutions from scratch. Standardisation of regimens for adults, paediatrics and neonates has enabled commercial manufacturers with specials licences to take a significant part of the TPN market. However, the greatest impact has been the introduction of technologies such as multicompartmental TPN bags, which enable manufacturers to provide macronutrients in standard quantities as terminally sterilised solutions in individual compartments of the bag. These presentations have long shelf-lives, often at room temperature, and are activated to permit mixing of components immediately before use. Many of the hospitals where TPN is still compounded prepare or purchase batches of 'base TPN' bags in which macronutrients (glucose, amino acids, lipid and water) are present in standard amounts. Standard TPN formulations are available with standard electrolyte concentrations or as electrolyte-free solutions to which patient-specific electrolytes can be added before administration. In all cases, it is necessary to add unstable components such as vitamins and trace elements prior to use.

Standard formulae are satisfactory for the majority of patients requiring TPN and there is no scientific or clinical evidence to support some of the very complex individualised preparations that have been used in the past. It must be recognised, however, that some patients (for example, renal patients) have specific needs and the NHS must retain the expertise and capacity to compound individualised TPN feeds in cases of genuine clinical need. The 2010 National Confidential Enquiry report A Mixed Bag addresses many of the clinical aspects of decision-making and use of TPN.[15]

Cytotoxics

The risk of occupational exposure to these mutagenic and potentially carcinogenic drugs has restricted the preparation of all cytotoxic doses to specialist facilities in the hospital pharmacy. The narrow therapeutic index, extreme toxicity and complexity of cytotoxic treatment regimens provide strong clinical justification for dose calculation and preparation by experienced staff using well-controlled systems. A close working relationship between clinical pharmacy and technical services staff is desirable for all aseptic work, but is essential in the case of cytotoxics.

Even with the use of oral agents, pressures on pharmacy cytotoxic services include increased demand, as more cancer patients receive chemotherapy and also an increasing trend towards outpatient-based administration of chemotherapy. This places immediate demands on the service to avoid lengthy patient waiting times and the risk of errors caused by untrained staff administering chemotherapy outside normal working hours. Strategies designed to offset these pressures include dose banding, which enables doses to be prepared as standard prefilled syringes, which are used in combination to provide the 'banded' dose.[16] This approach is, of course, dependent upon the stability of the reconstituted infusions. A recent survey reported that dose banding of chemotherapy is now widely accepted by UK oncologists and haematologists.[17]

The introduction of monoclonal antibodies or targeted therapies such as trastuzumab into chemotherapy regimens has also created additional workload. These are not conventional cytotoxic drugs and the occupational exposure risks are the subject of much debate.[18] However, given that targeted therapies are used to treat high-risk patients who are immuno-compromised, many pharmacists feel these infusions should be treated in the same way as conventional cytotoxic infusions.

Radiopharmaceuticals

Nuclear medicine provides important diagnostic and functional information on specific organs in addition to radiation therapy for certain disease states. Diagnostic scans are used in many specialities, including oncology, cardiology, surgery, neurology and renal medicine. Departments routinely perform investigations such as cardiac scans to evaluate the extent of heart disease, bone scans to detect metastatic disease and cell labelling to help evaluate whether infectious or non-infectious inflammatory conditions are present. As radiation detectors continue to improve and new ligands are developed, the number of clinical applications continues to expand. Lymph scanning is a case in point where technological advances have now enabled surgeons to use the scan to assist in staging of malignant melanomas and breast cancer.

Radiopharmacy is a specialised area of CIVAS with several unique characteristics. Radiopharmaceuticals have extremely short shelf-lives compared to other pharmaceuticals. Shelf-lives are frequently measured in the range of seconds, hours and days rather than weeks, months or years, and this requires that doses are prepared on the day of use using radionuclides obtained freshly from a technetium generator kept in the radiopharmacy.

Facilities and equipment

All aseptic manipulation must take place in EU grade A work zones.[8] These can be provided by horizontal or vertical laminar air flow cabinets or positive-pressure isolators. For hazardous drugs, such as cytotoxics and radiopharmaceuticals, the use of a negative-pressure isolator is recommended to provide protection not only to the product, but also the operator(s).[19] The grade A workstation must be located in a controlled background environment, usually of EU grade B, although some isolators may be located in an EU grade C or D background. Figure 6.4 shows horizontal laminar flow workstations used for IV additive work.

Automated filling equipment may be placed in the critical work zone providing it is fully validated. Figure 6.5 shows an automated system.

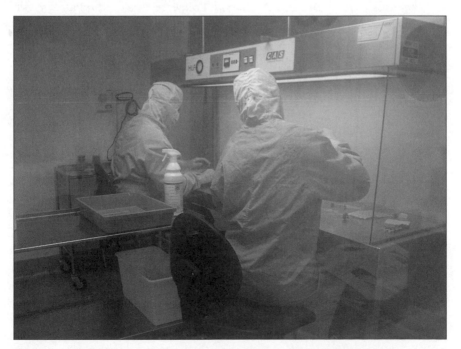

Figure 6.4 Horizontal laminar flow workstations used for intravenous additive work.

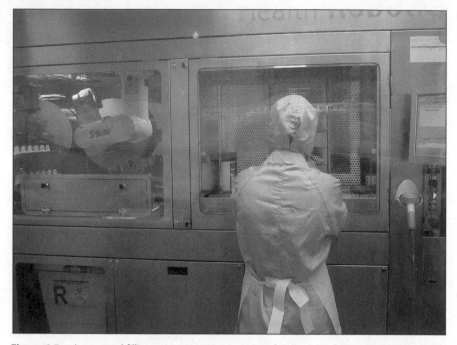

Figure 6.5   Automated filling equipment system, Imperial College Healthcare NHS Trust.

The *Rules and Guidance for Good Pharmaceutical Manufacture and Distribution*[8] and *Quality Assurance of Aseptic Preparation Services*[20] should be consulted for exact standards and requirements of facilities and equipment. Specialist guidance on isolator technology is also available.[21]

In addition to the critical aseptic handling areas, areas must be designated for setting up ingredients, producing batch documents and labels, and checking and packing the finished product. Handling radiopharmaceuticals requires additional equipment to protect the operator from ionising radiation and to monitor exposure levels. Also, tandem isolator systems are necessary to include the technetium (Tc99) generator in the controlled work area (Figure 6.6). Operators are required to wear body badges and finger badges in order to quantify the amount of exposure they have received. They must also follow systems of work which control exposure by either minimising the time spent directly exposed to the source of radiation or by maximising the distance from it. Such practices include working behind lead glass shields and the use of syringe and vial shields and lead housing for generators. These shields must also be accommodated within the isolator or class 2 cabinet workstation. Tongs are used to increase the distance between the operator and the doses. Dose monitors are also used to check for spillages and contamination and are subsequently used to ensure such incidents are cleared up appropriately. There are specific elements of operator training

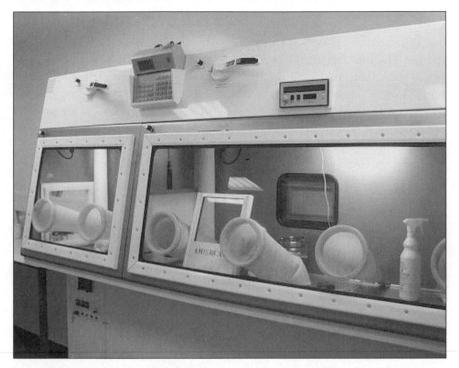

Figure 6.6   Radiopharmacy workstation at St George's Hospital, London.

which must be covered besides the routine pharmacy training. There are also local rules which must be read which cover the safe systems of working with radiation. The introduction of the robotic arm for manipulation of radio-pharmaceuticals should further increase operator safety.

Process

Wherever possible, all aseptic processes should be based on closed systems so that the product or the product fluid path has only minimal exposure to the environment. Product segregation is essential to prevent gross contamination and separate clean rooms and workstations should be used for cytotoxic drugs and radiopharmaceuticals. Operator technique is critical and all operators, processes and equipment must be fully validated.

The manipulation of cytotoxic drugs requires additional protective clothing and emergency procedures for spillage management. These are detailed in non-official UK guidelines.[19, 22] To avoid aerosol formation, venting needles and filters or purpose-designed fluid transfer devices must be used when adding and withdrawing liquids to and from vials. In the case of aseptic products, environmental monitoring and the use of routine media-fill simulations are more meaningful than sterility tests, which are designed to be used with terminally sterilised medicines. Support from an experienced QA department is essential not only for the validation of all aseptic processes but also for formulation and shelf-life issues with aseptic preparations. The additional risks associated with unintentional intrathecal administration of certain cytotoxic agents have led to additional guidance on the presentation, process and release of these products. With a few exceptions, all vinca alkaloid doses must now be presented as large-volume infusions (50 ml) to prevent the lethal intrathecal administration of these drugs.[23]

The processes involved in the preparation of radiopharmaceuticals require consideration of additional issues, including the prescribing and scheduling doses, which are often complex. Most doctors who request scans are not authorised to prescribe radioactive pharmaceuticals. Requests must therefore be authorised by the local Administration of Radioactive Substances Advisory Committee licence holder before they can be scheduled into the nuclear medicine clinic. To maximise the scanning capacity of a nuclear medicine department, doses need to be ready at the beginning of the working day. An on-site radiopharmacy can help facilitate this and enable the service to be more flexible when responding to urgent requests. In contrast to routine CIVAS work, radiopharmacy staff start dose preparation first thing in the morning and early starts of 7 a.m. are not unusual. Reconstitution of kits requires the addition of a radionuclide and saline to a ligand contained in a sterile vial. The resulting solution may need to be incubated for a set period to ensure the radionuclide has attached to the ligand. Simple QC analysis can be performed to confirm the radiochemical purity of the radiopharmaceutical. Poor-quality radiopharmaceuticals may expose patients to radiation unnecessarily and their treatment may be delayed while the investigation is repeated.

Education and training for hospital technical services

Technical services departments are expected to develop in-house training schemes for all grades of staff that fully cover all activities undertaken. All training must be fully documented and evidence of effectiveness of training must be supported by competency assessment. Observation of individual practice as a part of self-inspection schemes and operator validation data are important components of the assessment process. Training programmes should be reviewed regularly and updated in line with service and individual needs. Systems should be in place to identify staff who fail validation tests or are associated with poor QA monitoring data and repeated errors. Such individuals may need additional training and reassessment.

A number of formal education and training courses specialising in the pharmaceutical technical services are available in the UK. These include various short courses in specialised areas and postgraduate programmes leading to diploma or masters qualification, such as the Pharmaceutical Technology and Quality Assurance programme offered by Leeds University. The Technical Specialist Education and Training website is an excellent source of information for all types of courses (www.tset.org.uk).

Health and safety and environmental issues

In recent years, healthcare professionals have become increasingly aware of health risks in the workplace, partly because of the introduction of the Control of Substances Hazardous to Health Regulations.[24] In the case of technical services, particular risks identified relate to occupational exposure of hazardous materials, including solvents and powders used in classical manufacturing processes and cytotoxics and sensitising antibiotics handled by aseptic units. New pharmaceutical developments such as targeted toxins, gene therapy and viral vectors for drug delivery are entering clinical use. These new agents will present a particular challenge in aseptic preparation where measures to reduce or eliminate the risk of occupational exposure and cross-contamination of products must be adopted and validated. There is an urgent need to evaluate new 'closed-system' technologies for the safe handling of toxic agents. Some of these devices, for example the Tevadaptor and PhaSeal systems, are already in limited use, but given the additional cost of these technologies it is essential that evidence of their effectiveness in reducing occupational exposure is obtained. The use of environmental monitoring services is also recommended for cytotoxic compounding units.

Environmental issues are of increasing significance. Controls to prevent the discharge into the environment of genetic material, biologicals and radioactive substances are likely to become more stringent at a time when the medicinal use of such agents continues to increase. Collaborative research to develop safe handling and containment systems is essential, together with other measures to reduce the amounts of medical and plastic waste produced by the technical services activities.

The future

Competing pressures of resource limitations, staffing issues, workload, and complexity and regulatory controls require a clear, coherent strategy for the organisation and development of technical services.

Large-scale manufacturing activities (non-sterile and sterile manufacture) appear particularly vulnerable despite ongoing supply difficulties experienced by the pharmaceutical industry and problems in obtaining specialist medicines for which demand is low. Under local trust, and more recently foundation trust, management, the remaining classical manufacturing units seem either to struggle for investment and resource or, conversely, are viewed purely as income generation activities from which year-on-year increases in profit are required. This approach can only lead to increased costs of specials medicines for the NHS as a whole, inadequate capacity and the selection of product lines according to profitability rather than clinical need. There is an argument for taking these services under national rather than local control to support strategic planning and foster the cooperation required to provide a product portfolio based on clinical need rather than short-term profit. This may require a professional-led approach, rather than governmental; at the time of writing the NHS National Advisory Board for Manufacturing and Preparative Services is overseeing a number of projects to support standardisation of products in use and is considering how collaboration may be developed.

Aseptic services have faced significant workload increases and, despite some welcome innovations by the pharmaceutical industry, this trend is likely to continue. In terms of contribution to direct clinical care, pharmacy aseptic services rank alongside medical imaging, laboratory services, theatres and outpatient departments. The challenge faced by hospital pharmacy managers is to ensure that trusts recognise the value of aseptic services and resource them accordingly. Staff shortages have restricted the development of aseptic services in some areas. It is likely that recruitment of staff outside the traditional pharmacy disciplines is the only solution. This approach would need the provision of specific training programmes, ideally developed nationally with input from relevant stakeholders, but delivered at local or regional level. The use of computer-aided learning technology could, at least in part, assist with this. The availability of a comprehensive range of medicinal products, in clinically required presentations at affordable cost, is dependent upon a constructive and open relationship between hospital technical services departments and the pharmaceutical and medical device industries. Some national special-interest groups have already recognised this. However, the issue of guidance note 14 by the Medicines Control Agency (now the MHRA) has not helped relations with industry.[5] It can be argued that this document unwittingly supported the exploitation of hospital-led developments by industry for commercial gain.

To protect against this, technical services pharmacists must recognise the value of IPR in their developmental work. Revenue raised from the sale of IPR to industry could support further developmental activity and infrastructure.

Despite this concern, it is hoped that there will be strong hospital–industry collaboration. The introduction of dose banding for cancer chemotherapy has provided an excellent opportunity for some dose standardisation. Provided that extended shelf-life data can be obtained for prefilled syringes and infusions, these standard doses offer an opportunity for industry to provide ready-to-use doses with full marketing authorisation and reduce some of the pressure on hospital cytotoxic units. The concept of dose banding could also be applied to other therapeutic areas with similar benefits in terms of workload control, patient care and reduced wastage.[16] Such collaborations are essential if the requirements of National Patient Safety Agency alert 20, on injectable medicines, is to be fully implemented.[25]

The introduction and use of new technology in technical services are, in most parts of the UK, fragmented and uncoordinated. As a result, many aspects of the work, particularly in aseptic preparation, remain labour-intensive because the computer and robotic technologies required are either non-existent or poorly developed. Greater cooperation between centres at national and international level on specification, development and investment strategies will be required before the full benefits of the new technologies can be realised.

Acknowledgement

The author is grateful to Maria Connelly (Qualasept Ltd, trading as Bath ASU), for her help in preparing material on radiopharmaceuticals.

References

1. *British Pharmaceutical Codex*, 10th edn. London: Pharmaceutical Press, 1973.
2. Breckenridge A. *The Report of a Working Party on the Addition of Drugs to Intravenous Infusion Fluids*. HC(76)9. London: HMSO, 1976.
3. Department of Health and Social Security. *Health Services Management: Manufacture of Products in the NHS*. HC(84)3. London: HMSO, 1984.
4. Medicines Control Agency. *Guidance to the NHS on the Licensing Requirements of the Medicines Act 1968*. London: HMSO, 1992.
5. Medicines Control Agency. *The Supply of Unlicensed Relevant Medicinal Products for Individual Patients*. Specials MCA guidance note 14. London: The Stationery Office, 2000.
6. NeLM report re British Association of Dermatologists list of preferred specials. Available online at: http://www.nelm.nhs.uk/en/NeLM-Area/News/2008-October/08/British-Association-of-Dermatologists-issues-updated-list-of-preferred-specials/ (accessed 19 July 2010).
7. Report of the Advisory Group on the Risk Assessment of Unlicensed Relevant Medicinal Products (Specials) within the NHS. *Risk Assessment of NHS Manufacturing*. London: Department of Health, 2002.
8. *Rules and Guidance for Good Pharmaceutical Manufacture and Distribution*. London: Pharmaceutical Press, 2009.
9. *British Pharmacopoeia*. London: British Pharmacopoeia Commission, 2010.
10. Audit conducted by Research and Development Team of UK National CIVAS Group 2001. (unpublished data).
11. Audit Commission. *A Spoonful of Sugar – Medicines Management in NHS Hospitals*. London: Audit Commission, 2001.
12. Department of Health. *Pharmacy in England. Building on Strengths – Delivering the Future*. London: Department of Health, 2008.
13. Farwell J. *Aseptic Dispensing for NHS Patients*. London: Department of Health, 1995.
14. Gandy RJ, Beaumont IM, Lee MG *et al*. Risk management and the aseptic preparation of medicines. *Eur Hosp Pharm* 1998; 4: 114–119.

15. National Confidential Enquiry into Patient Outcome and Death. *A Mixed Bag – An Enquiry into the Care of Hospital Patients Receiving Parenteral Nutrition*. London: NCEPOD, 2010.
16. Plumridge RJ, Sewell GJ. Dose-banding of cytotoxic drugs: a new concept in cancer chemotherapy. *Am J Health-Systems Pharm* 2001; 58: 1760–1764.
17. Kaestner S, Sewell G. A survey of UK prescribers' opinions on chemotherapy dosing and dose-banding. *Clin Oncol* 2009; 21: 320–328.
18. Langford S, Fradgley S, Evans M *et al*. Assessing the risk of handling monoclonal antibodies. *Hosp Pharm* 2008; 15: 60–64.
19. Allwood M, Stanley A, Wright P (eds) *Cytotoxics Handbook*, 4th edn. Oxford: Radcliffe Medical Press, 2002.
20. Beaney A. *Quality Assurance of Aseptic Preparation Services*, 4th edn. London: Pharmaceutical Press, 2006.
21. Midcalf B, Phillips W, Neiger J *et al*. *Pharmaceutical Isolators*. London: Pharmaceutical Press, 2004.
22. MARCH guidelines. Available online at: www.marchguidelines.com (accessed 7 March 2010).
23. Department of Health. Health Service circular updated national guidance on the safe administration of intrathecal chemotherapy (issued under HSC 2008/001, 11 August 2008). Available online at: http://www.dh.gov.uk/en/Publicationsandstatistics/Lettersandcirculars/Healthservicecirculars/DH_086870 (accessed 23 July 2010).
24. Control of Substances Hazardous to Health regulations. Available online at: http://www.hse.gov.uk/coshh/ (accessed 10 March 2010).
25. National Patient Safety Agency. Promoting safer use of injectable medicines. Available online at: http://www.nrls.npsa.nhs.uk/resources/?entryid45=59812 (accessed 23 July 2010).

Further reading

Maltby P. The maze of regulations in radiopharmacy. *Hosp Pharm* 1999; 6: 42–45.
The Management and Awareness of Risks of Cytotoxics (MARC) programme. Available online at: http://www.marchguidelines.com/.
Rules and Guidance for Pharmaceutical Manufacturers and Distributors. London: Pharmaceutical Press, 2009.
MARCH guidelines: http://www.marchguidelines.com.
Needle R, Sizer T. *The CIVAS Handbook*. London: Pharmaceutical Press, 1998.
NHS Technical Specialist Education and Training (TSET): http://www.tset.org.uk.
Pharmaceutical Aseptic Services Group: http://www.civas.co.uk.
Pharmaceutical Isolator User Group: http://www.piug.org.uk.
UK Radiopharmacy Group: http://www.ukrg.org.uk.

7

Quality assurance

Ian M Beaumont

National Health Service (NHS) regional quality control (QC) laboratories were first established in 1966 following health memorandum HM(65)22.[1] This dealt with the QC of purchased drugs and dressings, giving guidance to NHS regions on setting up regional QC services. The aim was to ensure that the quality of the products procured through the regional purchasing system met a satisfactory standard. In the early 1970s the work of the laboratories was significantly extended following HSC(IS)128 *Application of the Medicines Act to Health Authorities*, which applied the principles of the *Medicines Act* to all pharmaceutical manufacturing operations undertaken by health authorities.[2] The circular required quality assurance (QA) and QC arrangements to be in place for all such activities and resulted in provision of QC laboratory facilities for each NHS manufacturing unit, located in most major pharmacy departments. It also resulted in them being subjected to regular inspection by the Medicines Inspectorate.[3, 4]

In 1984, health circular HC(84)3 introduced a policy of costing hospital pharmaceutical manufacturing operations and required the NHS to engage in manufacture only if there was no satisfactory commercial source or if it was significantly more economical to do so.[5] This, along with the increasing commercial availability of hospital requirements, resulted in the rationalisation of both manufacturing and QC laboratory facilities through the remainder of the 1980s and the 1990s. Some NHS regions took the view that QA and QC services should be provided centrally at regional level, in order to make the best and most cost-effective use of the specialist staff and laboratory resources; this resulted in regional QC services based within one or two large laboratories on hospital sites within their region.

Throughout the 1990s and early 2000s there was a very large increase in the number of pharmacy aseptic units preparing injections and other products, as well as an increase in the preparation of clinical trial materials. NHS executive letters EL(96)95 and EL(97)52 introduced requirements for regular internal and external quality audit of pharmacy aseptic preparation activities to ensure these services achieved appropriately high standards.[6, 7] The requirements established the role of the regional QA specialist in performing these external audits. These aseptic services, along with the remaining NHS manufacturing units, continue to require specialist QA and QC facilities, as well as pharmacists and other QA staff with substantial skills and knowledge in QA, good pharmaceutical manufacturing practice, QC, audit, pharmaceutical sciences and technology, formulation and stability.

In the early 2000s the Department of Health established the NHS Hospital Medicines Manufacturing and Preparative Services Implementation Board, which oversaw the review of hospital pharmacy manufacturing and associated QA services, and then managed a modernisation programme from 2004 to 2006. The programme included considerable capital investment in facilities for these services. A risk management programme involving product rationalisation followed, including implementation of autoidentification (bar coding) systems, and the launch of a national database (called Pro-File) of NHS-manufactured items.

Following publication of the NHS next-stage review *High Quality Care for All*[8] and the government's White Paper *Pharmacy in England: Building on Strengths, Delivering the Future* in 2008,[9] a new national strategy for NHS pharmaceutical services was developed and issued by the NHS Pharmaceutical Quality Assurance Committee. This gave details of the important roles that NHS pharmaceutical QA services now play as part of the pharmacy team in assuring the quality of medicines in the NHS from procurement or preparation/manufacture through to their final point of use by patients.

The NHS quality agenda and the role of the quality assurance pharmacist

Quality assurance

QA of pharmaceutical products and services is of prime importance. Patients rely on pharmacists providing medicines which are consistently safe, efficacious and of suitable quality. Quality itself has a number of definitions: dictionary.com has 19 different definitions for quality, many of which give a rather subjective view, one which is both comparative and difficult to quantify and measure.[10] The total quality management (TQM) approach describes quality as: 'meeting customer needs'.[11] TQM is a management philosophy which embraces all activities, through which the needs and expectations of the customer and the community are satisfied, and through which the objectives of the organisation are met; these aims are achieved in the most cost-effective way by maximising the potential of all employees in a continuing drive for improvement. This is a useful definition to apply to pharmacy services, and one that aims to ensure service objectives are entirely organised around meeting customer needs.

A third approach to defining quality, and the one most appropriate to be applied to pharmaceutical products, is the 'fitness for purpose' definition, as adopted in pharmaceutical manufacturing over many years. The *Rules and Guidance for Pharmaceutical Manufacturers and Distributors* (commonly called the *Orange Guide* because of the colour of its cover) states that the quality objective in manufacturing is to ensure that the products are 'consistently produced and controlled to the quality standards appropriate to their intended use and as required by the Marketing Authorisation or product specification'.[12] This definition can be applied in a quantitative sense, with quality parameters and limits being set against which all services or batches of products are tested and checked for compliance. Examples of this are product specifications comprising assays and service specifications comprising quantitative service parameters, such as length of waiting times for prescriptions.

'Quality assurance' is the term applied to all the arrangements which influence the quality of the products or services supplied. The *Orange Guide* defines it as 'the total sum of the organised arrangements made with the object of ensuring that medicinal products are of the quality required for their intended use'.[12] In pharmaceutical manufacturing it encompasses both good manufacturing practice (GMP) and QC. GMP is the part of QA which ensures that products are consistently produced and controlled to the quality standards appropriate to their intended use. QC is the part of GMP concerned with sampling, specifications and testing, and with the release of products for use. Sharp provides a detailed discussion of these concepts in his text on quality in manufacture of healthcare products.[13]

Clinical governance

A First Class Service: Quality in the New NHS introduced the concept of clinical governance to the NHS.[14] It defined the term as 'a framework through which NHS organisations are accountable for continuously improving the quality of their services and safeguarding high standards of care by creating an environment in which excellence in clinical care will flourish'. Chapter 12 will discuss governance and risk management in more detail. Pharmaceutical QA services have a long history of innovation and quality improvement of hospital pharmacy services at both local and national level. Many of the components of clinical governance have been well developed and in place for many years, for example, the issue of standards and guidance, QC and audit of manufacturing and aseptic services. Responsibility and accountability for quality of products prepared in licensed units have long been clearly placed with the quality controller. Quality improvement activities are a fundamental part of the QA pharmacist's role. Examples of this are audit, continuing professional development for QA and other pharmacy staff, the application of evidence-based good practice based on clear evidence provided through QC and monitoring data, and sound pharmaceutical research and development (R&D) work.

Risk management

Many aspects of pharmacy services have the potential to harm patients through errors or poor advice. Robust QA systems need to be in place to prevent this happening, especially for activities that carry the most risk. QA pharmacists have well-established systems for risk management of procurement activities and of licensed manufacturing and aseptic preparation services through systems of QC and audit.

Medication errors

In 2000 an expert group chaired by the Chief Medical Officer published a report entitled *An Organisation with a Memory*, which summarised the scale and nature of serious failures in NHS healthcare and made recommendations on how lessons should be learnt from errors and near-misses and how to minimise the likelihood of repeating these errors in the future.[15] This was followed in 2001 by *Building a Safer NHS for Patients*,[16] which set the NHS targets for implementing the recommendations from *An Organisation with a Memory*.[15] It established a national agency, the National Patient Safety Agency (NPSA), which has the remit of collecting and analysing information on adverse events in the NHS, assimilating other safety-related information, learning lessons and ensuring they are fed back into practice, producing solutions to prevent harm where risks are identified, specifying national goals and establishing mechanisms to track progress. The NPSA continues to produce and issue patient safety alerts, rapid response reports and guidance on design for patient safety and is discussed further in Chapter 12.

QA pharmacists have a key contribution to make towards achieving these targets, in assisting with the reporting, analysis and feeding back of information regarding medication errors, and in ensuring that appropriate systems of QA, QC and audit are in place throughout all areas of pharmacy practice.

The aims of NHS pharmaceutical quality assurance services

The quality of medicines and their management are vital for the NHS. There are important health gains to be achieved from the use of quality-assured, clinically effective medicines. It is also important to manage the potential risks of using medicines which may be of an inappropriate quality and could result in poor efficacy and safety. As part of a team effort, the overall management of medicines requires specialist input from QA pharmacists and other QA staff. They can contribute an in-depth knowledge of the pharmaceutical sciences, formulation and stability, QA systems and the QC of medicines. Therefore, the key aims of pharmaceutical QA services are assuring the quality of medicines and minimising the risk to NHS patients of receiving defective medicines. These aims are achieved by applying appropriate systems of QA, audit and QC to the purchasing, manufacturing and preparation of medicines in hospitals.

Pharmaceutical QA services include:

- development, issue, implementation and monitoring of standards and guidance relating to quality aspects of hospital pharmacy services and the management of medicines
- QA and QC of medicines purchased or manufactured prepared for hospital patients
- quality audit of pharmacy technical services
- investigation and testing of defective medicines
- advisory services on all aspects of pharmaceutical QA and QC
- R&D, especially in the areas of pharmaceutical formulation and stability studies
- QC of medical gas installations in hospitals
- training of pharmacy staff
- laboratory and environmental testing services.

NHS QA services are coordinated nationally by the NHS Pharmaceutical Quality Assurance Committee, which includes regional QA pharmacists from throughout the UK. In addition to coordinating QA services, the Committee also develops and issues policy, standards and guidance on a range of pharmaceutical QA issues. It operates a communications network at national and local levels, provides leadership and collective expert views, develops and promotes best practice and educational programmes and assists in maximising the efficient use of QA resources by sharing information. This information sharing includes the Analytical Information Centre database containing summarised test data from all regional laboratories, and reports of stability studies carried out in QC laboratories across the UK. The Committee has close working relationships with pharmaceutical advisers, the Medicines and Healthcare products Regulatory Agency (MHRA), the General Pharmaceutical Council, Royal Pharmaceutical Society and other key national bodies and agencies.

Development, issue, implementation and monitoring of standards and guidance

QA staff are actively involved locally and nationally in the development of pharmaceutical technical standards and guidance for application to pharmacy services. The NHS Pharmaceutical Quality Assurance Committee has produced guidance documents covering a wide span of topics.[17-22] Implementation and monitoring of national and local standards and guidance are carried out on an ongoing basis through QC, environmental monitoring and audit programmes in hospital pharmacy manufacturing units and in both licensed and unlicensed aseptic dispensing units.

Quality assurance and quality control of medicines

Hospital manufacturing units

The manufacture of medicines is a complex operation and must conform to GMP requirements of the MHRA.[12] These require a system of QA designed to build quality into each product at all stages of its manufacture. To this end, pharmaceutical QA services work closely with production staff and provide a series of checks, tests and controls throughout the manufacturing process as follows:

- pharmaceutical quality systems
- pharmaceutical risk management
- microbiological and chemical testing, where appropriate, of ingredients, labels and packaging components, in-process samples and finished products
- checking and approval of all standard operating procedures and production documents
- environmental monitoring in clean and aseptic areas, validating processes, equipment and procedures
- change control
- corrective and preventive actions
- product quality reviews
- the performance of sterilisers
- pharmaceutical development work, including formulation development, stability studies and manufacturing and analytical method development and validation
- planned quality auditing at regular intervals
- liaison with the MHRA.

Each manufacturing unit is required to be licensed under the *Medicines Act*, holding a manufacturer's specials licence. A requirement of the licence is that there must be a named production manager and named quality controller for the release for use of all products manufactured in the unit. This is a key role for QA pharmacists and other appropriately qualified and experienced QA staff. Before releasing each batch for use, the quality controller has to satisfy him- or herself that GMP, as laid down in MHRA guidance, has been complied with, that all manufacturing and QC processes have been validated, that all checks and tests have been carried out and are satisfactory, that all documentation is satisfactory and that all other factors which affect product quality are satisfactory. This requires QC staff who are fully trained and competent in the quality, safety and efficacy requirements for pharmaceutical products.

Purchased medicines

Hospital pharmacists purchase medicines either through a system of contracts or through local purchasing arrangements with suppliers (see Chapter 3). QA pharmacists have an important role in advising procurement staff on the quality and suitability of commercially manufactured pharmaceutical products purchased through the contracting system or purchased locally. Regional pharmaceutical QA services carry out work in assessing samples of products prior to contract awards. This includes medication error potential analysis, involving risk assessment of each product for its potential to lead to medication errors in use. It can also include laboratory testing for compliance with standards, and for bioequivalence where appropriate, and assessment of the packaging and labelling for correctness.

Holders of manufacturers' specials licences prepare unlicensed medicines or they may be imported from outside the UK. These products are frequently required for individual hospital patients with special needs when no suitable licensed equivalent is available.

Unlicensed medicines are not subject to the same controls as licensed medicines, and so special care needs to be taken during their purchase and use. The MHRA and regional QA pharmacists have issued guidance on these issues.[17, 22, 23] QA pharmacists have a key role in assessing and approving suppliers of specials, in evaluating and, if necessary, testing the products themselves before use. They can also make an important contribution in training and advising pharmacists and other users on risks associated with unlicensed medicines and the standards and controls to be applied.

Quality assurance of pharmacy services

Owing to their detailed knowledge and experience of the application of the principles of QA and GMP to manufacturing and aseptic dispensing activities, QA staff have developed their services in the past few years to encompass other areas of pharmacy services. A particular area is in extemporaneous dispensing activities. These carry a high risk to the patient if mistakes are made.[24] The risk of error can be reduced or eliminated by the application of appropriate QA and QC systems. QA pharmacists have, in some hospitals, introduced systems such as QC of dispensing ingredients, independent QC checking of documentation and testing and releasing of extemporaneously dispensed products. Further developments have included issuing guidance on standards, facilities and procedures for dispensing operations and the introduction of internal and external audit schemes. It is hoped that the application of quality systems to dispensing processes and other high-risk areas of pharmacy practice will become universal through-out pharmacy services in the near future.

Quality assurance of aseptic services

Aseptic preparation units in hospital pharmacies prepare a large range of injectable and other sterile products for individual patient use, including addi-tives to infusion solutions, total parenteral nutrition (intravenous feeding) solutions, prefilled syringes and cytotoxic drug injections (see Chapter 6). Many of these products have a narrow therapeutic range and carry a very high risk to the patient if they are not made up correctly or if they become contam-inated with microorganisms.[25] There are many reports in the literature describ-ing errors when injections have been made up by nursing or medical staff on the ward.[26–34] In order to minimise risks to patients, whenever possible these high-risk products should be prepared under pharmacy control in appropriate facilities where risk of contamination risks is known to be reduced.[35] This approach was confirmed by the Audit Commission's advice in *A Spoonful of Sugar*.[36] In 2007 the NPSA published patient safety alert 20 *Promoting Safer Use of Injectable Medicines*, which included a number of actions for healthcare organisations, including risk-assessing injectable medicine procedures and con-trols in all clinical areas, and developing an action plan to minimise high risks.[37] As a result, there has continued to be a large increase in the activity of pharmacy aseptic units, with high-risk aseptic preparation activities trans-ferring to pharmacy control. Guidance on standards for aseptic services is given in the fourth edition of *Quality Assurance of Aseptic Preparation Services*.[19] This describes standards for facilities, procedures and controls to be applied, and also includes useful guidance on the risks associated with aseptic prepa-ration, and the management of these risks.

A priority for pharmaceutical QA services is to work closely with these aseptic units to ensure the safety and quality of the products prepared. QA staff are routinely involved in assisting in the design of facilities, and in monitoring them using a series of regular environmental and personnel moni-toring techniques (see later in this chapter). They are involved in training aseptic unit staff and regularly issue advice and guidance on all aspects of QA in aseptic preparation. They are also involved in quality audit processes. In licensed units, the QA officer is named as the quality controller and has responsibility for releasing all products for use.

The continuing direct involvement of QA personnel with aseptic prepara-tion activities is a key future role for the QA service.

Quality audit

Quality audit is a systematic and independent examination to determine whether quality activities and related results comply with planned arrangements and whether these arrangements are implemented effectively and are suitable to achieve objectives.[38]

QA pharmacists have been involved for many years in the application of audits to license manufacturing units and other pharmacy technical services such as radiopharmacy. In the 1990s aseptic dispensing in unlicensed units was the subject of two NHS Executive Letters, EL(96)95 and EL(97)52.[6, 7] The former required hospitals to carry out an internal audit exercise and the latter set in place an ongoing system of external audits carried out by regional QA specialists every 12–18 months. These audits are reported directly to the chief executives of NHS trusts and to the commissioners of these services, with areas requiring action highlighted. The NHS Pharmaceutical Quality Assurance Committee has issued guidance on the training of auditors to undertake these audits.[20]

The audit system in pharmacy services is now firmly established as a key component of the NHS clinical governance agenda. Audit aims to improve quality continuously, and to assist in the identification and management of risks and in learning from errors and near-misses.

Advisory services and research and development

Advisory services

The QA specialists' knowledge of quality systems, pharmaceutical QA, audit and QC is utilised widely for advising pharmacists, other healthcare professionals, health authorities, hospital trusts and primary care trusts.

Research and development

The pharmaceutical QA specialist has a key role in catalysing innovation and ensuring its uptake, as described in the 2008 government White Paper.[9] As clinical practice changes there is a constant need for the development of new formulations and for determining their shelf-lives. R&D activity is therefore mainly focused around formulation and pharmaceutical development projects and stability studies, although much other R&D work around analytical method development and validation, method transfer, bioavailability and compatibility with packaging components is carried out. R&D activities undertaken in NHS QA services are co-coordinated through the R&D sub-committee of the NHS Pharmaceutical QA Committee.

There is a particularly heavy demand for R&D activities associated with aseptic preparation of medicines, often involving complex mixtures of drug substances and drug-packaging component interaction.

QA personnel are increasingly involved in clinical research and good clinical practice, in particular in providing qualified person support to clinical trials and the releasing for use of investigational medicinal products. In 2009 the NHS Pharmaceutical Quality Assurance Committee issued guidance on pharmacy clinical trial activities.[21]

Dedicated laboratory and controlled temperature and humidity storage facilities for both real-time and accelerated stability studies are usually available in the larger laboratories and regional QA centres.

Testing piped medical gas installations

Standards for medical gas installations in hospitals are laid down in a health technical memorandum (HTM02-01).[39] This covers the design, installation, validation, verification and maintenance of pipeline systems. Medical gases are classified as medicinal products under the *Medicines Act*, and the quality controller has responsibility for the QC of the medical gases supplied by the pipeline system. A register of quality controllers who are authorised to release medical gas pipeline installations for patient use is maintained by the NHS Pharmaceutical QA Committee.

QA personnel are regularly required to visit operating theatres, wards and other clinical areas where medical gas pipelines are used, to carry out testing of the identity, quality and purity of the gases prior to them being taken into use. The tests involve using portable equipment including paramagnetic oxygen analysers, infrared gas analysers, particle filter test units and chemical reagent tubes. A permit-to-work system is used for recording details of work performed.

QA staff are also involved in advising on suitable procedures for the handling, storage and control of medical gases.

Training pharmacy staff

QA staff are regularly involved in the provision of training on a wide range of QA issues to preregistration pharmacists and to other pharmacy personnel.

Defective medicines

Great care is taken to ensure that all medicines used in hospitals are of a suitable quality. However, occasionally defects are identified in medicinal products: this requires rapid and reliable action to determine the severity of the defect and its implications to the patient and to other patients who may be receiving treatment from the affected batch.

Defects may be reported by patients themselves, or by any healthcare professional. They may be relatively minor in nature, for example chipped tablets, or potentially very serious, for example suspected contamination of an intravenous injection. Systems are in place in all hospitals to communicate rapidly the details of the defect, and if appropriate to take the sample to the regional QA department for investigation.

In the laboratory, rapid response procedures are then initiated to investigate the defect, carry out laboratory testing if necessary, and to communicate the outcome of the investigation as appropriate. Serious defects are reported directly to the Defective Medicines Reporting Centre at the MHRA and, if it is considered necessary, a formal drug alert is sent to regional QA services to be communicated throughout the NHS.[40] In serious cases the affected batches are withdrawn from use.

Laboratory services

QC laboratory facilities can be divided into two specialist areas: pharmaceutical chemistry and microbiology.

Pharmaceutical chemistry facilities comprise areas for classical 'wet' chemical methods of analysis and gravimetric analysis, along with laboratory areas for a range of physical testing methods such as melting point, hardness, friability, disintegration and dissolution testing. Wet analysis includes aqueous and non-aqueous volumetric analysis (although burettes have now largely been replaced by computer-controlled autotitrator systems). Other chemistry laboratory areas are dedicated to instrumental methods of analysis, such as spectrophotometry (ultraviolet–visible, Fourier transform infrared and atomic absorption), polarimetry, refractometry, subvisual liquid particle counting and chromotography (thin-layer, gas and high-performance liquid chromatography). The use of high-performance liquid chromatography in pharmaceutical analysis has grown enormously over recent years owing to the ability of this technique to separate and quantify mixtures of components in aqueous formulations. It is also utilised very heavily in pharmaceutical development and in stability studies since it can separate and quantify active drugs and degradation products produced on storage. Liquid chromatography–mass spectrometry is also used, for example for analysing cytotoxic drug residues, and a number of other techniques are under development for the analysis of monoclonal antibodies and other drugs of biological origin.

Analytical methods used in the laboratories are primarily pharmacopoeial, taken from the *British Pharmacopoeia* or *European Pharmacopoeia* or from other international pharmacopoeias as appropriate. However, in many cases no suitable official monograph exists, so in-house specifications are developed and validated. The frequent changes in and development of new clinical treatments require the formulation and QC testing of new products and the ongoing development of new product specifications and analytical methods. This presents a variety of interesting challenges to laboratory staff, requiring a high level of scientific knowledge and the ability to apply it to new problems.

Samples entering the laboratory are many and varied, ranging from pharmacopoeial raw materials, in-process samples and finished products from hospital manufacturing units to samples of unlicensed medicines. These may have been purchased by hospitals from commercial holders of manufacturers' specials licences or may have been imported from anywhere in the world to meet a specific patient's need. Samples may also be of any licensed medicinal product being assessed for its suitability for purchase, or may be the subject of a defective medicines report, referred to the laboratory for investigation. In many cases (such as in the case of suspected defective medicines) the analysis and assessment of the product are required urgently. It is therefore essential that suitable laboratory resources and expertise are available to deal with these when required.

A key area of work of the laboratories is R&D, covering a range of activities including investigational medicinal products, new product formulation and pharmaceutical development, analytical method development and validation, and stability studies. In many laboratories this work runs alongside other QC work with the same staff carrying out QC testing and R&D activities, but in some larger regional laboratories a separate R&D section with its own dedicated laboratories is in place. These dedicated R&D laboratories are mainly equipped with chromatographic equipment, especially high-specification computer-controlled high-performance liquid chromatography equipment utilising mass spectrometer, diode array, fluorimetric, refractive index and other detectors, along with gradient elution programmers and autoinjectors allowing the equipment to be utilised 24 hours a day. Data generated are analysed by sophisticated data-handling software systems.

As a result of the wide variety of samples submitted for QC testing, along with the involvement in R&D activities, laboratory staff obtain a large breadth of experience in pharmaceutical analysis. As well as pharmacists, other laboratory staff are trained to graduate or higher level in chemistry, microbiology or an associated science. Opportunities exist for continuing professional development and many QC laboratory staff have undertaken external courses such as the MSc in Pharmaceutical Technology and Quality Assurance, run jointly by the NHS and Leeds University.

Pharmaceutical microbiology facilities comprise areas for carrying out a wide range of microbiological tests on pharmaceuticals and raw materials, such as total viable counts, incubation and reading of settle plates (and media from other environmental and personnel-monitoring techniques such as active air sampling, surface testing or finger dabs), organism identification, preservative efficacy testing and microbiological stability studies. There are also dedicated areas for carrying out endotoxin testing (using automated systems involving Limulus amoebocyte lysate) and dedicated aseptic facilities for sterility testing.

The quantity of work passing through the pharmaceutical microbiology laboratory has increased significantly over recent years, reflecting the large increase in activity of hospital pharmacy aseptic preparation and dispensing units and the publication of standards laying down high levels of monitoring.[19] Each aseptic unit is required to undertake a programme of sessional, daily, weekly and quarterly validation and monitoring tests, resulting in large numbers of settle plates and other microbiological media, along with samples of finished products for sterility testing or endotoxin testing. Microbiology laboratory facilities have therefore increased in size and capacity in response to this increasing demand.

A key element of the work of the pharmaceutical microbiologist is the interpretation of the significance of the results obtained from the various tests performed and their effect on the quality and safety of aseptically prepared and manufactured products. This requires a constant awareness of trends in results for each aseptic unit, and the ability to react quickly and issue advice and guidance to the pharmacist supervising aseptic preparation if problems are found. Modern Laboratory Information Management Systems (LIMS), utilising bar-coding and direct data entry by laboratory staff, coupled with automatic trend analysis and electronic reporting to the aseptic or manufacturing unit, facilitate these processes.

The standard of laboratory work performed is of prime importance in all hospital QC laboratories. QA and other pharmacists, in making critically important decisions regarding release of batches of medicines for use in patients, rely upon all results generated, and so it is essential that all results are valid. Pharmaceutical quality systems are in place to ensure this is the case, including systems for staff training, supervision and checking, method validation, calibration, traceability of standards, documentation, internal QC procedures and participation in interlaboratory testing schemes. The Pharmassure scheme has run successfully in this regard for many years, with a large number of hospital QC laboratories participating. Many laboratories follow an ISO 9000 quality system model.[41, 42] Some laboratories are accredited by the UK Accreditation Service (UKAS) for compliance with ISO IEC 17025 standards.[43] All laboratories associated with licensed manufacturing operations are subject to regular risk-based inspection by MHRA inspectors. The small number of laboratories associated with hospital units producing CE-marked medical devices are also subject to notified body inspection.

Environmental monitoring services

Specialist QC staff are involved in the monitoring of hospital pharmacy clean and aseptic environments used for the manufacture and aseptic dispensing of medicines, along with other hospital clean areas such as ultraclean ventilation systems in operating theatres, clean isolation rooms in bone marrow units and hospital sterilising and disinfecting units. Portable monitoring equipment consisting of a range of physical and microbiological equipment is used.

Physical testing has several components: first, airborne subvisual particle counting, using laser-equipped particle counters capable of counting particles as small as 0.3 μm. A second aspect is air velocity measurements using anemometers for calculating the rate of air exchange in clean rooms and for ensuring that devices such as laminar air flow cabinets and pharmaceutical isolators are operating within the required parameters. Air pressure differential monitoring between different categories of clean rooms is undertaken using portable manometers. Filter integrity testing is carried out using dispersed oil particle generators and photometric detection equipment to ensure that high-efficiency particulate air filters and their housings are not leaking. Finally, operator protection testing is carried out using potassium iodide discus equipment.

Microbiological monitoring comprises settle plate testing, active air sampling, surface swabbing, finger dabs and other techniques designed to monitor levels of environmental microorganisms in the clean aseptic area and to demonstrate whether acceptable levels are exceeded.

Owing to the specialised nature of this work, and the high cost of some of the test equipment, these services are often organised on a regional or group of hospitals basis.

The future

Because of the historical background, QA services have focused mainly on laboratory services and the provision of QA, QC and audit to technical areas of hospital pharmacy practice. All of these will remain important. Set against the NHS clinical governance agenda and the need to ensure high-quality pharmacy services are designed around the patient, the intention for the future is to widen the focus to encompass the QA aspects of pharmacy services in general. This will build on the considerable strengths of the service in terms of its expertise in the areas of QA, quality improvements, audit and risk management.

In line with the government's White Paper, *Pharmacy in England: Building on Strengths – Delivering the Future*,[9] QA services will continue to develop and play an increasing role in assuring the quality of pharmaceutical services and products for patients, especially in the development of more comprehensive systems for management of risks, and for learning from and preventing errors. There will be a greater input into assuring the quality of high-risk activities such as preparation and handling of aseptic products, clinical trial materials and unlicensed medicines, and increasing challenges in ensuring that appropriate QA arrangements are developed for the products of new technologies, such as gene therapy products and a rapidly increasing number of monoclonal antibody products.

The desire to see care, including diagnostic and higher-tech treatments, provided nearer to or in the patient's home brings a challenge to the QA team. It will be important to ensure there is no loss of quality as these services develop.

The present national network of QA staff, led by the NHS Pharmaceutical Quality Assurance Committee, is important in ensuring the coordination of laboratory work, elimination of duplication, unification of standards across the NHS and the dissemination of information. This will continue to develop. In 2008 the Committee published a new strategy for NHS Pharmaceutical Quality Assurance Services.[44] The strategy provides a national framework in which the service can continue to make an effective contribution to the rapidly expanding demands of risk management and clinical governance in delivering the patient safety agenda in the NHS. It sets out that, in working with others, there are seven strategic aims:

1   to support evidence-based use of medicines for patients by producing, assessing, interpreting and applying pharmaceutical QA and QC evidence, data and information
2   to develop clinical research and good clinical practice in clinical trials
3   to catalyse innovation in practice and promote its uptake
4   to contribute to the development and introduction of autoidentification and data capture to support safe medicines supply and administration
5   to quality assure NHS preparative services and manufacturing
6   to ensure the future availability and commissioning of specialised pharmaceutical QA services
7   to be recognised and represented in the General Pharmaceutical Council and the new pharmacy professional body.

In the NHS of the future, in which a comprehensive range of services is provided to meet the needs of individual patients, and where quality will be continuously improved and errors minimised, the QA pharmacist and NHS Pharmaceutical Quality Assurance Service will have a key role in delivering these objectives.

References

1. Ministry of Health. National Health Service. *Quality Control of Hospital. Supplies of Drugs and Dressings.* HM(65)22. London: HMSO, 1965.
2. Department of Health and Social Security. *Application of the Medicines Act to Health Authorities.* Health Service circular (interim series) HSC(IS)128. London: HMSO, 1975.
3. Sprake JM. The development of quality assurance in the Trent region, England. *J Clin Pharm* 1977; 2: 17–21.
4. Sprake JM. An increasingly attractive specialty. *Pharm J* 1980; 224: 600–601.

5. Department of Health and Social Security. *Health Services Management: Manufacture of Products in the NHS.* HC(84)3. London: HMSO, 1984.
6. Department of Health. *Aseptic Dispensing for NHS Patients.* Executive letter EL(96)95. London: The Stationery Office, 1996.
7. Department of Health. *Aseptic Dispensing for NHS Patients.* Executive letter EL(97)52. London: The Stationery Office, 1997.
8. Department of Health. *High Quality Care for All. NHS Next Stage Review Final Report.* London: Department of Health, 2008.
9. Department of Health. *Pharmacy in England: Building on Strengths, Delivering the Future.* London: Department of Health, 2008.
10. Dictionary.com. Available online at: http://www.dictionary.com (accessed 16 March 2010).
11. British Standards Institution. *BS7850-2: 1994. ISO 9004-4: 1993. Total Quality Management. Guidelines for Quality Improvement.* London: British Standards Institution, 1994.
12. Medicines and Healthcare products Regulatory Agency. *Rules and Guidance for Pharmaceutical Manufacturers and Distributors 2007.* London: Pharmaceutical Press, 2007.
13. Sharp J. *Quality in the Manufacture of Medicines and other Healthcare Products.* London: Pharmaceutical Press, 2000.
14. Department of Health. *A First Class Service: Quality in the New NHS.* London: The Stationery Office, 1998.
15. Department of Health. *An Organisation with a Memory – Report of an Expert Group on Learning from Adverse Events in the NHS Chaired by the Chief Medical Officer.* London: The Stationery Office, 2000.
16. Department of Health. *Building a Safer NHS for Patients. Implementing an Organisation with a Memory.* London: The Stationery Office, 2001.
17. NHS Pharmaceutical Quality Assurance Committee. *Guidance for the Purchase and Supply of Unlicensed Medicinal Products. Notes for Prescribers and Pharmacists*, 3rd edn. NHS Pharmaceutical Quality Assurance Committee, 2004.
18. Midcalf B, Phillips WM, Neiger JS *et al. Pharmaceutical Isolators.* London: Pharmaceutical Press, 2004.
19. Beaney AM. *Quality Assurance of Aseptic Preparation Services*, 4th edn. London: Pharmaceutical Press, 2006.
20. NHS Pharmaceutical Quality Control Committee. *Quality Audits and their Application to Hospital Pharmacy Technical Services.* Liverpool: Quality Control Committee, 1999.
21. NHS Pharmaceutical Quality Assurance Committee. *Pharmacy Clinical Trials Activities.* NHS Pharmaceutical Quality Assurance Committee, 2009.
22. NHS Pharmaceutical Quality Assurance Committee. *Quality Assurance and Risk Assessment of Licensed Medicines for the NHS.* NHS Pharmaceutical Quality Assurance Committee, 2004.
23. Medicines and Healthcare products Regulatory Agency. *The Supply of Unlicensed Relevant Medicinal Products for Individual Patients* (January 2008 revision). Guidance note no. 14. London: Medicines and Healthcare products Regulatory Agency, 2008.
24. Anonymous. Boots pharmacist and trainee cleared of baby's manslaughter, but fined for dispensing a defective medicine. *Pharm J* 2000; 264: 390–392.
25. Anonymous. Two children die after receiving infected TPN solutions. *Pharm J* 1994; 252: 596.
26. Ernot L, Thoren S, Sandell E. Studies on microbial contamination of infusion fluids arising from drug additions and administration. *Pharm Suec* 1973; 10: 141–146.
27. Cos GE. Bacterial contamination of drip sets. *NZ Med J* 1973; 77: 390–391.
28. Woodside W, Woodside WM, D'Arcy EM *et al.* Intravenous infusions as vehicles for infection. *Pharm J* 1975; 215: 606.
29. Deeks EN, Natsios GA. Contamination of infusion fluids by bacteria and fungi during preparation and administration. *Am J Hosp Pharm* 1971; 28: 764–767.
30. D'Arcy PF, Woodside ME. Drug additives, a potential source of bacterial contamination of infusion fluids. *Lancet* 1973; ii: 96.

31. Quercia RA, Hiels SW, Klimek JJ *et al.* Bacteriologic contamination of intravenous infusion delivery systems in an intensive care unit. *Am J Med* 1986; 80: 364–368.
32. O'Hare MCB, Bradley AM, Gallagher T *et al.* Errors in administration of intravenous drugs (letter). *Br Med J* 1995; 310: 1536–1537.
33. Cousins DH, Upton DR. Medication error 125: parenteral vial errors must stop. *Pharm Pract* 1999; 9: 220–221.
34. Cousins DH, Upton DR. Medication error 62: act now to prevent KCl deaths. *Pharm Pract* 1996; 6: 307–310.
35. Austin P, Marinos E. A systematic review and meta-analysis of the risk of microbial contamination of aseptically prepared doses in different environments. *J Pharm Pharmaceut Sci* 2009; 12: 233–242.
36. Audit Commission. *A Spoonful of Sugar – Medicines Management in NHS Hospitals.* London: Audit Commission, 2001.
37. National Patient Safety Agency. *Promoting Safer Use of Injectable Medicines.* Alert 20. London: NPSA, 2007.
38. ISO 19011 : 2002. Guidelines for quality and/or environmental management systems auditing. Geneva: International Standards Organization, 2002.
39. Department of Health. *Medical Gas Pipeline Systems.* Health technical memorandum HTM 02-01. London: Department of Health, 2006.
40. Medicines and Healthcare products Regulatory Agency. *A Guide to Defective Medicinal Products.* London: The Stationery Office, 2004.
41. BS EN ISO 9000. *Quality Management Systems. Fundamentals and Vocabulary.* London: British Standards Institution, 2005.
42. BS EN ISO 9001. *Quality Management Systems. Requirements.* London: British Standards Institution, 2008.
43. BS EN ISO IEC 17025. *General Requirements for the Competence of Testing and Calibration Laboratories.* London: British Standards Institution, 2005.
44. NHS Pharmaceutical Quality Assurance Group. *NHS Pharmaceutical Quality Assurance Strategy.* London: NHS Pharmaceutical Quality Assurance Group, 2008.

Further reading

Beaney AM. *Quality Assurance of Aseptic Preparation Services*, 4th edn. London: Pharmaceutical Press, 2006.
Medicines and Healthcare products Regulatory Agency. *Rules and Guidance for Pharmaceutical Manufacturers and Distributors 2007.* London: The Stationery Office, 2007.
Sharp J. *Quality in the Manufacture of Medicines and other Healthcare Products.* London: Pharmaceutical Press, 2000.

8

Medicines information

Peter Golightly and Christine Proudlove

Medicines information (MI) has developed as a specialty of hospital pharmacy within the UK National Health Service (NHS), and is mirrored by similar service developments in advanced healthcare systems in most of the developed world, including Europe, the USA and Australasia. However, the models adopted vary according to the health systems and practices in a particular country. Although most MI services are provided by pharmacists, as part a hospital pharmacy service, there are models where doctors, nurses and other technical staff have a more dominant role than in the UK. This chapter will focus on the provision and practice of MI in the UK, much of which is transferable to other countries.

History

The history and structure of MI services in the UK largely reflect those of the NHS in which it functions, and to which most of its activities are directed. Through the 1960s hospital pharmacy was undergoing a radical change, especially with the development of ward-based, patient-focused activities – clinical pharmacy. The pharmacist's traditional role of compounding and supply was being replaced by the provision of prescribing advice to doctors and nurses, and information provision directly to patients. The hospital pharmacist became the ward-based expert on medicines and therapeutics. However, this expansion of activity was accompanied by a parallel demand for high-quality and reliable information. Prior to this, information on medicines was acquired from personal knowledge or from standard reference sources. The requirement for information and advisory support to healthcare professionals with a medicines-related role was further stimulated by a number of simultaneous developments. The so-called therapeutic explosion in the 1960s and 1970s made available a vast array of new and potent medicines with increased efficacy and toxicity. Accompanying this was an 'information explosion' in which the availability of published, critically assessed, clinical information and evidence increased dramatically. This literature covered all aspects of medicines, including their pharmacology, pharmacokinetics, comparative clinical efficacy, toxicity, use in specific circumstances such as pregnancy, and the pharmaceutics of formulation and drug delivery. It is estimated that there are currently over 18 000 medical and pharmaceutical journals worldwide, the majority of which have the potential to include information on medicines, although many are not peer-reviewed nor of high quality. Of these only about 5400 are cited by Medline and 7000 by Embase (these data sources are discussed later). The establishment of these new roles for hospital pharmacists in the UK, including MI services, was formalised in the Noel Hall report.[1]

The demand for high-quality, evaluated, rapidly available, patient-oriented information, that was not from pharma industry, for all members of the healthcare team led to the development of drug information services, which were renamed MI services in the UK in 2000, to reflect better current terminology and links to medicines management.

Structure and activities

The first MI services in the UK were established at the London Hospital and Leeds General Infirmary in 1969, followed over the next 10 years by a UK-wide network of local and regional services.[2, 3] This was supported by recommendations from a working party of the Pharmaceutical Society of Great Britain.[4] Local MI centres were established in about 270 mainly acute hospitals, largely providing a service to their base hospital and associated local healthcare community. This number had reduced to approximately 220 by 2010 with rationalisation and health service reforms. Twenty regional MI centres, including national centres in Wales and Northern Ireland, and four regional centres in Scotland have subsequently been reduced to 15, again through a series of NHS reorganisations. These services have been brought together in a structured and coordinated national network (UK Medicines Information: UKMi), to which both local and regional services contribute skills, expertise, knowledge and resources. The network is coordinated and provided with strategic leadership by a national representative body, the UKMi Executive (previously known as the UK Medicines Information Pharmacists Group).

MI services in the UK have developed on a hierarchical basis in which all the levels of service provision provide mutual support through a network

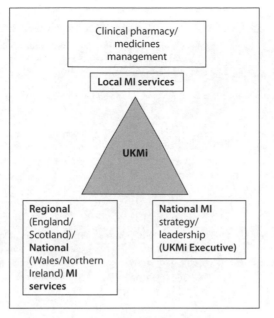

Figure 8.1 Structure of medicines information (MI) services in the UK.

that encourages and promotes effective provision of services. Support is for all levels of healthcare from point of care to national strategic development. Figure 8.1 summarises the structure and relationships. Each level undertakes a range of activities that is most appropriate to the users of the service, produces maximum benefit of scale and reduces duplication, at and between operational levels.

Table 8.1 sets out these activities. The development of these services has been well described and supported in the professional literature as well as being recognised by government and other official organisations.[5-17]

Aims and strategy

The aim of the MI service is to facilitate high-quality patient care, through the promotion of the safe, effective and economic use of medicines, by the provision of accurate, timely, appropriate, evidence-based and unbiased information and advice on all aspects relating to the use of medicines. This has been the core principle that has formed the framework of the service since its inception. By fulfilling these aims the service has achieved its current high level of use, acceptability and recognition amongst users and the broader NHS.

Table 8.1 Examples of activities of medicines information (MI) services in the UK

Locally	Regionally in England and Scotland; nationally in Wales and Northern Ireland	Nationally for whole National Health Service (NHS)
Advisory and information services for health professionals and patients tailored to individual and organisational needs		
Influence direct patient care Underpin clinical pharmacy services Support effective prescribing	Resource and expertise to support local services Support to primary care organisations on prescribing issues	Specialist advisory services (e.g. on medicines in pregnancy/lactation) Referral for NHS Direct/NHS24 patients
Clinical governance		
Risk management and prescribing guidelines Support for information governance Advice on medicines management, including support to D&TCs, formularies and PGDs	Quality assurance of local MI services Respond to commissioning and service issues as identified by service users	Develop standards for professional practice and resources to support practitioners within the UKMi network (e.g. MiDatabank) Implementation of a national research strategy
Education and training for healthcare professionals, including medicines information skills and therapeutics		
Preregistration and junior pharmacists Nursing and junior medical staff	MI workforce NHS Direct Training resources (MI Workbook, MiCAL)	
Other activities		
Facilitating adverse drug reaction reporting	Development and provision of content for the National electronic Library for Medicines, including a daily news service, and maintaining a library of high-quality evidence about medicines, e.g. Medicines Q&As Horizon scanning: predicting the impact of new medicines and national guidance Evidence-based evaluations of new medicines before and after launch	

D&TCs, drugs and therapeutics committees; PGDs, patient group directions.

To maintain the level and quality, core principles have been developed that underpin all the activities of the service. These are set out in Table 8.2.

As NHS changes have given opportunities to develop MI there have also been increased demands on the capacity of the MI service. In response, a 5-year UK-wide strategy, *Better Information for Managing Medicines*, published in 2000, established a framework for the provision and development of the service.[18] The strategy, approved and endorsed by health departments across the UK, was implemented throughout the service. The strategy

Table 8.2 Core medicines information principles

1 Apply evidence-based principles in the provision of impartial, evaluated, accurate and timely information. This will be in a suitable format, that is, pertinent to the user's needs and readily understood
2 Provide professional advice to support and influence clinical decisions with respect to patient care and to enable the individual to make a balanced choice
3 Keep abreast of developments in therapeutics, professional practice, technology and information sources to support continuing professional development within the specialty and to ensure that the service provided is as up to date as possible
4 Be readily accessible and responsive to user needs
5 Network with others to share information and experience at local, regional and national levels

was revised in 2007 to align it with prevailing NHS strategy. The revised MI strategy, *Effective Information for Managing Medicines*,[19] has five key strategic aims:

1 Reflect a patient-focused NHS.
2 Develop the service to healthcare providers.
3 Develop healthcare staff.
4 Support NHS commissioning and planning bodies.
5 Collaborate effectively with other organisations at national level.

Some of the main drivers for the development of the service through this strategy include the development of primary care trusts as the lead for healthcare provision and commissioning, the continued role of UKMi in the development of NHS Direct in England and Wales and NHS24 in Scotland, the expansion of new independent non-medical prescribers (nurses, pharmacists and others), the provision of guidance from national bodies such as the National Institute for Health and Clinical Excellence (NICE), Scottish Medicines Consortium (SMC) and All-Wales Medicines Strategy Group (AWMSG) and the need for effective management of new medicine entry. The development of evidence-based information technology platforms, especially the National electronic Library for Medicines (NeLM) and NHS Evidence, also influences the MI agenda, as they make information on medicines directly available to health professionals and the public.

Roles and skills

MI pharmacists undertake a wide range of roles and activities that encompass provision of information and advice on all aspects of medicines. These roles are applied at both a clinical level to facilitate individual patient care, and at a strategic level to facilitate decision-making processes in the production of medicines-related policies, the rational introduction and use of medicines (new and established) in the NHS, including the production of guidelines to ensure the appropriate, safe and cost-effective use of medicines. The MI pharmacist therefore must have the knowledge and skills to undertake these roles effectively. These skills fall into a number of broad categories, as shown in Table 8.3, and are the basis for a person specification for an MI pharmacist. However, these skills are not unique to an MI pharmacist; many will be possessed by clinical pharmacists. Of course, an effective MI pharmacist has to be, first and foremost, a competent clinical pharmacist with an in-depth knowledge of therapeutics, and should, where possible, continue to provide a local clinical pharmacy role to sustain his or her knowledge and to ensure MI outputs are clinically and patient-relevant. The MI pharmacist will then have to

Table 8.3 Skill requirements for a medicines information pharmacist	
Skill	**Scope**
Clinical	Knowledge and understanding of all aspects of drugs, therapeutic processes and procedures, disease pathology and management
Communications	Verbal: interrogating enquirers, determining the enquiry, obtaining appropriate and adequate background information, giving verbal responses, telephone techniques Written: writing reports, enquiry replies, bulletins; writing to the level of the recipient; converting data into concise and usable outputs; use of 'plain English'
Critical appraisal	Critically appraise and assess clinical and pharmaceutical literature, content and quality of commercial claims for medicines; working knowledge of medical statistics, including appropriateness and limitations; construction of clinical trials; pharmacoeconomics
Knowledge management	Resource utilisation, e.g. searching primary literature (Medline, Embase) databases, internet, in-house and library resources; interpreting data retrieved; determining cost-effective and quality resources; systems design for in-house storage and retrieval of data
Interpersonal	Ability to work on own initiative; to prioritise work, self-assess performance and work quality and manage time effectively
Information technology (IT)	Ability to use IT resources for acquiring and disseminating information and service outputs; understanding applications of IT; keyboard skills
Management	Managing resources and people
Training	Ability to train pharmacists and other professionals requiring these skills or knowledge, e.g. preregistration pharmacists, pharmacists, nurses, doctors

develop the other skills, in some cases to a higher level, in order to undertake the full MI pharmacist role.

Ethics and legal issues

All pharmacists should be aware of the legal and ethical principles governing the practice of the profession. There is no specific UK case law relating to the provision of MI by hospital pharmacists. The whole pharmacy profession is governed by the legal and ethical principles set out by its own regulatory body, and published in *Medicines, Ethics and Practice – A Guide for Pharmacists and Pharmacy Technicians*.[20] Although it contains no specific reference to the practice of MI, the section 'Code of Ethics and Professional Standards' does include statements which have direct applicability to the practice and provision of MI, including: (1) acting in the interests of patients and the public; (2) keeping up to date; and (3) respecting confidentiality. Specifically regarding information provision, the guide states: 'Be accurate and impartial when teaching others and when providing or publishing information to ensure that you do not mislead others or make claims that cannot be justified.'

MI pharmacists are also a source of advice on legal and ethical issues routinely confronting all pharmacists, as well as on all legal and ethical issues relating to the prescribing, supply and administration of medicines by other healthcare professions. UKMi has published guidelines that cover the legal and ethical issues confronting MI pharmacists in the course of their duties.[21] These are, again, issues that will need to be considered by all pharmacists, but which have a more immediate significance to an MI pharmacist. The main issues are identified in Table 8.4.

Clinical governance and risk management

Clinical governance, with its focus on quality, is an essential element of MI practice. The concept of clinical governance was introduced into the NHS by *A First Class Service: Quality in the New NHS*.[22] Subsequently, the Royal Pharmaceutical Society published a framework for clinical governance in pharmacy.[23] It identified four main components for achieving excellence:

1 clear lines of responsibility and accountability for overall quality of clinical care
2 a comprehensive programme of quality improvement activities (including audit, continuing professional development, research and development)
3 clear policies aimed at managing risks
4 procedures for identification of poor performance.

This approach has been reinforced following various reviews where quality of healthcare has been seen to fall below acceptable standards.

Table 8.4 Legal and ethical issues in medicines information (MI)

Issue	Details
Negligence and liability	An MI pharmacist has a duty to ensure that all information and advice supplied is as accurate and comprehensive as could reasonably be expected. If that information or advice, when acted on, causes loss or damage to a patient, the MI pharmacist may be liable in negligence. For the MI pharmacist to be shown to be negligent it must be established that the MI pharmacist had a duty of care towards the patient, that the duty of care was breached and that damage to the patient occurred. It is, therefore, incumbent on an MI pharmacist to keep up to date as far as is reasonable with current developments and knowledge, to use all reasonably available resources to provide the information required, to present that information in a usable and intelligible form and to act in a professional manner which is appropriate to the skills possessed and the service offered by an MI pharmacist. Working to defined standards with agreed minimum resources and complying with standards for safe systems of work and documentation are part of this process
Unlicensed and clinical trial medicines	MI pharmacists can provide information and advice about unlicensed medicines or unlicensed uses of medicines as long as the enquirer or user is clearly informed that this is the case
Proactive information	The same principles apply to written proactive information, for example, that supplied in bulletins or new-product evaluations. MI pharmacists should be able to demonstrate the process undertaken to produce the information. Disclaimers, although bringing to the attention of the information users their responsibilities in using that information, do not negate the liability of the MI pharmacist supplying the information. These issues apply to both hard copy and electronically published information
Defamation	MI pharmacists have a duty when providing information to ensure that information is accurate, fair and produced from demonstrable and quality evidence. Failure to do so, leading to unreasonable loss of commercial success of a medicine, could lead to the pursuance of defamation of product by a pharmaceutical company. However, a genuine error or omission would not normally be grounds for such an action

The UKMi network has implemented a comprehensive clinical governance programme and utilises a range of tools to support this programme. The tools are common to other areas of healthcare provision and include defined national practice standards, quality assurance programmes, training and competency frameworks. UKMi has also developed a research strategy.

Standards

National standards for MI services were first introduced in 1990. Since then they have been revised and expanded to cover all of the principal elements of the service. In defining the standards, account is taken of identified best practice, policy and regulatory developments, technology advancements and the requirements of commissioners, stakeholders and other organisations with which MI work. The current standards cover six core areas relevant to most MI centres and a seventh that is specific to those centres providing a national specialist service.

The first standard states that an MI centre must have appropriate space, facilities and resources to ensure the provision of a safe and efficient service. The elements of this standard include staffing levels, the working environment and the availability of appropriate equipment, facilities and information resources. Information resources that are considered to be essential to local and regional/national MI centres to enable them to provide a safe and robust enquiry-answering service are defined.

Provision of the enquiry-answering service has four associated standards. Achievement of these standards requires that the service is easily accessible and organised to allow prompt handling of enquiries, that it meets quantifiable and consistent criteria to measure user satisfaction and that it meets quantifiable and consistent criteria for assessing the quality of enquiry answers. The latter includes assessment of the analysis of the enquiry, the utilisation and interpretation of appropriate resources and the construction and delivery of an appropriate, timely and evidence-based answer that incorporates relevant practical, clinical advice and is tailored to a specific patient.

A further standard for enquiry-answering, and for the production of pro-active information, for example bulletins and guidelines, is adequate documentation of the process and adequate procedures for record management. These have always been important for provision of an efficient MI service to prevent duplication of work and allow information to be retrieved if follow-up is required (for example, complaint or legal case). However, with the call for greater transparency in decision-making, the implementation of the *Freedom of Information Act*[24] and the introduction of the NHS information governance framework[25] these are now imperative. The experience MI staff have developed in this area puts them in an excellent position to act as knowledge managers for the pharmacy department, advising on best practice for documentation and information storage.

The standard for publications and proactive work includes other elements relating to text production, proofreading and accuracy checking, and adherence to legal requirements such as copyright. The training standard covers the requirements for training of MI staff and training provided within MI centres. MI staff deliver a significant amount of training to other members of the pharmacy service, providing them with skills relating to problem-solving and critical appraisal that are transferable to all aspects of professional practice.

A relatively new standard relates to research and service development. It requires the manager of an MI service to develop the service and demonstrate its value through participation in audit, practice research and other similar activities. The standard reflects the launch of the UKMi national research strategy in 2006 with the aim of driving innovation, improving service quality and sharing good practice, as well as providing data relating to the impact of MI on the wider organisation.[26]

Risk management

The sixth standard relates to risk management, although this plays a major element in all the other standards. Hospital trusts have wider risk management programmes with which MI services will comply. In addition, MI centres in the UK should develop their own risk management plans, reviewed annually, to provide a framework for safe working. A risk management-based approach to quality-assuring written information has been suggested to address this approach, utilising broad risk management techniques.[27]

As part of the risk management standard, MI centres must have a specified set of standard operating procedures (SOPs). A number of these have been produced nationally for local adaptation. They are available on the UKMi website (www.ukmi.nhs.uk). This portfolio includes SOPs on handling and documenting enquiries, dealing with enquiries in the absence of an MI pharmacist, dealing with difficult callers and enquiries that might be considered for onward referral and adverse incident reporting.

An important component of clinical governance is learning from experience, both of success and failure. MI has established an incident-reporting scheme to record errors and near-misses occurring within the service, similar to those in place for dispensing and aseptic manufacture. The Incident Reporting in Medicines Information System (IRMIS) was introduced in 2005 and is held on a secure web-based database hosted by NHSnet. The scheme is intended to complement existing reporting schemes within NHS organisations and users are asked to report any incidents to their trust system in addition to IRMIS. The aim of the system is to enable the network to collate data on anonymous reports, identify common themes and look at ways to avoid future incidents. Quarterly reports are distributed to all MI staff and are used as a learning tool within individual centres, at local meetings and on national training courses. Recurrent incidents include confusion over drug names and calculation errors. The system has also identified errors within manufacturers' information and published resources. These have been incorporated into UKMi guidance on risk issues with commonly used MI sources.

Monitoring standards

MI centres are recommended to undertake regular peer review sessions. These focus principally on enquiry-answering and provide opportunities to identify poor practice systematically and also to provide opportunities for learning and sharing, and as such, form an element of MI staff's continuing professional development. In addition, the aim is that all MI centres are externally audited against relevant national standards every 3 years. An audit tool has been developed to document the standards that centres have achieved, to identify improvement over time and also to provide a pathway for achieving excellence.

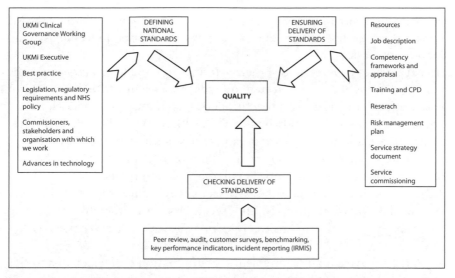

Figure 8.2 A quality framework for medicines information (MI) services.

The framework developed in the UK for achieving quality within MI services through implementing an appropriate clinical governance process is outlined in Figure 8.2.

In addition to improving their own performance, MI pharmacists are well placed to contribute to a wider clinical governance agenda within the NHS by supporting evidence-based practice across pharmacy and the wider trust, for example supporting formularies and contributing to educational programmes and knowledge management systems.

Customers and users

The historical user base of MI services has been principally drawn from hospital healthcare professions, mainly from pharmacy, medicine and nursing. Clinical pharmacists are often the largest user group of a local MI service because ward-based clinical pharmacists have a high profile in problem-solving and facilitating optimum patient care. Therefore, they act as the primary contact for medicines-related issues, for which MI services provide their first-line back-up. However, there are many situations in which a clinical pharmacist is not available for dealing with such issues, such as in less acute clinical areas and outpatient clinics, when direct contact by the doctor or nurse with the MI service is appropriate. More recently, independent non-medical prescribers – nurses and pharmacists – have emerged to take over some traditional medical prescribing. MI services have a significant role in training and supporting the prescribing activities of these new groups. There are also many other hospital-based healthcare professions that have an interaction with drug therapy and who therefore may need to utilise the MI service; such groups include dieticians, physiotherapists, psychologists and laboratory services.

MI services have expanded their activities to include primary care. The majority of this activity is directed towards those groups with direct patient care responsibilities, general practitioners, community pharmacists, nurses (community, practice, midwives) and health visitors. However, professional advisers in primary care organisations, such as primary care trusts, also require MI services support to facilitate safe and cost-effective prescribing. This more strategic role is largely being provided from regional MI services. It is important that MI services recognise the critical nature of the link between primary and secondary care, thereby facilitating the transparent and seamless treatment of patients, wherever they receive their care.

Patients have a high requirement for information on medicines and this is provided in a number of ways. All patients, whether in hospitals or in the community, should receive a patient information leaflet with any licensed, dispensed medicines. This, in many circumstances, is augmented with counselling from a hospital or community pharmacist. NHS Direct (England and Wales) and NHS24 (Scotland) are telephone and internet services established to provide the general public with instant information on any aspect of healthcare, including medicines. Although these services have trained staff and limited resources to deal with medicines-related issues, they utilise MI services to deal with more complex clinical issues.[28–30] In addition, in the UK, local MI services are providing medicines/patients telephone helplines for patients who have received medicines, either as inpatients or outpatients, so that specific enquiries regarding their hospital-dispensed medication, or more general issues, can be resolved.[31, 32] These services therefore are aimed at improving both safety and concordance.

Other groups, such as the police, coroners, self-help groups and the media, also have a requirement to use MI services, although there are specific guidelines for dealing with such groups which address issues such as confidentiality. Different professional groups, and levels and specialties within these groups, have differing requirements of the service, both in term of reactive clinical problem-solving and educational and current awareness services, and this is an important feature for MI services to recognise.

Activities

The activities of MI services can arbitrarily be divided into two main groups, reactive and proactive, although this presents an oversimplified picture.

Reactive

The reactive service is mainly focused on enquiry-answering for the broad range of users of the service described previously. Most enquiries to the MI service are directly related to individual patient care, although many are concerned with developing policy and guidelines, pharmacy practice, pharmaceutical issues, pharmaceutical and medicines research and teaching support. The service will answer enquiries on any aspect of the prescribing, supply, formulation and administration of medicines, where possible from an evidence-based perspective. Common types of clinical enquiry are listed in Table 8.5.

Table 8.5 Common enquiry types	
Enquiry type	**Includes**
Administration	Route and timing, techniques and equipment
Adverse effects	To all medicines, including OTCs and alternative therapies and in all clinical situations (e.g. pregnancy) but excluding poisoning
Alternative therapies	Homeopathic, herbal, aromatherapy and ethnic therapies
Availability	In the UK or abroad for foreign travel
Clinical choice	Best treatment choice, including most appropriate drug in a therapeutic class, for a specified patient or policy
Indications/contraindications	For what, and in what situations, a drug can be, or should be, used
Dosage	Including in children and in specialist clinical situations, e.g. with renal and kidney disease
Drug abuse	Often in conjunction with drug abuse specialists
Identification	Generic, OTC, herbal, homeopathic, veterinary and foreign medicines
Incompatibilities	Normally in intravenous formulations
Interactions	With other drugs, including OTCs, food and laboratory tests
Pharmaceutics	Formulation, excipients, stability and analysis
Pharmacoeconomics	Including cost-effectiveness
Pharmacology/ pharmacokinetics	Mechanism of action and adverse effects and factors associated with metabolism, distribution and excretion
Poisoning/overdose	Normally referred to the Poisons Information Service
Use in specific situations	Pregnancy, breast-feeding, with liver or renal disease, with porphyria

OTC, over-the-counter.

Providing an effective response to a clinical problem is a multiple-stage process and requires a wide range of skills and knowledge. The main components of the enquiry-answering process can be simplified as:

- contact with the enquirer
- identification of the problem
- acquiring appropriate and adequate background information
- establishing the urgency of the enquiry and prioritising with other enquiries
- retrieval, utilisation and critical appraisal of information relevant to the enquiry. This may include referral to a subject specialist if appropriate
- preparing the response
- presentation of response in most appropriate form, e.g. letter or verbally
- documenting the whole process
- feedback and follow-up if necessary to determine outcome and need for further information.

Guidelines and standard procedures have been established nationally to facilitate this process being undertaken to a consistent and high-quality level across the UK. Enquiry-answering is the main activity on which various quality control and audit processes are performed to ensure that the service is meeting its objectives, within a clinical governance framework, in facilitating safe and effective medicines use in patients.

Proactive

The proactive part of the service includes a wide range of outputs, which can be partly or wholly produced by the MI service. The involvement of individual local MI services in these activities varies, depending on both local need and service resourcing. Proactive outputs aim to provide support to prescribing policy and strategy construction, guideline production and implementation, and education, knowledge and professional development support. These activities include bulletins and newsletters; standardised, evidence-based answers to common questions (over 200 'Medicines Q&As' are published on NeLM and updated regularly); current awareness publications; horizon-scanning and evidence-based appraisals of new medicines; and vital tools in strategic medicines management and part of proactive MI outputs.

Support for decision-making on new medicines

New medicines can offer benefits to patients and to the NHS. However, whilst new medicines may result in potential savings in some parts of the care pathway, they are often more expensive than established drug therapies. Not all new medicines have advantages over existing therapy and generally, where the benefits exist, they are incremental rather than significant. As a result, the NHS has to manage the introduction of new medicines carefully, taking into account their clinical and cost-effectiveness. A number of bodies have been established in the UK to help the NHS manage this process by conducting technology appraisals. In England (and Wales), NICE assesses an increasing number of newly licensed medicines. Where NICE appraises a medicine positively, the NHS is required to adopt the medicine and make funding available for the indications for which it has been approved. In Scotland the equivalent body is SMC; in Wales, the AWMSG provides guidance in addition to that provided by NICE. The SMC and the AWMSG make recommendations for the use of new medicines within their populations but these do not have the statutory enforcement of NICE Technology Appraisals.

Where there is no national guidance, the decision on the introduction and funding of a new medicine has to be made locally by a trust medicines management committee (drug and therapeutics committee or area prescribing committee). Lord Darzi's *Next Stage Review*.[33]] and *The NHS Constitution*[34] acknowledged that patients should have access to the most clinically and cost-effective medicines and have the right to 'expect rational local decisions on funding of new drugs and treatments'. The robustness of the evidence base on which these committees make their decisions is therefore of great importance. Chapter 11 deals with these issues in greater depth.

In many hospitals, the MI staff support their medicines management committee by providing the evidence on which the committee will make a decision. In some cases, where no other evaluation is available, the trust MI pharmacist may critically appraise the evidence for the committee. However, wherever possible, MI pharmacists will use evaluations produced by credible other bodies, including those produced by the UKMi network, as part of the UKMi 'new product portfolio' of resources.[35]

Information on newly launched medicines

The UKMi evaluations of new products are published under the title of *New Medicines Profiles* (http://www.ukmi.nhs.uk/Med_info/profile.asp). Medicines considered for evaluation include the first or second new medicine in a therapeutic class, and medicines with major new indications or major new formulations. The aim of the profiles is to assess the available evidence on efficacy and safety of a drug and to review its place in therapy and any risk management issues. The evaluations are written to strict criteria to ensure quality and accuracy, and comments are invited from relevant clinicians and from the pharmaceutical manufacturer before publication. In addition to supporting the needs of decision-making committees, they are also intended to support the information needs of clinicians and prescribers.

In order to prevent duplication of work and to extend the range of medicines for which evaluations are available, UKMi takes account of the work produced by other organisations, including the National Prescribing Centre (NPC) and the London New Drugs Group (LNDG) when deciding if a *New Medicines Profile* is to be written.

Planning for new medicines

Advanced notice and planning for the introduction of new medicines are essential if NHS organisations are to allocate resource appropriately. The number of high-cost treatments, the *NHS Constitution*[36] and increasingly vocal interest groups make the task of allocating resources one of the most politically sensitive and complex issues facing the NHS.

Prescribing Outlook, New Medicines is a UKMi resource (produced with input from the SMC and the AWMSG) that provides advance information to NHS organisations on around 30–50 new medicines (and new licensed indications) with market launches anticipated in the next 18–24 months.[37] It is a signposting document (as opposed to an evaluation document) giving brief details of likely indications, pharmacology, available clinical trial results and estimates of potential uptake.

The content of *Prescribing Outlook, New Medicines*[37] is not comprehensive but focuses on medicines with potential for significant clinical, financial or service delivery implications for the NHS. A number of criteria are applied to those medicines considered for inclusion to help prioritise those likely to have the largest impact, including whether:

- the drug is expected to provide significant improvement in disease management
- the drug is 'first in class'
- there are limited other drug/non-drug alternatives
- the cost of the medicine will be high
- the target population is large
- there are likely to be significant service implications, e.g. there may be increased monitoring requirements
- the medicine or disease area is considered an NHS priority
- the medicine has significant additional indications in the advanced pipeline stage
- the medicine is in the EU licensing process
- there is likely to be significant media interest.

For more detailed evaluations of medicines in development, the NPC, in collaboration with UKMi, publishes evaluations of key new medicines – around six per year – under the *On the Horizon* title. Recently the collaboration has started to publish 'blog-style' *On the Horizon* commentaries evaluating the design and outcome of individual clinical trials of medicines likely to be launched in the next year or so.

The pressure on prescribing budgets is not solely associated with new medicines: a significant pressure arises from the issue of new national guidance, such as that produced by NICE, or the impact of major clinical trials on clinical practice. UKMi produces a further resource, *Prescribing Outlook, National Developments,* which aims to provide the NHS with advanced warning of such prescribing pressures.[38] It includes information on relevant documents, target populations, potential financial implications for the NHS and issues that need to be considered by commissioners and providers of services.

A further UKMi planning resource is *Prescribing Outlook – Cost Calculator,* which is based on the other two *Prescribing Outlook* documents.[39] It is an Excel spreadsheet that allows crude calculations of potential costs of prescribing changes for a local population, facilitating budgetary prediction. *Prescribing Outlook* is published annually in the autumn to meet the NHS planning timetable for the following year. The value of *Prescribing Outlook* to NHS organisations as a horizon-scanning tool has been highlighted by the Audit Commission.[17]

Early horizon scanning

While the resources discussed above support NHS organisations' short-term planning needs, there is also a need for a longer-term view of new medicines that are in the development pipeline. UKMi maintains a database, NewDrugsOnline (NDO) that tracks drugs from the phase IIb/III development stage to product launch. NDO is used to inform the content of *Prescribing Outlook*; it also drives the work plan of other organisations, such as LNDG.

NDO can be accessed by NHS staff who have a budgetary planning role relating to medicines. Although the full content is only available to those who are registered users of the database, as it contains information which has been provided by pharmaceutical companies on a confidential basis, much of the public domain information is made freely available through the NHS website portal, NHS Evidence.

NDO contains around 1000 monographs relating to medicines in development, including significant licence extensions to existing therapies. It is updated daily with information from a number of sources, including medical news feeds, journals and company and licensing authority press releases. The content is also informed through direct one-to-one meetings with all major pharmaceutical companies in the UK. The database can be used to meet a variety of needs, including allowing planners to keep up to date with developments in between annual publications of *Prescribing Outlook*. In addition, it is used, for example, by clinical pharmacists to update directorate staff on developments in their speciality, by medicine management committees for forward-planning purposes, by specialist commissioners to identify medicines that may fall within their jurisdiction and by those involved in clinical trial work. The advanced search facility of the database allows complex reports to be run to fulfil individual requirements.

The *Next Stage Review* recognised the importance of horizon scanning in facilitating an increase in the rate of appropriate uptake of new medicines by the NHS.[33] Under the auspices of the Ministerial Industry Long-term Leadership Strategy Group, the Department of Health and the Association of the British Pharmaceutical Industry proposed the development of a national horizon-scanning database, populated with information by the pharmaceutical industry, to support directly organisations, such as UKMi, that have an NHS horizon-scanning role. The database, known as UK Pharmascan, was launched in mid-2010. UKMi will be using this database to improve and advance its own early planning resources for new medicines.

Specialist information services

There are a significant number of specialised medicines-related subjects that are frequently referred to due to their nature, which MI pharmacists therefore have to address routinely. Some of these subject areas are of a clinical nature, for example drug use in pregnancy, whilst some are of a pharmaceutical nature, for example medicines that are latex-free. As they are in subject areas that are frequently encountered, a network of MI services providing a specialist information advisory service in some of these areas has been established over the past 25 years (summarised in Table 8.6).

This network provides several distinct advantages. Firstly, in clinical areas, it enables the establishment of a depth of understanding and expertise that would not be feasible in every MI service. This includes more comprehensive coverage of the evidence base for that subject, and establishment of clinical 'expert' contacts to augment the information provided. Secondly, for non-clinical subjects, it enables the compilation of comprehensive databases of specialised product information, often with the collaboration of the pharmaceutical industry. In all cases it provides either a single contact source for users or a single back-up source for MI services, and it reduces a substantial amount of work duplication. The quality of the information is also significantly enhanced. These specialised services were originally based on regional MI centres, but have expanded to encompass the specialties able to be provided from local MI centres based in specialist hospitals or in hospitals providing a high-level specialty in its clinical portfolio. The availability of some of these services is restricted to MI pharmacists only, whilst others have a more open availability and may be wholly or partly web-enabled.

Table 8.6 Specialised medicines information (MI) services in the UK	
Subject	**MI service provider**
Alternative medicine	Welsh (Cardiff)
Drugs in:	
Lactation	Trent (Leicester)/West Midlands (Sutton Coldfield)
Cardiothoracics	Brompton Hospital (London)
Dentistry	North West (Liverpool)
Liver disease	Yorkshire (Leeds)
Oncology	Royal Marsden Hospital (London)
Porphyria	Welsh (Cardiff)
Pregnancy and teratology	Northern and Yorkshire DTC (Newcastle)
Psychiatry	Maudsley Hospital (London)
Renal failure	South West (Bristol)
Drugs of abuse	Wessex (Southampton)
Fridge stability of medicines	North Thames (Northwick Park)
Latex in injections	Nottingham (Queens Medical Centre)
HIV/AIDS	Chelsea and Westminster Hospital (London)
Toxicology and poisoning	Northern and Yorkshire DTC (Newcastle)/Northern Ireland (Belfast)

DTC, drugs and therapeutic centre; HIV, human immunodeficiency virus; AIDS, acquired immunodeficiency syndrome.

National electronic Library for Medicines

NeLM (www.nelm.nhs.uk) is the largest MI portal for healthcare professionals in the UK NHS. It aims to promote the safe, effective and efficient use of medicines. This free service has been in operation since 1998 and is updated daily. The site has a wide range of information products, including news, evidence-based reviews on drugs and drug therapy and material to support health promotion. It also provides a facility for sharing practice. Much of the current content is provided by UKMi.

Current awareness services offered by NeLM include a personalised daily e-mail newsletter and a wide range of rich site summary (RSS) feeds on specific topics. The Medicines A–Z facility uses codes from the NHS Dictionary of Medicines and Devices (dm+d: http://www.dmd.nhs.uk/) to present on a single page evidence about an individual medicine which is held in NeLM, integrated with links to further information in external sources, including the *British National Formulary* (BNF), the electronic Medicines Compendium (eMC) and the National Injectable Medicines Guide (Medusa: password-protected NHS website).

NeLM also incorporates selected content from the former Pharm-line bibliographic database to create an area of NeLM dealing with the broad area of medicines management and pharmacy practice.

The current NeLM is the result of a series of transformations as the site has been redeveloped to provide a comprehensive medicines knowledge base. It will store and link to a wide range of MI products procured or produced by the NHS. The vision is to build a system for the integration of knowledge for utilisation at local health community level. Some NeLM content can already be retrieved using the NHS Evidence search interface.

Other NHS or related organisations that produce medicines information which is available through the NeLM portal include:

- NPC
- NICE
- Medicines Healthcare product and Regulatory Authority
- Department of Health
- SMC.

In addition, information from professional bodies such as the Royal Pharmaceutical Society and the British Medical Association and independent organisations such as the eMC is also available via NeLM.

The objectives of the NeLM are:

- to develop a 'one-stop' platform from which users can easily find medicines information that matters in a simple and coherent manner
- to establish a mechanism for aggregating medicines knowledge to support electronic prescribing and similar applications
- to produce local medicines knowledge bases for health communities to support local prescribers. These will reflect local practice while integrating with national resources of MI.

Information resources

MI services require access to a wide range of published information sources to fulfil all the activities outlined. Many activities may require access only to standard reference books or systems that provide relatively static, unchanging information. However, as the role of the MI pharmacist has developed, the information sources required have become more evidence-based and current, often with use of the primary literature as the main source of information. Whilst textbooks will remain a valuable source of information, their limitations (cost, currency, completeness) restrict their importance and are changing the way in which information and clinical evidence are accessed and utilised. Most core, standard information sources are now available electronically, commonly via the internet, which makes them not only more accessible but increasingly more cost-effective to use.

MI services in the UK have established a minimum information resources standard, that is, a collection of core information resources that all MI services must either hold in house or to which they must have immediate and unrestricted access. The resources contained in this minimum standard are continually reviewed and updated for new editions, new titles and obsolescence. The current information resource standard contains reference and textbooks, journals and electronic databases and is common for all MI services. In addition, larger local MI centres, regional MI services and specialist MI services will have a requirement for a wider range of resources which will partly be defined by national standards and partly by service need. One basic premise of information resource use is that only the most recent editions of resources should be used. Out-of-date resources could lead to unreliable and erroneous information that could result in harm to a patient, or even a legal challenge.

There are also a large number of important resources that are freely accessible and considered useful to NHS MI services, including free paper resources (for example, BNF, *Drug Tariff*) and freely accessible websites via the internet or via national library arrangements. Full current lists of recommended and important free information resources can be found at www. ukmi.nhs.uk.

Expanding internet and intranet publishing will increasingly make many of the remaining paper-based resources more readily available, often in a form that is 'free to end-user', although this will inevitably include current users of MI services. The implications of this shift in the balance of information access and utilisation will have to be taken into account by service providers, including MI services.

In addition to published resources, MI services will also use in-house collections of commercial and published literature, in-house databases and collections of past outputs (past enquiries, frequently asked questions, bulletins, reports, and so on) to augment information access.

Utilising information technology

MI services are heavily dependent on all aspects of information technology and electronic communications, both to acquire and to disseminate information. Online resources have been outlined and provide the dominant platform for evidence-based information on medicines, medicine management and pharmacy practice. Electronic and web-based internet and/or intranet applications are predicted to continue to develop and expand in the foreseeable future. This presents both threats and opportunities to MI services. The main threat, as already described, is that information is becoming more directly and readily available, and in more useful formats and outputs, to the end-user, including healthcare professionals and patients. The quality, accuracy and validity of many of these 'accessible' sources are, however, open to question, with no guidance to users either to increase their awareness of the inherent issues or to help them make judgements about quality, appropriateness and contextual interpretation. The opportunities, however, are for MI services to produce and present quality information that will assist patients and healthcare professionals to make valid judgements on the use of medicines that maximise safety and effectiveness. The positive aspects of these information platforms must also be fully utilised, both to communicate within the MI network and to disseminate information to patients and healthcare staff, through increasingly popular features including, at the time of writing, RSS news feeds, blogs and podcasts, personal customisation of online resources, web conferencing and webinars, online learning and assessment.

Developments in the functionality and accessibility of hardware and gadgets will also influence how MI will adapt to its users by making evidence-based information and decision support more rapidly available to the user for application at the point of care. Similarly, electronic prescribing will have an impact on how MI services engage with prescribing and patient care. Some of the basic decision-making processes of electronic prescribing will be embedded in the decision support and clinical knowledge systems inbuilt into electronic prescribing packages. Whilst this may remove some of the basic clinical problem-solving tasks currently undertaken by clinical and MI pharmacists, the need for patient-specific customised information and solving more complex problems will be a crucial role for the MI pharmacist. Validation of the information contained in e-prescribing systems will also need to be undertaken to ensure prescribing and patient care are not compromised.

Established methods of electronic information communication, such as websites and e-mail, are now taken for granted in day-to-day practice. Over the past decade the intuitive nature of their use, their immediate access to information and users, and their ready availability in most work and home settings have radically and fundamentally changed the way in which MI services function.

MI services in the UK have used new technologies and electronic communication to enhance service access, delivery and processes, although the potential for further developments, as outlined, is enormous, largely constrained only by the need for investment. Apart from the NeLM, developments in MI include the following:

- MiDatabank: this is a Windows software application that enables MI services to record, manage and store their enquiries. MiDatabank was developed specifically for the UKMi network, and has now been adopted as the UK national standard. It is used by over 200 MI centres processing more than 500 000 enquiries per year. It is also being used internationally. One of its crucial features is to provide an audit trail of the complete enquiry-answering process. One of the future objectives of MiDatabank is to facilitate sharing enquiry-related research and answers between MI centres nationally and internationally through web-based applications.

- The national MI website, www.ukmi.nhs.uk, provides a one-stop resource for MI in the UK, containing a wide range of information, including training and research resources and a single source of all strategic, clinical governance and operational policies and MI guidelines. It also gives access to all the major clinical outputs of the national UKMi network. The national MI website is augmented by a UK-wide e-mail discussion group, MI-UK, which supports information-sharing.

Workforce and training

As with most areas of professional practice, the most important resource of MI services is its staff. MI services are normally managed by experienced clinical pharmacists with specialist training to develop the additional skills, competencies and knowledge required. Training in MI skills and techniques begins at the preregistration stage, with most pharmacy graduates undergoing specific MI training before registration; this also meets the core statutory requirements for pharmacists' competencies. After registration this is augmented by further training, both formally and through placements in established MI centres. Developing clinical and problem-solving skills supports MI-related skill development, useful in ward and more formal MI service settings.

Pharmacists undertaking more formal work in an MI service are then normally exposed to more formal MI training on a national basis. In the UK, a structured training programme is in place, starting with a national introductory MI training course that introduces the pharmacist to the range of skills and activities relevant to an MI specialist. Entry to this course requires a basic level of predetermined competencies acquired through structured work experience. This level of training aims to enable the trainee to:

- understand and apply the skills, knowledge and resources to provide clinically oriented MI
- apply the basic principles of searching electronic sources of information, in particular Medline, Embase and the internet
- know the strengths and weaknesses of the key MI databases
- apply basic statistical tests to clinical trial data
- identify the key components of clinical trial design and apply these to critical appraisal of the literature
- know the necessary verbal communication skills required to deliver an effective MI service

- identify legal and ethical problems that may be encountered when providing MI
- understand the principles of clinical governance, and in particular risk management and quality, and apply these to the provision of MI.

This training is supported by the availability of a national MI workbook.[40]

More advanced training to develop skills, knowledge and effective use of resources is then provided to suit the needs of the individual and the service.

The whole training strategy is supported by a national competency framework for MI, introduced in 2001.[41] The aim of this is to identify the competencies that individuals working in MI either have, or need to develop, in order to perform their work effectively now and in the future. The framework is used to:

- facilitate continuing professional development at an individual level
- help managers and MI pharmacists identify ongoing training and development needs
- provide a framework to support local recruitment and appraisal processes.

As competencies for all aspects of clinical pharmacy practice are developed, MI competencies will be aligned and integrated into more general, national competency frameworks, at both standard and advanced practice levels, to reflect the MI provider role of all clinical pharmacists.

Although pharmacists have been the principal professional component of the MI workforce in the past, other professional groups are now being developed, and actively deployed, in MI services to support and provide some of its activities. In particular, experienced pharmacy technicians are now in the service, as they are in many other areas of clinical pharmacy practice. Appropriate technicians, once identified, are trained through a rigorously controlled programme which includes core training, in-house work, supervised work experience, development of a personal work evidence portfolio, continuous assessment, a probationary period and subsequent accreditation as an MI technician. Accredited technicians can then assume some responsibilities within the enquiry-answering process. Currently, there are seven common enquiry types, for which MI technicians can have a substantive responsibility, although the final responsibility for the overall process remains with the MI pharmacist. These are:

1 tablet and capsule identification
2 availability of medicines
3 formulation and stability (excluding parenteral)
4 interactions
5 adverse effects

6 complementary medicines

7 travel medicine.

Routine activity within these seven designated subject areas is covered by the accreditation process. However, MI technicians can be involved in other enquiry types and other MI activities as long as adequate training has been undertaken and risk management issues assessed.

The future development of MI technicians' activities and responsibilities will be an important feature of future service development which will take account of skill mix, recruitment and clinical competence issues. Other professional groups, including information scientists, life science graduates, librarians and others, may also have roles to fulfil in future MI services which are yet to be defined.

Conclusion

This overview considers the provision of NHS@MI services in the UK, although services exist, in both public and private healthcare sectors, across the world, especially in those countries with well-developed healthcare systems and economies. The UK is thought to have the most highly developed and efficient MI services and network: this has been due to its public sector funding and investment, the opportunities available in the developing NHS over the past 30 years and the enthusiasm, commitment, skills and competence of its practitioners, all made possible through the strong leadership and vision behind the UK-wide infrastructure and network, UKMi. At the time of writing it is clear that the NHS faces a significant financial challenge and this necessitates organisational change and changes in how services are delivered. Their value, and value for money, will be scrutinised. MI will not be immune from these challenges, but is well placed to respond to the requirements of both health professionals and patients, although the research evidence on the contribution MI makes is difficult to produce and has been limited.[42] Organisational changes will concentrate on increasing the focus of commissioning, decision-making and financing on the primary care sector, especially general practitioners – for England, this strategy is defined in a Department of Health White Paper, *Equity and Excellence: Liberating the NHS*.[43] MI services will need to adapt to this new culture and take advantage of the new opportunities that will be presented to support local health communities.

MI is a key component of, and a crucial contributor to, the medicines management agenda across the NHS. MI services in the UK are frequently cited as a role model for healthcare systems outside the UK, but the unique nature of the NHS has been the main factor in the way in which MI services have developed as a self-supporting network with operational and strategic roles at local and national levels.

Advances in information technology are changing the way in which MI services both gather and disseminate information. The advent of electronic prescribing will add to the changes that MI services will have to encompass and support. No matter how powerful and extensive information technology-driven health information becomes, these developments will only be additional tools to the MI practitioner – tools to increase the efficiency and effectiveness of service delivery and enhance user accessibility. MI practitioners – pharmacists and technicians – will still be the ultimate source of quality, critically assessed and tailored evidence-based information on medicines. To achieve this the service must remain constantly vigilant to NHS changes and seize the opportunities for new 'customers'. MI must also respond to developments in information technology and to new providers in the healthcare information market with which it will develop collaborative and partnership arrangements, and to new therapeutics and medicines-related healthcare technologies. Underpinning all this will be the users of the service, from bedside to boardroom and from practitioner to commissioner, who are treating patients and devising healthcare policy.

References

1. Hall N, chair. *Report of the Working Party Investigating the Hospital Pharmaceutical Service*. London: HMSO, 1970.
2. Anonymous. Leeds hospital plans full time pharmacy service. *Pharm J* 1971; 207: 561.
3. Rogers M, Barrett C. The drug information centre at the London Hospital. *Pharm J* 1972; 209: 37–39.
4. Anonymous. Report of the working party on drug information services. *Pharm J* 1974; 213: 297–301.
5. Leach FN. The regional drug information service: a factor in healthcare? *Br Med J* 1978; 178: 766–768.
6. Anonymous. Getting the information we need – how drug information centres can help. *Drug Ther Bull* 1978; 16: 41–43.
7. Smith JC, McNulty H. The national drug information network. *Pharm J* 1982; 228: 67–69.
8. Proudlove CR, Smith JDC, Breckenridge AM. Medical awareness and usage of a regional drug information service. *Pharm J* 1983; 230: 394–396.
9. Hands D, Judd A, Golightly PW *et al*. Drug information and advisory services – past, present and future. *Pharm J* 1999; 262: 160–162.
10. Jenkins P. Secretary of State views the pharmaceutical scene and outlines his policy. *Pharm J* 1979; 223: 240.
11. Audit Commission. *A Prescription for Improvement – Towards more Rational Prescribing in General Practice*. London: HMSO, 1994.
12. Department of Health. *Memorandum of Understanding on Appraisal of Health Interventions*. London: Department of Health, 1999.
13. Audit Commission. *A Spoonful of Sugar – Medicines Management in NHS Hospitals*. London: Audit Commission, 2001.
14. Audit Commission. *Acute Hospital Portfolio: Medicines Management – Review of National Findings*. London: Audit Commission, 2002.
15. National Prescribing Centre. *PCT Responsibilities Around Prescribing and Medicines Management – A Scoping and Support Guide*. Liverpool: National Prescribing Centre, 2003.
16. Smith J. *Building a Safer NHS for Patients – Improving Medication Safety*. London: Department of Health, 2004.

17. Audit Commission. *Managing the Financial Implications of NICE Guidance*. London: Audit Commission, 2005.

18. UK Medicines Information Pharmacists Group. *Better Information for Managing Medicines – A Strategy for Pharmacy's Medicines Information in the NHS*. London: UKMIPG, 2000.

19. UKMi Executive. *Effective Information for Managing Medicines – A Strategy for the UK Medicines Information Network in the NHS*. London: UKMi, 2007.

20. Royal Pharmaceutical Society of Great Britain. *Medicines, Ethics and Practice – A Guide for Pharmacists and Pharmacy Technicians*, 33rd edn. London: RPSGB, 2009.

21. UKMi. Legal and ethical aspects of medicines information. Available online at: http://www. ukmi.nhs.uk/activities/clinicalGovernance/default.asp?pageRef=10 (accessed 30 July 2010).

22. Department of Health. *A First Class Service: Quality in the New NHS*. London: The Stationery Office, 1998.

23. Royal Pharmaceutical Society of Great Britain. *Achieving Excellence in Pharmacy Through Clinical Governance*. London: RPSGB, 1999.

24. *Freedom of Information Act*. Available online at: http://www.legislation.gov.uk/ukpga/2000/36/contents.

25. Department of Health. *NHS Information Governance: Guidance on Legal and Professional Obligations*. London: Department of Health, 2007.

26. UKMi. Available online at: http://www.ukmi.nhs.uk/filestore/ukmiar/ResearchStrategy2006-webversion_1.pdf.

27. Wills S, Stephens M. How safe is information about medicines? A risk assessment framework. *Clin Governance* 2007; 12: 29–37.

28. Jamieson H, Joshua A. Pharmacy support to NHS Direct: what is needed and what is delivered? *Pharm J* 2002; 268: 289–291.

29. Radia H, Lee P, Wright DJ *et al*. Medicines information enquiries received by the NHS Direct Online enquiry service: what do patients want to know? *Int J Pharm Pract* 2004; 12 (suppl): R57.

30. Wills S, Campbell F. To evaluate the impact of written answers to frequently asked questions about medicines, prepared by pharmacists, for NHS Direct nurses. *Pharm J* 2007; 278: 140–141.

31. Raynor DK, Sharp JA, Rattenbury H *et al*. Medicine information help lines: a survey of hospital pharmacy-based services in the UK and their conformity with guidelines. *Ann Pharmacother* 2000; 34: 106–111.

32. Joseph A, Franklin BD, James D. An evaluation of a hospital-based patient medicines information helpline. *Pharm J* 2004; 272: 126–129.

33. Lord Darzi. *High Quality of Care for All: NHS Next Stage Review*. London: The Stationery Office, 2008.

34. Department of Health. *The NHS Constitution for England*. London: Department of Health, 2010.

35. Davis H. Is the information out there? What the UKMi new medicines portfolio offers. *Pharm J* 2005; 274: 19–20.

36. *The NHS Constitution*. Available online at: http://www.nhs.uk/choiceintheNHS/Rightsandpledges/NHSConstitution/Documents/nhs-constitution-interactive-version-march-2010.pdf.

37. UKMi. *Prescribing Outlook, New Medicines*. London: UKMi, 2009.

38. UKMi. *Prescribing Outlook, National Developments*. London: UKMi, 2009.

39. UKMi. *Prescribing Outlook – Cost Calculator*. London: UKMi, 2009.

40. UKMi. UKMi training workbook, 6th edn, 2009. Available online at: http://www.ukmi.nhs.uk/activities/manpowerTraining/default.asp?pageRef=16 (accessed 4 August 2010).

41. Picton C. *A Competency Framework in Medicines Information*. London: UKMIPG, 2001.

42. Hands D, Stephens M, Brown D. A systematic review of the clinical and economic impact of drug information services on patient outcome. *Pharm World Sci* 2002; 24: 132–138.

43. Department of Health. *Equity and Excellence: Liberating the NHS*. London: Department of Health, 2010.

Further reading

National electronic Library for Medicines (NeLM): http://www.nelm.nhs.uk.

UKMi website: http://www.ukmi.nhs.uk for:

- directory of local and regional MI centres
- information about UKMi and UKMi executive
- UKMi strategy
- access to information on MI services and activities, including clinical governance, workforce development, new products, research and specialist services
- news about MI activities and outputs.

UKMi workbook (see section on UKMi website: http://www.ukmi.nhs.uk).

9

Clinical pharmacy

Damian Child, Jonathan Cooke and Richard Hey

Introduction

Managing medicines safely, effectively and efficiently is central to the delivery of high-quality care that is focused on the patient and gives value for money.[1] Over the past two decades, growing evidence from within and outside the UK has demonstrated the positive impact of clinical pharmacy services on patient outcomes; the Department of Health recognised that pharmacists' clinical skills and expertise are an integral part of delivering better services to patients in the 2008 pharmacy White Paper, and reinforced this in 2010, identifying their role in optimising the use of medicines.[2, 3] Examples include reductions in medication-related adverse events, lower treatment costs, better patient outcomes, reduced length of stay and reduced readmission rates.[4–6]

However, simply attempting to develop and implement best practice as opportunities permit is becoming increasingly unacceptable as the regulatory framework surrounding medicines management becomes more demanding. In addition to working towards delivery of numerous national recommendations, hospitals are also now required to register with the Care Quality Commission and meet the medicines management standards detailed in its essential standards of quality and safety (see Chapter 1). The standards detail regulations, outcomes and prompts to protect patients against the risks associated with the unsafe use and management of medicines, in accordance with regulation 13 of the *Health and Social Care Act 2008 (Regulated Activities) Regulations 2010*.[7] Compliance with the standards can only be achieved with the delivery of high-quality clinical pharmacy services.

What is clinical pharmacy?

Clinical pharmacy is defined as the area of practice in which pharmacists provide patient care that optimises medication therapy and promotes health, wellness and disease prevention.[8] The practice of clinical pharmacy embraces the concepts of both pharmaceutical care, first introduced by Hepler and Strand,[9] and medicines management, which encompasses the entire way in which medicines are selected, procured, delivered, prescribed, administered and reviewed to optimise the contribution that medicines make to producing informed and desired outcomes of patient care.[10]

Hepler and Strand's definition of pharmaceutical care, 'the responsible provision of drug therapy for the purpose of achieving definite outcomes which improve the patient's quality of life', included pharmacist input in the design, implementation and monitoring of a therapeutic plan, in collaboration with the patient and other healthcare professionals, and helped to change the focus of clinical pharmacy activities from processes to therapeutic outcomes. Despite widespread acceptance, use of the term 'pharmaceutical care' in the UK does not always follow the rigorous definition of Hepler and Strand, but is often used simply to imply a patient-focused approach to clinical pharmacy practice.[11] In some respects, the term 'clinical pharmacy' is somewhat outdated as the National Health Service (NHS) recognises that the term 'clinician' refers to all healthcare staff involved with the care of patients. Pharmacy, by definition, is a clinical profession and thus clinical pharmacy is a patient-centred service where the pharmacist is a key member of the multidisciplinary clinical team.[12]

The history of clinical pharmacy in the UK

Clinical pharmacy is now practised in all healthcare settings, but its main origins lie in the hospital sector. Until the mid-1960s, hospital pharmacists were mostly engaged in traditional pharmaceutical activities such as dispensing and manufacturing.[11] Then, the increasing range and sophistication of medicines available, awareness of medication errors and the widespread use of ward-based prescription charts brought pharmacists out of the dispensary and on to the wards in increasing numbers.

This was initially described as 'ward pharmacy' and was mostly a post hoc process with the emphasis on the safe and timely supply of medicines in response to medical and nursing demands. However, the service quickly evolved into something significantly more proactive, seeing pharmacists interacting with patients and other healthcare professionals and directly intervening in the patient care process.[13] The growth in these services over the 1970s and 1980s was said to represent a change in hospital pharmacy from product orientation to patient orientation and was formally acknowledged as 'clinical pharmacy' in the 1986 Nuffield report.[14] The report welcomed these changes and recommended an increased role for hospital pharmacists through the development of clinical pharmacy services.

The recommendations made in the Nuffield report were officially recognised in a 1988 Health Services circular that outlined the main aims of the Department of Health with respect to hospital pharmacy:

the achievement of better patient care and financial savings through the more cost-effective use of medicines and improved use of pharmaceutical services obtained by implementing a clinical pharmacy service.[15]

A number of key areas where pharmacist input could assist other clinicians and benefit patients were highlighted, including contributing to prescribing decisions, monitoring and modifying drug therapy, counselling patients and involvement in clinical trials. The document acknowledged that, by helping to ensure patient safety and appropriate use of medicines, clinical pharmacy services could prove to be cost-effective.

As clinical pharmacy services expanded, there was increasing specialisation, with the expertise of individual pharmacists in certain therapeutic areas contributing to more significant developments in service provision. The speed of progress was demonstrated in a review undertaken in the early 1990s, which showed that the majority of NHS hospitals in the UK provided clinical pharmacy services and most hospital pharmacists participated in ward-based clinical pharmacy activities.[14] However, the range of clinical pharmacy services varied enormously, from almost 100% of hospitals having pharmacists who monitored drug therapy to less than 10% for services such as infection control, clinical audit or medical staff education. Since then, the widespread development of clinical pharmacy services has continued, with significant expansion in the number and range of services provided at most hospitals.

Wide variations in the extent and nature of hospital clinical pharmacy services were also noted in the Nuffield report and large differences still exist across much of the UK.[10] This lack of uniformity applies not just to clinical pharmacy, but also covers almost every aspect of hospital pharmacy services. The absence of specific directions from government and from the pharmacy profession, coupled with the varying degrees of success with which individual pharmacy managers in each hospital have been able to develop services, has allowed diversity to flourish with wide variations in the proportion of time spent on clinical pharmacy activities, ranging from less than 30% of pharmacist time at some hospitals to over 70% of pharmacist time at others.[10] The Audit Commission recommended that hospitals undertake reviews of their staffing levels and consider whether there were adequate resources to provide all aspects of clinical pharmacy services, so it is likely that the national figures on implementation of clinical pharmacy services will be changing for some time.

One of the differences between hospital and community pharmacy is the location of the patient and how this affects the dynamics of providing clinical pharmacy services. Most hospitals provide their pharmaceutical services to patients on (but not exclusively) wards of various kinds. Thus, in order to deliver care the pharmacist needs to visit the ward and interact with the patient, doctor, nurse and others, as well as have access to consult and contribute to the patient's medical records.

Clinical pharmacist presence on wards allows dialogue with patients and professionals in addition to ensuring supplies of medicines are adequate for patients' needs, and that medicines are stored appropriately and safely. Pharmacy technicians, assistants and others work with ward staff to provide effective supply of commonly used items and, with the pharmacists, are increasingly leading the introduction of the reuse of patients' own drugs (PODs) schemes to reduce waste and, where appropriate, patient self-medication to support concordance.

The importance of communicating requests for medicines and the need to record administration of medicines have led to the universal usage of the ward prescription chart. Various reports on the value of recording the prescription and administration of medicines emanated from situations where there was no record of them having been given. Requiring nurses and doctors to record the administration of medicines offered the rudiments of an audit trail for medicines.

The design and use of these charts have consumed much time and energy from a variety of clinicians in order to produce a hybrid document that serves the multiple purposes of conveying: (1) patient details such as identification, age, weight, gender and allergies; (2) prescribing details such as medicine, form, dose, route and frequency of administration and previous medicines; and (3) medicine administration details including who administered (nurse, doctor, patient), when and by which route. It also serves to indicate when a medicine has not been given. An alert from the National Patient Safety Agency on reducing harm from omitted and delayed medicines in hospital requires all healthcare organisations to identify a list of critical medicines where timeliness of administration is crucial.[16] It also requires them to ensure that medicine management procedures include guidance on the importance of prescribing, supplying and administering critical medicines, timeliness issues and what to do when a medicine has been omitted or delayed. Incident reports should be regularly reviewed and an annual audit of omitted and delayed critical medicines should be undertaken to ensure that system improvements to reduce harms from omitted and delayed medicines are made. Figure 9.1 is an extract from a typical hospital inpatient medicines chart.

The Welsh NHS took this one step further in 2004 with the introduction of a new all-Wales prescription chart, accompanied by prescription-writing standards and an e-learning tool installed on the intranet systems of hospital trusts and included in medical degree teaching.[17]

PATIENT DETAILS		ALLERGIES, INTOLERANCES & ADRs	OTHER CHARTS IN USE	
NAME :			ANTICOAGULANTS	
AGE / D.O.B. :			INSULIN	
HOSPITAL NUMBER :			INTRAVENOUS	
WARD : CONSULTANT :			DIALYSIS	
WEIGHT : HEIGHT : SA :			OTHER	

PLEASE INDICATE REASON WHY DRUG IS DISCONTINUED (If appropriate)

ADR = Adverse Drug Reaction, DOS = Dose Change, Dup = Duplication, END = End of Course, INE = Ineffective, REW= Rewritten.

REGULAR DOSE PRESCRIPTIONS	Times	Date	Date	Date	Date	Date	Date	Date	Date	Date	Date	Date	Code
PLEASE INDICATE TIMES OF ADMINISTRATION													

DRUG			
DOSE	ROUTE	STOP DATE	
ADDITIONAL INSTRUCTIONS		PHARM.	
SIGNATURE / PRINT NAME		DATE dd / mm / yy	

DRUG			
DOSE	ROUTE	STOP DATE	
ADDITIONAL INSTRUCTIONS		PHARM.	
SIGNATURE / PRINT NAME		DATE dd / mm / yy	

DRUG			
DOSE	ROUTE	STOP DATE	
ADDITIONAL INSTRUCTIONS		PHARM.	
SIGNATURE / PRINT NAME		DATE dd / mm / yy	

DRUG			
DOSE	ROUTE	STOP DATE	
ADDITIONAL INSTRUCTIONS		PHARM.	
SIGNATURE / PRINT NAME		DATE dd / mm / yy	

DRUG			
DOSE	ROUTE	STOP DATE	
ADDITIONAL INSTRUCTIONS		PHARM.	
SIGNATURE / PRINT NAME		DATE dd / mm / yy	

Figure 9.1 Hospital inpatient prescription sheet.

The important sets of prescription form data are essential for the efficient and effective delivery of pharmaceutical care to the patient and also form the basis for the development of electronic prescribing systems within the NHS.[18] This is discussed further in Chapter 15.

Prescription monitoring

The core of pharmacists' contribution to appropriate prescribing and medication use is made whilst undertaking near-patient clinical pharmacy activities. Checking and monitoring patients' prescriptions on hospital wards is frequently the starting point for this process and on most hospital wards the prescription card and clinical observation charts (temperature, pulse rate, blood pressure, and so on) are typically kept at the end of the patient's bed. This allows the clinical pharmacist to interact with the patient whilst reviewing the contents of the prescription.

The prescription is reviewed for medication dosing errors, appropriateness of administration route, drug interactions, prescription ambiguities, inappropriate prescribing and many other potential problems. Formal assessments of prescription charts in hospitals have shown that there are wide variations in the quality of prescribing and pharmacists are able to identify and resolve many clinical problems. Patients can be questioned on their medication histories, including allergies and intolerances, efficacy of prescribed treatment, side-effects and adverse drug reactions (ADRs). The routine presence of medical and nursing staff on the ward allows the pharmacist to communicate easily with other members of the healthcare team who value the prescription-monitoring service that clinical pharmacists provide.[19, 20] Patients' notes are also accessible, to enable the pharmacist both to check important information that may affect their healthcare and to record details of any clinical pharmacy input made.

Prescribing advice to medical and nursing staff

Prescribing advice can be provided by medicines information pharmacists within the pharmacy department or by pharmacists undertaking their clinical pharmacy duties in patient areas such as outpatient clinics or the wards. This latter role may also include attendance at medical ward rounds. The advice given can include help with choice of medicine, dose, method of administration, side-effects, interactions, monitoring requirements and many other aspects of medicines use. Studies examining prescribing advice given by clinical pharmacists have shown high rates of acceptance from medical staff, demonstrating that the role is both valued and effective.[21, 22]

Medication errors and adverse drug reaction reporting

Despite the important role of clinical pharmacy services, patients receiving drug therapy may still experience unintended harm or injury as a result of medication errors or from ADRs. Adverse events (from any cause) occur in around 10% of all hospital admissions and medication errors account for one-quarter of all the incidents that threaten patient safety.[23] A study commissioned by the General Medical Council identified a mean prescribing error rate of 8.9 per 100 medication orders.[24]

Contributing to the avoidance or resolution of adverse medication events is an important part of any hospital pharmacist's clinical duties. This requires a multisystem approach, often incorporated into a hospital's clinical risk management strategy. Important lessons can be learned from analysis of medication-related incidents and from near-misses (that is, those that do not develop sufficiently to result in patient harm or are detected prior to patient harm). Chapter 12 considers these issues in further detail.

Even when the prescribed and administered treatment is correct and no errors have occurred, a small proportion of patients can still suffer from ADRs. Clinical pharmacists have an important role to play in the detection and management of ADRs and, more recently, directly reporting ADRs to the Committee on Safety of Medicines via the Yellow Card scheme. Their involvement can help to increase the number of ADR reports made, particularly those involving serious reaction.[25, 26] However, even in hospitals with formal ADR schemes, gross underreporting of reactions still remains a major problem.[27]

Medication history-taking and medicines reconciliation

Taking a medication history from patients and prescribing on admission have traditionally been done by junior doctors, but published work suggests that pharmacists are able to take more accurate medication histories than medical staff.[28–30] The crucial role of clinical pharmacists in undertaking medicines reconciliation for patients on admission to hospital has been endorsed by the National Institute for Health and Clinical Excellence (NICE) and the National Patient Safety Agency.[31] The guidance recognised the increased risk of morbidity, mortality and economic burden to health services caused by medication errors and noted that errors occur most commonly on transfer between care settings, particularly at the time of admission, with unintentional variances of up to 70%. It recommended that pharmacists should be involved in medicines reconciliation as soon as possible after hospital admission, noting this is a cost-effective intervention. Reconciliation was defined as:

- collecting information on medication history (prior to admission) using the most recent and accurate sources of information to create a full and current list of medicines

- checking or verifying this list against the current prescription chart in the hospital, ensuring any discrepancies are accounted for and acted on appropriately
- communicating through appropriate documentation any changes, omissions or discrepancies.

With the increasing use of information technology, access to patients' summary care record from their general practitioner surgery offers a timely and accurate method for obtaining this important information. The pharmacist can also question patients on concordance with prescribed treatment, check their own medicines to ensure suitability for reuse in hospital of POD and self-medication schemes and help to identify whether or not an admission is due to prescribing errors or ADRs. Pharmacy technicians are increasingly involved in supporting these roles.[31] This is discussed further later in the chapter.

A report commissioned by NICE included economic evaluation modelling of several different methods of medicines reconciliation and stated that: 'in terms of effectiveness, the pharmacist-led reconciliation intervention is predicted to prevent the most medication errors. This reduction is shown to reduce costs associated with errors by £3002 [per 1000 prescription orders] compared to the baseline scenario'.[32]

For planned admissions to hospital (for example, elective surgery), the medication history-taking role can be moved to an earlier stage in the patient care process. Preadmission clinics have traditionally been used to assess patients' suitability for surgery, but are also increasingly used to make other preparations for admission. Clinical pharmacists can work alongside medical and nursing staff, to help ensure that full and accurate details of medication are recorded and that either patients bring their own medication with them on admission or that medicines not routinely stocked by the hospital pharmacy can be ordered in advance.[33, 34] For patients on clearly defined treatment pathways, early discharge planning and advance preparation of discharge medication can also help to reduce delayed discharges and this can also involve pharmacists prescribing the discharge medication.[35]

Patient education and counselling, including achieving concordance

One of the key themes of the 2010 White Paper is empowering patients to take an active role in managing their own care.[4] This is also one of the themes of many of the NHS–National Institute for Health Research collaborations for leadership in applied health research and care that focus on translating research into practice.[36]

Helping patients to understand their medicines and how to take them is a major feature of clinical pharmacy. Patient compliance, defined as adherence to the regimen of treatment recommended by the doctor, has been a concern of healthcare professionals for some time.[37] Adherence to treatment, particularly for long-term chronic conditions, can be poor and tends to worsen as the number of medicines and complexity of treatment regimens increase. NICE noted that between a third and half of all medicines prescribed for long-term conditions are not taken as recommended and estimated that the cost of admissions resulting from patients not taking medicines as recommended was between £36 million and £196 million in 2006–2007.[38, 39]

In recent years, use of the term 'compliance' in the context of medication has been criticised because it implied that patients must simply follow the doctor's orders, rather than making properly informed decisions about their healthcare. The term 'concordance' has been proposed as a more appropriate description of the situation.[40]

Concordance is a new approach to the prescribing and taking of medicines. It is an agreement reached after negotiation between a patient and healthcare professional that respects the beliefs and wishes of the patient in determining whether, when and how medicines are taken.

This change in approach aims to optimise the benefits of treatment by helping patients and clinicians collaborate in a therapeutic partnership. However, if patients are to make informed choices, then the need for comprehensive patient education becomes more pressing.

Concordance with treatment is dependent on a complex interplay of beliefs, trust and understanding, with non-adherence falling into two overlapping categories:[38]

1   intentional: the patient decides not to follow the treatment recommendations
2   unintentional: the patient wants to follow the treatment recommendations, but practical problems prevent the patient from doing so.

Many surveys have found that patients often know little about the medicines they are taking. Several studies examining patient counselling and education have shown that clinical pharmacists can help to improve patients' knowledge of their treatment.[41, 42] The contribution made can also improve patient adherence to treatment.[41, 43] Improved adherence should lead to improved outcomes and evidence has been collected to demonstrate this.[41, 43, 44]

In addition to providing face-to-face education and counselling on medicines, clinical pharmacists can also help patients by contributing to the preparation of written material and audiovisual demonstrations, or by using computer programs.[45–48]

How patients take their medicines is a crucial component of whether the desired outcomes will be achieved. Key to this is the health beliefs of individuals and the relationship with their healthcare providers that are necessary in order to ensure this happens. Society is moving away from a paternalistic approach to healthcare to a more empowered one. Thus, whereas a course of treatment used to be accepted obediently by patients, treatment is now negotiated and options, risks and benefits are discussed and, where necessary, consent is obtained. Thus there is a greater need for information and education of patients and/or carers in order for them to be able to make informed decisions about their treatment. Indeed, the 2010 White Paper emphasised the importance of patient involvement, and included the phrase 'nothing about me, without me'.[4]

Self-administration schemes

Schemes which allow patients to self-administer their medicines whilst in hospital have been attempted in selected groups or settings.[49, 50] The schemes have several purposes:

- a diagnostic role – checking to see if patients can cope with their medicines regimen
- an educational role – giving diminishing levels of support prior to discharge, allowing patients to gain skills and confidence with their medicines
- an empowering role – allowing patients to provide self-care as they would at home.

Schemes may also allow nursing staff to focus on other issues and mean that access to medicines is improved. This is particularly important where timing of doses can affect patient experience or safety, for example insulin use or analgesia. However, whilst these schemes may seem attractive, evidence of their benefits is limited and considerable effort may be required to assess patients' suitability.[51] Clinical pharmacists and pharmacy technicians can support nursing staff in establishing and running self-administration schemes. A POD scheme, though not essential, can be a useful precursor to such schemes.

Integrated medicines management

'Integrated medicines management' is a term that has been used to describe bringing together several elements of clinical pharmacy services which have been shown to be effective in dealing with medicines management problems, delivering additional input at key phases of a patient's stay: admission, inpatient monitoring and counselling and discharge. By focusing additional clinical pharmacy input to selected patients (that is, those taking at least four medicines, those on defined high-risk medicines, patients 65 years or older and on antidepressants, and those with a previous admission within the last 6 months), reduced length of stay and a decreased rate of readmission have been demonstrated, providing efficiency savings to the health economy in addition to improved clinical outcomes for patients.[6]

Pharmacokinetics and therapeutic drug level monitoring

Pharmacokinetics addresses the absorption, distribution, metabolism and excretion of drugs in patients. A sound knowledge of the pharmacokinetic profiles of different drugs enables the pharmacist to assess the dosing requirements for certain drugs in patients in extremes of age and in the presence of impairment of kidney and liver function. Clinically important drug interactions and adverse reactions can sometimes be predicted. Dosing calculations of aminoglycoside antibiotics are usually made by employing pharmacokinetic principles.

A number of medicines in common use have a narrow therapeutic index; that is, the difference between the lowest effective dose and a potentially toxic dose can be quite small. In many cases it is necessary or desirable to undertake therapeutic drug level monitoring (TDM) to ensure that patients can be treated safely. TDM services include the measurement of drug levels in the patient's blood and the application of clinical pharmacokinetics to optimise drug therapy. There is a wide range of medicines that fall into this category, but TDM services typically include aminoglycoside antibiotics, anticonvulsants, immunosuppressants, digoxin, lithium and theophylline. Monitoring drug levels in patients can also provide an important indicator as to whether they are taking their medicine. Clinical pharmacy input into TDM services can range from the provision of simple advice to other clinicians on when to take samples and how to interpret results, to fully fledged services that may include collection and laboratory analysis of the blood sample.[52-54]

Anticoagulant services

Clinical pharmacy input into anticoagulant therapy is now a widely accepted part of clinical practice in many hospitals. Some anticoagulant services were initially set up as collaborative ventures with medical staff, but pharmacists now manage many services. Although the exact nature of services provided by the pharmacist may vary slightly from hospital to hospital, the role of the pharmacist in anticoagulation has been clearly established: (1) ensuring complete documentation and referral information is present; (2) interviewing patients and assessing factors that may affect anticoagulant control, particularly disease states and drug interactions; (3) monitoring and adjusting anticoagulant doses to maintain the international normalised ratio within agreed therapeutic targets; (4) identifying clinical problems that require referral to a physician; (5) patient counselling and education; (6) providing a regular point of contact for patients with concerns about their treatment; (7) day-to-day clinic management training and education for physicians and pharmacists; and (8) research and audit. Clinical pharmacists can provide high-quality cost-effective anticoagulant services for both hospital inpatients and outpatients. Evaluations of services provided show that pharmacist anticoagulant control is at least as good as, and in some cases better than, that achieved by medical staff.[55, 56] However, the introduction of new oral antithrombin and Xa inhibitors, which do not require the same level of laboratory monitoring, are increasingly likely to offer a viable alternative to these traditional anticoagulant services.

In more recent years, the use of anticoagulants for prevention of venous thromboembolism (VTE) has become much more important as the risks to patients have become better recognised. NICE published a clinical guideline on VTE across all adult specialties in January 2010.[57] In England, from April 2010, the national Commission for Quality and Innovation payment framework includes reducing avoidable death, disability and chronic ill health from VTE as one of two national goals.[58] These documents seek to ensure that appropriate risk assessments have been carried out on admission to hospital so that patients can be identified for thromboprophylaxis, and mechanical measures, where necessary. This is not restricted to those involved in anticoagulant services and so clinical pharmacists from all disciplines will play a significant part in ensuring compliance with the national guidance. The particular contribution that pharmacy can make is set out in *Venous Thromboembolism Prevention, a Patient Safety Priority,* published by the Department of Health along with the All-Party Parliamentary Thrombosis Group.[59]

Personalised medicine

The fact that not all patients respond to the expected benefits of medicines and some have disproportionately adverse effects from them is leading to the development of personalised medicines services. Good clinicians have always tailored treatment to individual patients' needs, but this typically relied on trial and error. Personalised medicine can start from using biomarkers rather than clinical outcomes as surrogate markers of effectiveness and a new specialty of pharmacogenetics that aims to assess phenotypic differences in responding to and handling drugs that may account for a significant proportion of the variation in patient response. A Parliamentary Office of Science and Technology review noted that:

> Personalised medicine holds both promise and cause for concern. Selective treatment may limit access to those most likely to benefit, whereas following a 'one size fits all' approach to medical research and development may have benefited the widest number of potential patients. Nevertheless, explaining the environmental, genetic and other biological sources of human variation will alter the way diseases are diagnosed, drugs are developed, and the matching of therapeutic cells and tissues to patients.[60]

However, economic considerations, regulation of biological tests and the speed of clinical education and training will all influence the rate and degree to which personalised medicine will be incorporated into drug development and clinical practice.

Education and training

As hospital clinical pharmacy services expanded, there was a growing recognition of the need for postgraduate training for pharmacists. Postgraduate courses in clinical pharmacy started at Bradford, London and Manchester universities in the 1970s and others quickly followed.[61–63] This included the development of part-time courses, which resulted in a significant increase in the numbers of pharmacists being able to receive postgraduate training in clinical pharmacy. The majority of UK NHS hospitals now employ clinical pharmacists with advanced postgraduate qualifications and many clinical pharmacists also contribute to the teaching on postgraduate courses. The training and education that hospital pharmacists receive are covered in more detail in Chapter 17. Clinical pharmacy services also include the regular provision of training and education for other healthcare staff at most hospitals – a service that is valued highly.[13]

Medicines formularies

The role of the pharmacist in the development of medicines formularies is covered in more detail in Chapter 11. Pharmacists providing clinical services are responsible for ensuring that prescribers' practices comply with formulary recommendations. Clinical pharmacists' detailed knowledge of medicines and the regular contact they have with doctors, nurses and patients mean that they are ideally placed to influence prescribing on the wards. A key feature of successful medicines rationalisation is the ongoing communication between prescribers and pharmacists who encourage self-audit and peer review.[64]

Clinical outcomes

In 1966 Donabedian published his seminal work that described three distinct aspects of quality in healthcare: (1) outcome; (2) process (healthcare technologies); and (3) structure (resources for delivery of care).[65] He concluded that: 'Outcomes, by and large, remain the ultimate validation of the effectiveness and quality of medical care'. Standardised mortality rates have become a crude outcome measure but are used to describe a healthcare organisation's overall success. Other recent outcome measures include meticillin-resistant *Staphylococcus aureus* bacteraemia rates and *Clostridium difficile* infections which have a direct relevance to antimicrobial stewardship (AMS). More recently, patient-reported outcome measures (PROMs) have been advocated as a relevant outcome measure to describe patients' satisfaction in their healthcare provider.[66] Four elective procedures were initially proposed for PROMS data evaluation – hernia repair, hip and knee replacement and varicose veins – but a growing range of long-term conditions including diabetes, asthma, chronic obstructive pulmonary disease, epilepsy, heart failure and stroke are being added. These long-term conditions have medication effectiveness at their core and will offer considerable potential for clinical pharmacy involvement. At the time of writing, in England, consultation has begun on how an outcomes-based approach can be built into the routine running of the NHS. It will be interesting to see how medicines use and the role of clinical pharmacists can contribute to this agenda.

Professional and clinical audit

The range and complexity of healthcare services being provided to patients mean that there is now a need to look more critically at the effectiveness of what is being delivered.[67] Professional self-examination in healthcare dates back more than a century, but the widespread implementation of clinical audit started in earnest in the early 1990s.[68] This resulted from a number of important factors: (1) public expectations that professionals can deliver and maintain high standards of care; (2) government pressures to make healthcare professionals more accountable; and (3) the need to enhance and maintain professional credibility.

Clinical pharmacists can be involved in many different types of audit. These may range from topics including audit of clinical services themselves (for example, clinical pharmacy interventions) or may examine which treatments are used and how they are implemented within the framework of drug use evaluations. Audit aims to improve patient outcomes by examining how current clinical practice compares to agreed standards of care, implementing any changes necessary and then re-examining practice to ensure that real improvements have been made.

The most obvious benefits of good clinical audit include improvements in the quality of service and treatment. In addition, enhanced professional standing, improved communication with colleagues, increased knowledge, improved work satisfaction, publication opportunities and even promotion have all been put forward as other positive aspects that should encourage healthcare staff to get involved.

Clinical audit is pivotal in patient care: it brings together professionals from all sectors of healthcare to consider clinical evidence, promote education and research, develop and implement clinical guidelines, enhance information management skills and contribute to better management of resources – all with the aim of improving the quality of care of patients.[69]

Outpatient clinical pharmacy services

The traditional role of outpatient prescription dispensing is being replaced in many hospitals by clinical pharmacy input into the clinics themselves. This practice follows the logic that hospitals should only dispense medicines to those outpatients in immediate need and the Audit Commission has recommended that primary and secondary care should work together to limit the practice of outpatient dispensing to eliminate much of the confusion that is commonly generated when two doctors are prescribing to the same patient.[10] This allows hospitals to utilise some of the resources saved to implement more beneficial pharmacy services and many hospitals pharmacists now actively manage medication for selected outpatients, including those on anti-coagulation (see above), lithium, rheumatology medication, lipid-lowering agents, transplant medicines and many others.[70–73]

Primary–secondary care interface

Community-based pharmacy services are covered in Chapter 14. However, good-quality clinical pharmacy does not begin and end at the traditional barriers between hospital and community practice. The overall aim of such services is to provide patients with a smooth transition as they move between the primary and secondary care sectors during admission to, or discharge from, hospital, a process often described as 'seamless care'. The efficient and accurate transfer of information is an essential part of this process if unintended changes in medication are to be avoided. This needs to involve good communication links between other hospital colleagues, general practitioners and community pharmacists in addition to direct patient contact.[74] Other clinical pharmacy services that can contribute to seamless care include patient follow-up and domiciliary visiting, coordinating appropriate use of compliance aids, the availability of telephone helplines for patients and the establishment of joint primary–secondary care treatment protocols managing intravenous medication at home, out-of-hours services and influenza pandemic planning.[75, 76]

The role of pharmacy technicians in clinical pharmacy services

The role of pharmacy technicians is already well established in departmental activities such as dispensing and aseptic services. However, the expansion of clinical pharmacy services in hospital would not be possible without the additional support that can be provided by hospital pharmacy technicians. In a similar manner to the way in which ward pharmacy services provided by pharmacists evolved into clinical pharmacy, pharmacy technicians' roles are becoming increasingly clinical in nature and can include a wide range of activities.[31, 77–79] Current activities undertaken by pharmacy technicians, in collaboration with pharmacists, include:

- medication supply
- checking medication in POD schemes
- patient counselling and education, including the provision of patient aids where appropriate, as well as medication charts and monitored-dose systems to aid compliance
- supporting patient self-medication
- medicines information
- discharge planning for patients, including communication with primary care colleagues where appropriate
- involvement in clinical trials and good clinical practice governance
- preparation of medicines formularies and guidelines
- training and education
- liaison with clinical teams on medicines management and expenditure
- AMS.

Whilst this last subject will be addressed under strategic medicines management (Chapter 11), it is important to note that AMS was the first ever clinical pharmacy programme to receive national, ring-fenced, governmental funding. The importance of AMS is highlighted in national reports and is enshrined within statute in the *Health and Social Care Act 2008*.[80, 81] Guidance for compliance with criterion 9 states that healthcare providers 'have and adhere to policies, designed for the individual's care and provider organisations that will help to prevent and control infections'. Notably:

- Local prescribing should, where appropriate, be harmonised with that in the *British National Formulary*. Local guidelines for primary and secondary care should be observed.

- All local guidelines should include information on a particular drug's regimen and duration.
- Procedures should be in place to ensure prudent prescribing and AMS. There should be an ongoing programme of audit, revision and update. In healthcare this is usually monitored by the antimicrobial management team.

Antimicrobial stewardship

A systematic team approach to AMS should be adopted in all healthcare institutions in order to ensure optimal use and minimum toxicity in the use of antimicrobials. Evidence-based standards should be agreed and form the basis of an education programme for all users. Audit of the effectiveness of AMS should be regularly undertaken and fed back to users for review and action.

Where empirical use is considered a stepwise approach should be adopted:

Is there an infection?

Before an antimicrobial is selected the following questions should be asked:

- Is there an infection present? Physical and biomarkers must be considered and, whilst many of these are non-specific, a number together can indicate an infection is present. For example, CURB-65 is such a cluster of markers commonly used in the diagnosis of community-acquired pneumonias. It is an objective scoring system based on presence or absence of confusion, blood urea, respiratory rate, blood pressure and patient age.[82]
- What is the likely organism?
- Is it susceptible to antibacterial agents?
- Will the selected agent reach the site of infection at the required concentration?
- Is the route of administration appropriate?
- Is the duration of treatment appropriate?
- Is there a stop/switch strategy?

Which antimicrobial?

The choice of agent depends on a number of factors but the general principles behind selection are: (1) only use an agent that is likely to work in the infection being treated; (2) ensure that it is one that has the narrowest antibacterial spectrum; and (3) ensure that the dose, route and duration of therapy are optimised. Ideally, a laboratory sensitivity report should drive selection but intuitive choice can be made from likely portal of entry. Once a sensitivity report has been received then appropriate switching to a narrow-spectrum agent should be promoted. Intravenous to oral switching should be made as soon as possible using explicit agreed criteria. This can reduce both cost and complications and allow patients to be discharged more quickly.

Surgical prophylaxis – reducing surgical site infections

Surgical site infections have been shown to compose up to 20% of all health-care-associated infections. At least 5% of patients undergoing a surgical procedure develop a surgical site infection; surgical site infections can double the length of time a patient stays in hospital and thereby increase the costs of healthcare by up to £7000. If the timing of your first dose of antimicrobial surgical prophylaxis is right then the likelihood of acquiring a surgical site infection is markedly reduced. Giving the first dose of antibacterial surgical prophylaxis within 60 minutes prior to incision reduces surgical site infections to a minimum.

Services linked to clinical specialties

In much the same way that clinical specialties are firmly established in medicine and surgery, the same is now true for clinical pharmacy. This has been helped by the manner in which clinical specialties have been managed in hospitals, often divided into divisions or directorates along clinical lines, to which a pharmacist can be attached. Part of the responsibilities for such pharmacists will be strategic, managerial and financial: (1) appropriate governance and risk management procedures; (2) monitoring and auditing the use of medicines; (3) supporting the management of the medicines budget; and (4) contributing to the preparation of business cases for new drugs. The UK Clinical Pharmacy Association is a good source of information on pharmacy input to specific clinical specialties and has a number of active special interest groups accessible via its website.[83]

Ongoing development of clinical pharmacy services

Optimising the use of medicines in hospitals is central to the delivery of high-quality patient care. Medication errors in hospitals are still unacceptably common and medicines continue to become increasingly complex and more costly. In addition, this is likely to become a significant issue with payment by results non-elective reimbursement systems, which may result in hospitals not being paid for suboptimal clinical outcomes of care.

The future of medicines management is inextricably linked with clinical pharmacy, with much of the value that pharmacists can add being information provision and monitoring quality. Although there is still a long way to go, the Healthcare Commission noted that many positive improvements have been made since the 2001 report from the UK Audit Commission's investigation into medicines management in hospitals.[1] Despite the significant progress that has been made in recent years, the Department of Health recognises that there are further challenges requiring attention, and progress in some areas has been slow:[2]

- ensuring the more effective use of medicines
- people who need urgent access to medicines are not always getting them when needed
- accessing the right medicines at the right time – of crucial importance for people at all stages of their lives, but particularly in end-of-life care
- preventing admissions that could be avoided with proper medicines use
- there are still too many problems with medicines when people leave hospital and return home.

Pharmacy services in the future will need to be designed around the needs of patients, not organisations, integrated with other healthcare services, with an emphasis on the need to bring care as near to the patient's home as possible. There needs to be a greater contribution of the skills hospital clinical pharmacists have developed to the whole patient pathway, making care truly seamless. Clinical pharmacy must also be designed to make the best use of staff and their skills and take advantage of modern technologies. Although computers and automated dispensing systems can help undertake some of this work, there are limitations to the possible achievements of technology and there is no substitute for direct contact with patients. Clinical pharmacy services in hospital have changed significantly over the past few decades, but re-engineering the way in which patient care is delivered is an ongoing process. Many of the changes are designed to free up hospital pharmacists' time to focus even more on the delivery of clinical care. Despite their limitations, the use of electronic prescribing and automated dispensing systems can help pharmacists to devote more of their time to patient care. Revision and further expansion of the pharmacy technician and pharmacy assistant roles also need to play a major part in this strategy.

The long-term vision for clinical pharmacy is a service contributing to a health service that offers patients fast and convenient care, that is available when they need it, tailored to their individual requirements and delivered to a consistently high standard. Delivering a successful clinical pharmacy service will bring major benefits to patients and pharmacists alike, but effective medicines management involves the whole organisation and requires multidisciplinary team working supported by an effective strategy. However, the Healthcare Commission found evidence that a significant proportion of healthcare professionals do not understand how pharmacy staff can contribute to the care of patients.[1] It is essential to address this gap to ensure that all healthcare staff and patients gain the maximum benefit from their pharmacy service.

References

1. Healthcare Commission. *The Best Medicine. The Management of Medicines in Acute and Specialist Trusts. Acute Hospital Portfolio Review.* London: Healthcare Commission, 2007.
2. Department of Health. *Pharmacy in England. Building on Strengths – Delivering the Future.* London: Department of Health, 2008.
3. Department of Health. *Equity and Excellence: Liberating the NHS.* London: Department of Health, 2010.
4. Kucukarslan S, Peters M, Mlynarek M *et al.* Pharmacists on rounding teams reduce preventable adverse drug events in hospital general medical units. *Arch Intern Med* 2003; 163: 2014–2018.
5. Bond C, Raehl C, Franke T. Interrelationships among mortality rates, drug cost, total cost of care and length of stay in United States hospitals: summary and recommendations for clinical pharmacy services and staffing. *Pharmacotherapy* 2001; 21: 129–141.
6. Scullin C, Scott M, Hogg A *et al.* An innovative approach to integrated medicines management. *J Eval Clin Pract* 2007; 13: 781–788.
7. Care Quality Commission. *Guidance about Compliance. Essential Standards of Quality and Safety.* London: Care Quality Commission, 2010.
8. American College of Clinical Pharmacy. The definition of clinical pharmacy. *Pharmacotherapy* 2008; 28: 816–817.
9. Hepler C, Strand L. Opportunities and responsibilities in pharmaceutical care. *Am J Hosp Pharm* 1990; 47: 533–543.
10. Audit Commission. *A Spoonful of Sugar – Medicines Management in NHS Hospitals.* London: Audit Commission, 2001.
11. Calvert R. Clinical pharmacy – a hospital perspective. *Br J Clin Pharmacol* 1998; 47: 231–238.
12. Department of Health. *A First Class Service, Quality in the New NHS.* London: The Stationery Office, 1998.
13. Cotter S, Barber N, McKee M. Professionalisation of hospital pharmacy: the role of clinical pharmacy. *J Soc Admin Pharm* 1994; 11: 57–67.
14. Clucas K, chair. *Pharmacy: A Report to the Nuffield Foundation.* London: Nuffield Foundation, 1986.
15. Department of Health. *Health Services Management. The Way Forward for Hospital Pharmaceutical Services.* HC(88)54. London: HMSO, 1988.
16. National Patient Safety Agency. Rapid response report NPSA/2010/RRR009. Reducing harm from omitted and delayed medicines in hospital. Available online at: http://www.nrls.npsa.nhs.uk/alerts/?entryid45=66720. (accessed 16 March 2010).
17. Anonymous. New all-Wales drug chart looks set to increase patient safety. *Hosp Pharm* 2005; 12: 184–185.
18. NHS Executive. *Information for Health. An Information Strategy for a Modern NHS 1998-2005.* London: The Stationery Office, 1998.
19. Bentley A, Green R. Developing pharmaceutical services; the nursing view. *Br J Pharm Pract* 1981; 3: 4–9.
20. Cavell G, Bunn R, Hodges M. Consultants' views on the developing role of the hospital pharmacist. *Pharm J* 1987; 239: 100–102.
21. Cairns C, Prior F. The clinical pharmacist: a study of his hospital involvement. *Pharm J* 1983; 320: 16–18.
22. Trewin V, Town R. Pharmacist effectiveness at case conferences. *Br J Pharm Pract* 1986; 8: 298–304.
23. Department of Health. *Building a Safer NHS for Patients. Implementing an Organisation with a Memory.* London: The Stationery Office, 2001.
24. Dornan T, Ashcroft D, Heathfield H *et al. An Indepth Investigation into Causes of Prescribing Errors by Foundation Trainees in Relation to their Medical Education.* EQUIP study. Final report to the General Medical Council. Manchester: University of Manchester School of Pharmacy and Pharmaceutical Sciences and School of Medicine, 2009.

25. Winstanley P, Irvin L, Smith J *et al*. Adverse drug reactions: a hospital pharmacy-based reporting scheme. *Br J Clin Pharmacol* 1989; 28: 113–116.
26. Lee A, Bateman D, Edwards C *et al*. Reporting of adverse drug reactions by hospital pharmacists: pilot scheme. *Br Med J* 1997; 315: 519.
27. Green C, Mottram D, Rowe P *et al*. Adverse drug reaction monitoring by United Kingdom hospital pharmacy departments: impact of the introduction of 'yellow card' reporting for pharmacists. *Int J Pharm Pract* 1999; 7: 238–246.
28. Dodds L. An objective assessment of the role of the pharmacist in medication and compliance history taking. *Br J Pharm Pract* 1982; 4: 12–24.
29. Hebron B, Jay C. Pharmaceutical care for patients undergoing elective ENT surgery. *Pharm J* 1998; 260: 65–66.
30. Gleason K, Groszek J, Sullivan C *et al*. Reconciliation of discrepancies in medication histories and admission orders of newly hospitalized patients. *Am J Health-Syst Pharm* 2004; 61: 1689–1695.
31. National Institute for Health and Clinical Excellence. *NICE Patient Safety Guidance 1. Technical Patient Safety Solutions for Medicines Reconciliation on Admission to Hospital*. London: National Institute for Health and Clinical Excellence, National Patient Safety Agency, 2007.
32. Karnon J, Campbell F, Czoski-Murray C. Model-based cost-effectiveness analysis of interventions aimed at preventing medication error at hospital admission (medicines reconciliation). *J Eval Clin Pract* 2009; 15: 299–306.
33. Hick H, Deady P, Wright D *et al*. The impact of the pharmacist on an elective general surgery pre-admission clinic. *Pharm World Sci* 2001; 23: 65–69.
34. Oliver S, Ashwell S. Pharmacists prescribing take home medication. *Pharm J* 2000; 265: 22.
35. Department of Health. *Pharmacy in the Future – Implementing the NHS Plan*. London: The Stationery Office, 2000.
36. National Institute for Health Research website: http://www.nihr.ac.uk/infrastructure/Pages/infrastructure_clahrcs.aspx.
37. Bloom B. Daily regimen and compliance with treatment. *Br Med J* 2001; 323: 647.
38. National Institute for Health and Clinical Excellence. *Medicines Adherence. Involving Patients in Decisions about Prescribed Medicines and Supporting Adherence*. NICE clinical guideline 76. London: NICE, 2009.
39. National Institute for Health and Clinical Excellence. *NICE Costing Statement. Medicines Adherence: Involving Patients in Decisions about Prescribed Medicines and Supporting Adherence*. Accompanying medicines adherence clinical guideline 76. London: NICE, 2009.
40. Royal Pharmaceutical Society of Great Britain. *From Compliance to Concordance: Towards Shared Goals in Medicine Taking*. London: RPSGB, 1997.
41. Varma S, McElnay J, Hughes C *et al*. Pharmaceutical care of patients with congestive heart failure: interventions and outcomes. *Pharmacotherapy* 1999; 19: 860–869.
42. Johnston M, Clarke A, Mundy K *et al*. Facilitating comprehension of discharge medication in elderly patients. *Age Ageing* 1986; 15: 304–306.
43. Goodyer L, Miskelly F, Milligan P. Does encouraging good compliance improve patients' clinical condition in heart failure? *Br J Clin Pract* 1995; 49: 173–176.
44. Al-Eidan F, McElnay J, Scott M *et al*. Management of *Helicobacter pylori* eradication – the influence of structured counselling and follow-up. *Br J Clin Pharmacol* 2002; 53: 163–171.
45. Sandler D, Mitchell J, Fellows A *et al*. Is an information booklet for patients leaving hospital helpful and useful? *Br Med J* 1989; 298: 870–874.
46. McElnay J, Scott M, Armstrong A *et al*. Audiovisual demonstration for patient counselling in the use of pressurised aerosol bronchodilator inhalers. *J Clin Pharm Ther* 1989; 14: 135–144.
47. Daly M, Jones S. Preliminary assessment of a computerised counselling program for asthmatic children. *Pharm J* 1991; 247: 206–208.
48. Raynor D, Booth T. Blenkinsopp A. Effects of computer generated reminder charts on patients' compliance with drug regimens. *Br Med J* 1993; 306: 1158–1161.
49. Wood S, Calvert R, Acomb C *et al*. A self-medication scheme for elderly patients improves compliance with their medication regimens. *Int J Pharm Pract* 1992; 1: 240–241.

50. Lowe C, Raynor D, Courtney E *et al.* Effects of a self-medication programme on knowledge of drugs and compliance with treatment in elderly patients. *Br Med J* 1995; 310: 1229–1231.
51. Wright J, Emerson A, Stephens M *et al.* Hospital inpatient self-administration programmes: a critical literature review. *Pharm World Sci* 2006; 28: 140–151.
52. Bourne J, Farrar K, Fitzpatrick R. Practical involvement in therapeutic drug monitoring. *Pharm J* 1985; 234: 530–531.
53. Brown A. Establishment of a pharmacy-run TDM service. *Br J Pharm Pract* 1986; 8: 154–159.
54. Campbell D. A clinical pharmacokinetics service. *Hosp Pharm* 1999; 6: 206–208.
55. Booth C. Pharmacist-managed anticoagulation clinics: a review. *Pharm J* 1998; 261: 623–625.
56. Boddy C. Pharmacist involvement with warfarin dosing for inpatients. *Pharm World Sci* 2001; 23: 31–35.
57. National Institute for Health and Clinical Excellence. *Reducing the Risk of Venous Thromboembolism (Deep Vein Thrombosis and Pulmonary Embolism) in Patients Admitted to Hospital.* Clinical guideline 92. London: NICE, 2010.
58. Department of Health. *Using the Commissioning for Quality and Innovation (CQUIN) Payment Framework – An Addendum to the 2008 Policy Guidance for 2010/11.* London: Department of Health, 2010.
59. Ayra R (ed.) *Venous Thromboembolism Prevention, A Patient Safety Priority.* London: King's Thrombosis Centre, 2009.
60. Parliamentary Office of Science and Technology. Postnote. Personalised medicine. 2009; 329: 1–4: available online at: http://www.parliament.uk/documents/upload/postpn329.pdf (accessed 30 March 2010).
61. University of Bradford PGCert/PGDip/MSc in Clinical Pharmacy (Hospital) Course Prospectus 2006. Bradford: University of Bradford, 2006.
62. Anonymous. Postgraduate education for hospital pharmacists. *Pharm J* 1978; 220: 525–526.
63. Noyce P, Hibberd A. Launch of the London MSc in clinical pharmacy. *Pharm J* 1980; 225: 4733–4734.
64. Baker J. Seventeen years' experience of a voluntary based drug rationalisation program in hospital. *Br Med J* 1988; 297: 465–469.
65. Donabedian A. Evaluating the quality of medical care. *Milbank Memorial Fund Q* 1966; 44: 166–206.
66. Devlin N, Appleby J. *Getting the Most out of PROMS. Putting Health Outcomes at the Heart of NHS Decision Making.* London: King's Fund, 2010.
67. *Moving to Audit: What Every Pharmacist Needs to Know about Professional Audit.* Dundee: Postgraduate Office, Ninewells Hospital and Medical School, 1993.
68. Davies H. Developing effective clinical audit. *Hosp Med* 1999; 60: 748–750.
69. Teasdale S. The future of clinical audit: learning to work together. *Br Med J* 1996; 313: 574.
70. Dean J, Acomb J. A pharmacist managed lithium clinic. *Hosp Pharm* 1995; 2: 150–152.
71. Jones S, Pritchard M, Grout C *et al.* A rheumatology drug monitoring clinic. *Pharm J* 1999; 263: 25.
72. Williams H . Pharmacist-led lipid management clinic. *Pharm J* 1999; 263: 26.
73. Morlidge C. Pharmacist-run renal medication review clinics. *Br J Renal Med* 2001; 6: 25–26.
74. Care Quality Commission. *National Study. Managing Patients' Medicines after Discharge from Hospital.* London: Care Quality Commission, 2009.
75. Brown J, Brown D. Pharmaceutical care at the primary–secondary interface in Portsmouth and South East Hampshire. *Pharm J* 1997; 258: 280–284.
76. Child D. How well do you collaborate across the primary/secondary care interface? *Pharm Manage* 2009; 25: 3–7.
77. Colaluca A, Glet R, Smith D *et al.* Inpatient counselling – a technician's role. *Br J Pharm Pract* 1988; 10: 334–340.
78. Dosaj R, Mistry R. The pharmacy technician in clinical services. *Hosp Pharm* 1998; 5: 26–28.
79. Edwards L. The role of the directorate liaison technician. *Hosp Pharm* 2001; 8: 115–116.

80. Department of Health and Health Protection Agency. *Clostridium difficile – How to Deal with the Problem*. London: Department of Health and HPA, 2008.
81. Department of Health. *The Health and Social Care Act 2008: Code of Practice for the NHS on the Prevention and Control of Healthcare Associated Infections and Related Guidance*. London: Department of Health, 2009.
82. Lim W, van der Eerden M, Laing R *et al*. Defining community acquired pneumonia severity on presentation to hospital: an international derivation and validation study. *Thorax* 2003; 58: 377–382.
83. UK Clinical Pharmacy Association website: http://www.ukcpa.org/.

Further reading

Department of Health. *Pharmacy in England. Building on Strengths – Delivering the Future*. London: Department of Health, 2008.
Healthcare Commission. *The Best Medicine. The Management of Medicines in Acute and Specialist Trusts. Acute Hospital Portfolio Review*. London: Healthcare Commission, 2007.
National Institute for Health and Clinical Excellence, National Patient Safety Agency. *NICE Patient Safety Guidance 1. Technical Patient Safety Solutions for Medicines Reconciliation on Admission to Hospital*. London: National Institute for Health and Clinical Excellence, National Patient Safety Agency, 2007.

10

Pharmacist prescribing

Marie Brazil

Pharmacists share a common history with general practitioners (GPs). In 1815 the *Apothecaries Act* saw the professions divide to become either apothecaries, who later became GPs, or chemists and druggists, who today are known as pharmacists. The pharmacist has long been the first port of call for the public on matters of health, be that due to convenience or, in the past, a less costly alternative to medical practitioner care. So perhaps we can say that the profession has now regained its past prescribing rights.

To 'prescribe' was defined in the *Review of Prescribing, Supply and Administration of Medicines* of March 1999, also known as the second Crown report and widely acknowledged as the document that launched non-medical prescribing in the UK in its present form.[1] The detail is as follows:

> Prescribe: in the strict legal sense, as used in the *Medicines Act*: to order in writing the supply of a prescription-only medicine for a named patient.

But commonly used in the sense of:

> To authorise by means of an NHS prescription the supply of any medicine (not just a prescription-only medicine) at public expense.

And occasionally

> To advise a patient on suitable care or medication (including medicine which may be purchased over the counter).

The third definition confirms that pharmacists have a long history of prescribing, when we consider the large number of medicines sold over the counter. The range of these medicines available over the counter has increased over recent years with rescheduling from prescription-only medicines (POM) to pharmacy only (P). Pharmacists have had a tradition of allowing timely and appropriate access for patients to medicines and care through their efforts. This has become a founding principle of expanding prescribing rights outside the traditional groups. This chapter will focus on the first two definitions of prescribing, where the recent changes have been seen.

The journey towards non-medical prescribing started in the 1980s: the first milestone was the Cumberledge report (1986) recommending 'a limited list of items and simple agents' that could be prescribed by community nurses to streamline care.[2] Informed by the first Crown report of 1989, independent prescribing for nurses came into being in 1992, again from a limited formulary.[3] The list of medicines that could be prescribed, in defined circumstances, was published in the *Nurse Prescribers' Formulary*.[4] The first Crown report also recommended that nurses could supply medicines within group protocols, with the second report a decade later remodelling these protocols as patient group directions. Group protocols allowed nurses (or other healthcare professionals) to supply medicinal products to patients according to a strict protocol signed by a registered doctor or dentist.

The road to pharmacist prescribing, as we know it today in hospital practice, owes much to those pharmacists who practised and promoted clinical pharmacy in the 1980s. They demonstrated the important contribution pharmacists can make to the care of patients, instigating pharmaceutical care, and they were commended in the second Crown report for their professionalism. In the early work around pharmacist prescribing, community and primary care pharmacy was perceived as the obvious area of practice. However, the challenges relating to sharing the medical record with community pharmacists, that have not been resolved, make this difficult. This has led to the majority of active pharmacist prescribers practising in primary care clinics or within hospital pharmacy where shared records are the norm.[5, 6]

Between 1998 and 1999, the committee established at the request of the Department of Health to review prescribing, supply and administration of medicine led a consultation exercise engaging all areas of the National Health Service (NHS) and the varied professions involved in the provision of healthcare. The information gathered was used to inform a two-part report under the chairmanship of Dr June Crown, past-president, Faculty of Public Health Medicine and the chairman of the Advisory Group on Nurse Prescribing 1988–1989. As noted earlier, the first Crown report established group protocols which this later review modified to become patient group directions. The second part of this later report focused on non-medical prescribing. The report, published in 1999, recommended that pharmacists be given prescribing rights.[1] However, the initial recommendation was that this should be in a 'dependent' capacity (now termed supplementary prescribing), which is supported by a medical prescriber. Evidence, submitted under the consultation exercise, from other countries that already had pharmacist prescribers demonstrated those pharmacists involved in prescribing can often focus more time on patient concerns regarding their treatment, thus supporting greater concordance with therapy.

The second report from the Crown review set out its recommendations with the overriding principle that any changes to the roles of professionals 'must at the very least maintain, and preferably enhance, patient safety' and 'bring about demonstrable benefits to patient care'.[1] The need for the review was driven by changes in the roles of medical professionals and the increased complexity of care. It also noted the increase expertise of patients themselves in the management of their conditions, especially patients with long-standing disease states. It set out that changes in care should improve the convenience of services for patients as well as enabling them to be more involved in their treatment and in the control of their own health. To this end the extension of prescribing rights outside the traditional doctor and dentist model was proposed. The concept of two classes of prescribers was also proposed: independent and dependent prescribers, with the definitions shown in Text box 10.1. The concept of a dependent prescriber was later replaced with that of the supplementary prescriber but essentially this was just a change of nomenclature.

Box 10.1 Prescriber definitions from Crown II[1]

The independent prescriber

Responsible for the assessment of patients with undiagnosed conditions and for decisions about the clinical management required, including prescribing. At present, doctors, dentists and certain nurses in respect of a limited list of medicines are legally authorised prescribers who fulfil the requirements for independent prescribers and this should continue. Certain other health professionals may also become newly legally authorised independent prescribers.

The dependent prescriber (now known as supplementary prescriber)

Responsible for the continuing care of patients who have been clinically assessed by an independent prescriber. This continuing care may include prescribing, which will usually be informed by clinical guidelines and will be consistent with individual treatment plans; or continuing established treatments by issuing repeat prescriptions, with the authority to adjust the dose or dosage form according to the patient's needs. There should be provision for regular clinical review by the assessing clinician.

Supplementary prescribing

Supplementary prescribing involves a partnership between a medical practitioner (independent prescriber) who establishes the diagnosis and initiates treatment, a supplementary prescriber who monitors the patient and prescribes further supplies of medication and the patient who agrees to the supplementary prescribing arrangement.[7]

A clinical management plan is drawn up for each patient which includes demographic data, the condition to be treated, the treatment with medicines and information detailing when the patient should be referred back to the independent prescriber. Figure 10.1 provides an example template for a clinical management plan; other examples are available online.[8] Prescribing information included in clinical management plans can refer to an agreed limited amount of information and dosage adjustments that the supplementary prescriber can make or, more usually, to a locally or nationally agreed clinical guideline or pathway, for example, the British Thoracic Society's asthma guidelines.[9]

The supplementary prescribing model is the one initially recommended for pharmacists by the Crown report and subsequently put into statute in 2003.[10] The profession found this model to be somewhat unwieldy and pursued independent prescribing; this was made possible in May 2006.

Supplementary prescribing is championed as the efficient model for the management of long-term therapies within primary and secondary care. It has been used in hospital practice to establish pharmacists within outpatient clinics and provided a sound basis on which to build prescribing practice for pharmacists. A supplementary prescriber, using a clinical management plan, may prescribe a wide range of items, summarised in Text box 10.2.[9]

Independent prescribing

Since May 2006, after an amendment to the *Prescription Only Medicines (Human Use) Order 1997*,[11, 12] pharmacists have been able to train as independent prescribers. Once qualified and the appropriate addition to the register made, they are able to prescribe from the entire *British National Formulary*. Text box 10.3 sets out the range of medicines at the time of writing. Independent prescribing allows pharmacists greater autonomy; they can assess and manage patients and their medicines regimen within their specified area of competence. The advantage of this type of prescribing is that a pharmacist assessing a patient for a long-term condition is also able to diagnose and treat or refer for treatment a newly presenting complaint. Whilst working as an independent prescriber the pharmacist may choose to prescribe under a supplementary prescribing

Name of patient:	Patient medication sensitivities/allergies		
Patient identification e.g. ID number, date of birth:			
Independent prescriber(s):	Supplementary prescriber(s)		
Condition(s) to be treated	Aim of treatment		

Medicines that may be prescribed by SP:			
Preparation	Indication	Dose schedule	Specific indications for referral back to the IP

Guidelines or protocols supporting clinical management plan:

Frequency of review and monitoring by:	
Supplementary prescriber	Supplementary prescriber and independent prescriber

Precess for reporting ADRs:

Shared record to be used by IP and SP:

Agreed by independent prescriber(s)	Date	Agreed by supplementary prescriber(s)	Date	Date agreed with patient/carer

Figure 10.1   Example of a clinical management plan. SP, supplementary prescriber; IP, independent prescriber; ADRs, adverse drug reactions.

Box 10.2 *Medicines available to pharmacist supplementary prescribers*

Pharmacist supplementary prescribing

Any general sales list, pharmacy or prescription-only medicine prescribable at National Health Service expense. This includes the prescribing of:

- antimicrobials
- 'black triangle' drugs and those products suggested by the *British National Formulary* to be 'less suitable' for prescribing
- controlled drugs (except those listed in schedule 1 of *The Misuse of Drugs Regulations 2001* that are not intended for medicinal use)
- products used outside their UK-licensed indications (known as 'off-label' use). Such use must have the joint agreement of both prescribers and the status of the drug should be recorded in the clinical management plan
- unlicensed medicines

Box 10.3 *Medicines available to a pharmacist independent prescriber*

A pharmacist independent prescriber can prescribe any licensed medicine for any medical condition, including:

- UK-licensed products used outside their UK-licensed indications (i.e. 'off-label' use) (pharmacist prescribers, like all prescribers, must accept professional, clinical and legal responsibility for that prescribing and should only prescribe 'off-label' where it is accepted clinical practice)
- unlicensed drugs

At the time of writing, controlled drug prescribing is under review.

arrangement, moving between the two practices, as required, to meet the patient need.

General principles of prescribing

The actions of the pharmacist prescriber, both supplementary and independent, are governed by the *Code of Ethics for Pharmacists and Pharmacy Technicians* (published by the Royal Pharmaceutical Society of Great

Britain (RPSGB)) and they must work within their area of competence.[13] The RPSGB has also produced *Professional Standards and Guidance for Pharmacist Prescribers*.[14] This guidance states that the consultation that leads to a prescribing decision must include some fundamental elements:

* the prescriber must explain his or her role to the patient/carer
* he or she must obtain the patient's consent to prescribe – this is usually done verbally
* the decision to prescribe must be a shared decision with the patient
* the prescribing decision must be recorded within the patient's record
* wherever possible, the prescribing decision should be evidence-based and in accordance with national or local guidelines; deviation can occur if it is recorded and explained but must be in the patient's best interest.

An area of concern for many pharmacists is the dispensing of prescriptions they themselves have written. The RPSGB professional standards discourage this practice unless in an emergency situation.

Current prescribing practice

The second Crown report and the architects of non-medical prescribing saw its use mainly in the primary care setting. The hope was that information technology (IT) solutions would allow pharmacists in health centres and community pharmacies to share records and thus facilitate prescribing partnerships. However, this IT solution is not yet available in community pharmacy, a decade after this vision of pharmacist prescribing was described. The inclusion of pharmacists within the multidisciplinary team caring for hospital patients has perhaps allowed them to take on the role of prescriber with greater ease. There are still barriers to setting up prescribing practice within the hospital setting but, where an institution is supportive and resources are available, the skills of the pharmacist can be capitalised upon to improve patient care. The greatest success of pharmacist prescribing has been within outpatient clinics, on admissions units and within services utilising complex medicine regimens requiring expert monitoring.

Although numerous pharmacists have been trained as prescribers, not all of these individuals use their qualification in practice. A recently reported study noted that only 25% of pharmacists, interviewed and practising in Northern Ireland, who had trained as supplementary prescribers before September 2006 currently used their prescribing rights.[5] The ability to become an independent prescriber was, and still is, hoped to correct the disparity between training and utility. Another recent review of prescribing in the north-east supports the view that not all qualified prescribers are using their skills.[6, 15, 16] However, it did find that 67% of trained pharmacist prescribers had used their prescribing rights, the majority of them practising within secondary care.

Pharmacist prescribing seems to be used most commonly in a clinic setting and often in the management of chronic disorders. Independent prescribing has been used to facilitate prescribing on admission to and discharge from hospital.[17] However, further research is required to see if, as many practitioners believe, this form of pharmacist prescribing is of greater benefit in all areas of clinical practice. Many obstacles are cited in the literature to explain why there is a disparity between those who have trained to prescribe and those who use the qualification, but common themes appear: logistics, lack of strategic implementation and lack of funding.[5, 6, 15] Within hospital practice the easy access to support from the multidisciplinary team is often given as a positive encouragement to establishing pharmacist prescribing.[18] Where strong relationships exist between a medical team and a pharmacist or pharmacists, the pharmacists appear more likely to take on a prescribing role. Thus we can see that the innovation may be driven by individuals rather than the vision of the organisation.

Clinical governance

'A framework through which NHS organisations are accountable for continuously improving the quality of their services and safeguarding high standards of care by creating an environment in which excellence in clinical care will flourish' is how clinical governance was defined by the Department of Health.[19] It can be argued that non-medical prescribing sits easily with this approach, as it uses appropriately trained individuals to provide excellent care and it helps to improve patient services. Non-medical prescribing is based firmly on a foundation of competence; prescribers are required by their registering body to maintain their competence within their area of expertise and their competence to prescribe.

Pharmacists are instructed by the *Code of Ethics*:[13]

At all stages of your professional working life you must ensure that your knowledge, skills and performance are of a high quality, up to date and relevant to your field of practice.

Although independent prescribers have the ability to prescribe any item from the entire *British National Formulary*, it is embedded in non-medical prescribing education that practitioners must have a full knowledge of the medicine they prescribe and the disease they are treating. In practice, pharmacist prescribers work to a personal formulary based around their area of practice. A further fundamental part of any pharmacist prescriber's practice must be the participation in continuing professional development and reflection upon how new learning influences prescribing practice. Discussion groups have been set up for prescribing pharmacists to allow them access to other prescribers for advice and support.[9]

The National Prescribing Centre has developed a competency framework to aid pharmacist prescribers, those who commission their services and provide governance.[20] The framework is divided into three main areas: (1) the consultation; (2) prescribing effectively; and (3) prescribing in context. The areas of competency are set out in Table 10.1. The framework can be used by individuals to inform their continuing professional development or by an organisation to ensure quality.

It is incumbent on individual prescribers to apply clinical governance principles to their practice; however, the organisation within which they conduct that practice also has a duty of care to both the patient and the prescriber.[21] Organisations have established non-medical prescribing committees to provide a governance framework for prescribers to work within. Committees vary in their practice. However they:

- keep a register of non-medical prescribers operating within their organisation
- ensure that the relevant organisational policies include and incorporate non-medical prescribing
- agree and approve clinical management plans and personal formularies.

They also have a role in agreeing which staff groups and individuals will be supported by the organisation to train as non-medical prescribers. With the involvement of the organisation in the selection of candidates for training it is hoped that prescribers will utilise those skills once gained, as their position in the service will already be established.

Within the clinical governance arena we have seen the emergence of quality being allied to waste reduction within patient services. Pharmacist prescribers are using their knowledge of medicines regimens and their expertise in individualising patients' medicines to reduce medication errors within healthcare and this can only improve the quality of care offered to those patients.

Table 10.1 National Prescribing Centre prescribing competencies

The consultation	Clinical and pharmaceutical knowledge Establishing options Communicating with patients
Prescribing effectively	Prescribing safely Prescribing professionally Improving prescribing practice
Prescribing in context	Information in context The National Health Service in context The team and individual context

Education

All non-medical prescribing programmes training pharmacists must be accredited by the RPSGB. The RPSGB has outlined a curriculum for pharmacist prescribers, which at present requires them to have 2 years' postregistration experience of patient care.[22] This document sets out the aims and objectives shown in Text box 10.4. All candidates require a designated medical practitioner (DMP) to assist in their learning and to assess their competence during their practice-based experience. This 'clinical practice' takes the form of 12 days of supervision by the DMP and runs alongside 26 days of taught course content. The clinical practice element of the training programme is for trainees to hone their diagnostic and consultation skills. Trainees observe other prescribers and are observed in turn to verify their competence. This practical learning within trainees' organisation is also valuable for them in understanding the processes and policies of prescribing from the perspective of a prescriber rather than simply their role as pharmacist. The trainee enters into a learning partnership with the DMP and the higher education institute providing the accredited training programme. A learning contract is drawn up to ensure the goals are explicit and that all participants acknowledge what is required of them. A record of learning is kept throughout the training course with reflective practice as its cornerstone. Only after the trainee's DMP is satisfied with his or her practice and fulfilment of the agreed learning agreement can he or she be signed off as a competent prescriber.

Box 10.4 Prescribers' training course

Aim

To enable pharmacists to practise and develop as prescribers and to meet the standards set by the Royal Pharmaceutical Society of Great Britain

Learning outcomes

Being able to:

- understand the responsibility the role of independent prescriber entails, be aware of their own limitations and work within the limits of their professional competence – knowing when and how to refer/consult/seek guidance from another member of the healthcare team

- develop an effective relationship and communication with patients, carers, other prescribers and members of the healthcare team
- describe the pathophysiology of the condition being treated and recognise the signs and symptoms of illness, take an accurate history and carry out a relevant clinical assessment where necessary
- use common diagnostic aids, for example, stethoscope, sphygmomanometer
- use diagnostic aids relevant to the condition(s) for which the pharmacist intends to prescribe, including monitoring response to therapy
- apply clinical assessment skills to inform a working diagnosis, formulate a treatment plan, prescribe one or more medicines if appropriate, checking to ensure patient safety, and monitor response to therapy, review the working/differential diagnosis and modify treatment or refer/consult/seek guidance as appropriate
- demonstrate a shared approach to decision-making by assessing patients' needs for medicines, taking account of their wishes and values and those of carers when making prescribing decisions
- identify and assess information sources, advice and decision support, show how they will use them in patient care, taking into account evidence-based practice and national/local guidelines where they exist
- recognise, evaluate and respond to influences on prescribing practice at individual, local and national levels
- prescribe safely, appropriately and cost-effectively
- work within a prescribing partnership
- keep accurate, effective and timely records and keep other prescribers and healthcare staff informed
- demonstrate an understanding of the public health issues related to medicines use
- demonstrate an understanding of the legal, ethical and professional framework for accountability and responsibility in relation to prescribing
- work within clinical governance frameworks including prescribing practice audit and personal development
- participate regularly in continuing professional development (CPD) and maintain a record of their CPD activity

The future

It is anticipated that in the near future the skills required for prescribing will be included within the undergraduate pharmacy degree programme, possibly with prescribing rights awarded on registration. This has caused some disquiet among qualified staff who must demonstrate their competence and experience prior to undertaking their training as prescribers. The Modernising Pharmacy Careers Programme Board has addressed this issue and, at the time of writing, the proposal is that newly registered pharmacists will focus on optimising prescribing rather than initiating new prescriptions.[23, 24] It is envisaged that input will be at admission and discharge in hospitals and via repeat dispensing using prescribing partnerships as supplementary prescribers. The structure afforded by such an approach will allow newly qualified pharmacists to gain experience and expertise whilst ensuring quality can be maintained. As pharmacists progress through their career, independent prescribing rights may be gained after appropriate training; however, other pharmacists may wish to remain within the partnership framework afforded by supplementary prescribing. These changes will steadily increase the cohort of prescribing pharmacists and allow organisations to plan services that utilise these individuals.

When non-medical prescribing was envisaged it was intended to have a demonstrable benefit to patient care. Improving access to healthcare has been at the forefront of a number of recent initiatives. The *High Quality Care for All, NHS Next Stage Review*, chaired by Lord Darzi, echoed that sentiment and included the following objective: 'ensuring timely access'.[25]

There was a strong message that people can still find it difficult to access services:

> Improving access is a priority articulated in every vision, across every pathway of care. Each region will continue to improve the quality of access by reducing waiting times for treatment.[25]

The provision of timely and cost-effective care, further founding principles of non-medical prescribing practice, can only serve as drivers for its expansion. The pharmacist prescribers who have qualified and are using their skills are encouraged to disseminate good practice by both the RPSGB and the National Prescribing Centre. As new prescribers train they are using regional experts and early adopters as resources to inform and shape their practice. Sharing practice, publishing audit and research around prescribing services allows us to demonstrate benefit to patients and to the NHS. Encouraging and mentoring new prescribers and junior pharmacists is an important role for established prescribers and 'buddy' schemes exist in some organisations and networks. As the pool of pharmacist prescribers increases and the understanding of their role and value within organisations grows, the profession can truly address provision of timely, cost-effective care with this additional skill set.

Pharmacists have been comfortable with their role as the providers of quality advice; it has been part of our profession's public perception for many years. That advice has been used to inform countless prescribing decisions but the transition from adviser to practitioner is considered a large step. As professional boundaries overlap our experience of scrutinising others prescribing can inform our practice. As we move towards prescribing being as fundamental to pharmacists' practice as advice-giving has always been, we are cementing our role as the medicines expert within the healthcare team.

References

1. Department of Health. *Review of the Prescribing, Supply and Administration of Medicines.* Final report. London: The Stationery Office, 1999.
2. Department of Health and Social Security. *Neighbourhood Nursing – A Focus for Care.* London: HMSO, 1986.
3. Department of Health. *Report of the Advisory Group on Nurse Prescribing.* London: HMSO, 1989.
4. Joint Formulary Committee. *British National Formulary. Nurse Prescribers' Formulary.* London: British Medical Association and Royal Pharmaceutical Society, 1998.
5. Lloyd F, Parsons C, Hughes CM. 'It's showed me the skills that he has': pharmacist's and mentors' views on pharmacist supplementary prescribing. *Int J Pharm Pract* 2010; 18: 29–36.
6. Baquir W, Clemerson J, Smith J. Evaluating pharmacist prescribing across the north east of England. *Br J Clin Pharmacol* 2010; 2: 147–149.
7. Pharmacist prescribing. Royal Pharmaceutical Society of Great Britain website: http://www.rpsgb.org.
8. Clinical management plans website: http://www.cmponline.info.
9. British Thoracic Society and Scottish Intercollegiate Guidelines Network. Management of chronic asthma advice. Available online at: http://www.brit-thoracic.org.uk.
10. Medicines and Healthcare products Regulatory Agency. Available online at: http://www.mhra.gov.uk/Howweregulate/Medicines/Availabilityprescribingsellingandsupplyingofmedicines/ExemptionsfromMedicinesActrestrictions/Supplementaryprescribing/index.htm.
11. *Prescription Only Medicines (Human Use) Order 1997.* Available online at: http://www.statutelaw.gov.uk/content.aspx?LegType=All+Legislation&title=Prescription+Only+Medicines+(Human+Use)+Order&Year=1997&searchEnacted=0&extentMatchOnly=0&confersPower=0&blanketAmendment=0&sortAlpha=0&TYPE=QS&PageNumber=1&NavFrom=0&activeTextDocId=2871854&parentActiveTextDocId=2871854&showAllAttributes=0&hideCommentary=0&showProsp=0&suppressWarning=1.
12. Department of Health. Independent pharmacist prescribing. Available online at: http://www.dh.gov.uk/en/Healthcare/Medicinespharmacyandindustry/Prescriptions/TheNon-MedicalPrescribingProgramme/Independentpharmacistprescribing/DH_4133943.
13. Royal Pharmaceutical Society of Great Britain. *Code of Ethics for Pharmacists and Pharmacy Technicians.* London: RPSGB, 2010.
14. Royal Pharmaceutical Society of Great Britain. *Professional Standards and Guidance for Pharmacist Prescribers.* London: RPSGB, 2007.
15. Baquir W, Smith J. Why pharmacist prescribing appears to be floundering. *Br J Clin Pharmacol* 2010; 2: 150–151.
16. Baquir W. Evaluating pharmacist prescribing across the north east of England. *Br J Clin Pharmacol* 2010; 2: 147–149.
17. Thakkar K, Jani B. Pharmacist prescribing in an acute medical unit. *Br J Clin Pharmacol* 2009; 1: 253–254.
18. All Party Pharmacy Group. *Pharmacist Prescribing: A Report to Health Ministers.* London: All Party Pharmacy Group, 2001.

19. Department of Health. *Clinical Governance, Quality in the New NHS.* London: The Stationery Office, 1999.
20. National Prescribing Centre. *Maintaining Competency in Prescribing. An Outline Framework to Help Pharmacist Prescribers*, 2nd edn. Liverpool: National Prescribing Centre, 2006.
21. Royal Pharmaceutical Society of Great Britain. *Clinical Governance Framework for Pharmacist Prescribers and Organisations Commissioning or Participating in Pharmacist Prescribing (GB Wide).* London: RPSGB, 2007.
22. Royal Pharmaceutical Society of Great Britain. *Outline Curriculum for Training Programmes to Prepare Pharmacist Prescribers.* London: RPSGB, 2006.
23. Modernising Pharmacy Careers Programme Board. Note of meeting held on Tuesday 29 September 2009. Available online at: http://www.mee.nhs.uk/pdf/1Approved%20MPCPB %20minutes%20290909.pdf (accessed 9 August 2010).
24. Modernising Pharmacy Careers Programme Board. Note of meeting held on Thursday 12 November 2009. Available online at: http://www.mee.nhs.uk/pdf/1MPCPB%20Approved %20minutes%2012%20November.pdf (accessed 9 August 2010).
25. Department of Health. *The High Quality Care for All, NHS Next Stage Review.* Final Report. London: Department of Health, 2008.

Further reading

Department of Health FAQ pharmacist prescribing: http://www.dh.gov.uk/en/Healthcare/ Medicinespharmacyandindustry/TheNon-MedicalPrescribingProgramme/ Independentpharmacistprescribing/DH_4133943.
Royal Pharmaceutical Society of Great Britain. *Pharmacist Prescriber Pack.* London: RPSGB, 2010.
RPSGB pharmacist prescribing: http://www.rpsgb.org.uk/worldofpharmacy/currentdevelop-mentsinpharmacy/pharmacistprescribing/index.html.

11

Strategic medicines management

Ray Fitzpatrick

Medicines are central to most healthcare interventions, particularly in hospital, since 97% of patients in hospital are taking medicines.[1] However, the use of medicines carries risk, both clinical and financial.

Clinical risk

The sixteenth century physician Paracelsus is quoted as saying that 'the only thing that differentiates a medicine from a poison is the dose'. This view is just as pertinent today as it was then, with medication-related incidents the third highest incident type reported to the National Patient Safety Agency.[2] Furthermore, it has been estimated that 1000 deaths per year are due to medication errors or adverse events.[3] Although today's medicines are subject to rigorous safety checks as part of the licensing procedure they still represent a significant clinical risk, since the use of medicines as a healthcare intervention has grown significantly over the past decade. In 1998, there were, on average, 10.5 prescription items dispensed in the community per head of population per year, whereas in 2008 this had risen to 16.4 – growth of over 50%.[4]

Financial risk

In 2009 the National Health Service (NHS) in England spent £12.3 billion on medicines.[5] Hospital prescribing accounted for 30.9% of this expenditure, and whilst the total cost of medicines rose by 5.6% overall, in hospitals the cost rose by 13.2%.[5] This is not surprising, as hospital patients are becoming older and have more complex health problems. Furthermore, newer medicines are more complex and expensive. Indeed, it has been estimated that there

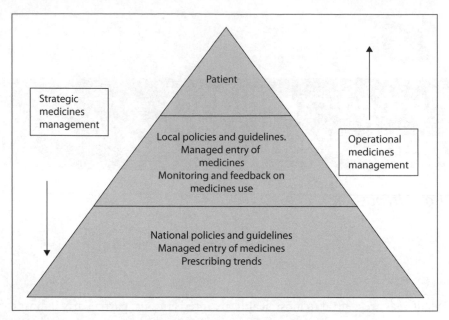

Figure 11.1 The medicines management pyramid.

are now more biopharmaceuticals entering the marketplace than conventional medicines.[6] In the author's own hospital high-cost medicines excluded from tariff now account for over half of the total medicines budget. As a result, growth in hospital prescribing costs doubled between 2001 and 2007 compared with a 50% increase in primary care.

Therefore, medicines management can be seen as risk management. The author's definition of medicines management is 'influencing the availability and policies on medicines at an organisational level as well as the prescription, use and administration of medicines at an individual patient level'. This can be best described pictorially by the medicines management pyramid shown in Figure 11.1. As shown in this diagram, medicines management processes centred on the patient can be considered operational and those dealing with policies and guidelines are strategic. This chapter will focus on the strategic elements of this definition, with the emphasis on financial aspects. Chapter 12 will focus on the clinical risks.

History

The hospital pharmacist's role in medicines management was recognised as long ago as 1955 in the Linstead report on hospital pharmacy.[7] In this report the role of the hospital pharmacy included:

- to assist in the development of new methods of treatment
- to promote economy in the use of medical supplies

- to assist in efficient prescribing by advising upon the nature and properties of medicaments, and selection of the most suitable substances and the form in which they should be prescribed.

These principles remain true today, particularly as both the range and complexity of medicines have increased enormously. In the intervening years, milestone reports such as the Nuffield report in 1986,[8] the Department of Health circular on clinical pharmacy in 1988,[9] *Pharmacy in the Future* in 2000[10] and the Audit Commission report on medicines management in hospital reinforced the role of the hospital pharmacist at the centre of medicines management.[3] More recently, the General Medical Council's own research identified that almost 10% of prescriptions written by junior doctors contained errors: these were only prevented from reaching the patient by other healthcare staff, primarily hospital pharmacists.[11]

Although systems to manage prescribing have a longer history in hospital than in primary care, more attention has focused on primary care prescribing costs with more central initiatives (for example, practice detailed prescribing information (PDPI) data (previously called PACT data), primary care trust (PCT) pharmaceutical advisers and general practice incentive schemes). This is not surprising since in 2000 the majority of NHS expenditure on medicines was in primary care. However, we have noted that more recently secondary care prescribing costs have been the larger area of growth.

Strategic medicines management in practice

In describing various approaches to implementing strategic medicines management in practice, it is appropriate to discuss the issue in the context of the medicines management pyramid shown in Figure 11.1. As can be seen from the diagram, there are three key elements to strategic medicines management:

1 managed entry of new medicines
2 prescribing policies and guidelines
3 monitoring and feedback on medicines use.

Managed entry of new medicines

At a national level the entry of new medicines is controlled in the licensing process by the Medicines and Healthcare products Regulatory Agency (MHRA); only medicines with an appropriate product licence may be marketed in the UK. However, the MHRA licence is primarily concerned with whether a new medicinal product works and is no less safe than existing medicines. The MHRA licensing process makes no judgement on the cost-effectiveness of a new medicine. The establishment of the National Institute for Health and Clinical Excellence (NICE) in England in 1999 was an attempt to introduce a system to assess the cost-effectiveness of new and established medicines. NICE is discussed further in the section on prescribing policies and guidelines, below.

The cornerstone of any system to manage the introduction of new medicines at health economy or trust level is the medicines formulary.

Formularies

In the 2007 review of acute trusts medicines management systems, 88% of trusts reported they had a formulary – a published list of preferred medicines to be used within the organisation.[1] A view many hospitals take is that prescribing information is contained in the *British National Formulary*, and the purpose of a local formulary is to inform the prescribing doctor what medicines are available for prescription within the organisation or health economy. Historically, formularies have been applied to junior doctors, whereas consultants have been allowed to prescribe outside this restricted list. However, with increased management control, rising drug expenditure and the advent of clinical governance, some hospital formularies have been applied rigorously to all grades of staff, including consultants.[12] Clearly, when implementing such a policy it is necessary to make arrangements for the exceptional clinical situation, since a limited range of medicines may not be sufficient to cover every clinical situation.

Deciding the content of the formulary is usually the responsibility of the hospital drug and therapeutics or medicines management committee. It is important that such decisions are evidence-based and transparent if the formulary is to improve prescribing and be owned by prescribers. When considering the evidence for new medicines, a number of questions need to be addressed:

- What is the safety profile of the medicine?
- Is it better or worse than existing medicines?

Clearly, an application would fail if the new medicine had significantly more side-effects than the current standard treatment unless there were exceptionally large benefits. Therefore, newer 'black triangle' medicines may require a more cautious approach.

In addition:

- What is the efficacy of the new medicine?
- Are there any advantages over what is already available? Often benefits are marginal and need to be balanced against cost.

Finally:

* What are the financial implications of the new medicine to the organisation or health economy?

Hospitals must consider the cost to primary care if treatment is to be continued. In particular 'loss-leading' should be avoided, where a pharmaceutical company sets the price in hospital artificially low in order to get a drug used, whereas the drug is very expensive in primary care.

One way of ensuring both primary and secondary care issues are considered when making formulary decisions is to have a joint hospital–primary care formulary covering a whole health economy.

In order to inform formulary decisions, the published evidence about the new medicine should be reviewed by someone with critical appraisal skills. This is often a medicines information pharmacist or, in larger hospitals, a dedicated formulary pharmacist.

Formularies are an effective way of controlling the introduction of new medicines in hospital, because the hospital pharmacy controls the medicines supply chain. However, in primary care, formularies can only be advisory, since the suppliers (the community pharmacy) are independent contractors. PCTs use a variety of methods to encourage compliance with formularies. These can include PCT medicines management teams amending practice computer systems, and prescribing targets in the GP quality outcomes framework scheme.

The Healthcare Commission recommended that formularies be linked to evidence-based guidelines.[1]

Medicines management committees

Drug and therapeutic (D&T) committees have been established in most hospitals in the UK for many years.[13] Their role in facilitating the development of formularies was endorsed in the Department of Health circular, HC (88)54, issued in the late 1980s.[9] In a survey of hospitals in 1994, 97% indicated they had a D&T committee.[14] More recently, in the Healthcare Commission's review of acute hospitals medicines management, all trusts reported they had such a committee.[1] D&T committees or, as a number are now called, medicines management committees are a multidisciplinary group reporting to the chief executive, medical director or management board and their remit is to look at prescribing issues in the trust. Table 11.1 shows the range of activities reported by D&T committees.

D&T committees have played an important role in controlling the introduction of new medicines and managing medicines policies in hospitals for over 30 years. However, with the establishment of PCTs in 2002, and more recently their changing role as commissioners of services, it has become clear that there needs to be a joined-up approach to effective

Table 11.1 Activities at drug and therapeutic (D&T) committees[33]

Activity	% D&Ts undertaking
Evaluating medicines	over 90%
Developing medicines policy	circa 90%
Reviewing treatment guidelines	85–90%
Considering financial effectiveness of medicines	80–85%
Overseeing errors and incidents	75–80%
Medicines risk management analysis	circa 75%
Medication alerts	circa 70%
Medicines spend versus budget	65–70%
Training for medicines for staff groups	50–55%
Implementation and training on new medicines	50–55%

medicines management across health economies. This can be effectively achieved through area prescribing committees, either undertaking the role of individual organisations committees or as an umbrella committee into which the various organisations committees feed, and which takes the final decision on health economy formulary. The latter is more likely, since within a health economy there may be a mixture of acute, mental health and social care trusts. Furthermore, the establishment of clinical networks, particularly cancer networks, which have their own therapeutics committees, adds to the potential plethora of decision-making committees around medicines, and requires overall coordination, particularly in relation to formulary decisions.

Funding new medicines

A further complication in managing the introduction of new medicines into a hospital, and ultimately a health economy, is the development of PCTs as commissioners of health services and the NHS tariff system (Chapter 1 discusses the payment by results system). The tariff has various prices within it for particular treatments depending on whether there are complications and varying lengths of stay. Table 11.2 is an example of the 2008–2009 tariff payments for respiratory-related treatments. Usually the tariff payment includes the cost of medicines used; the hospital is expected to fund the medicines treatment from the tariff payments it receives.

Medicines budgets in most hospitals have been devolved to clinical directorates so applications for the introduction of new medicines from consultants

Table 11.2 Extract from payment by results tariff with costs per stay

HRG code	HRG name	Elective spell tariff (£)	Non-elective spell tariff (£)
D21	Asthma w cc	2280	1875
D22	Asthma w/o cc	1108	1166
D23	Pleural effusion w cc	2500	3189
D24	Pleural effusion w/o cc	2159	2434
D25	Respiratory neoplasms	1118	3003
D31	Sleep-disordered breathing	628	1630
D33	Other respiratory diagnoses >69 or w cc	1493	1670
D34	Other respiratory diagnoses <70 w/o cc	1498	890
D37	Pulmonary oedema	2203	2137
D39	Chronic obstructive pulmonary disease or bronchitis w cc	1546	2360
D40	Chronic obstructive pulmonary disease or bronchitis w/o cc	609	1752
D41	Unspecified acute lower respiratory infection	2005	2059
D42	Bronchopneumonia w cc	3443	3340
D43	Bronchopneumonia w/o cc	2121	2058

HRG, health resource group; w, with; w/o, without; cc, complications and comorbidities.

usually require financial sign-off by the directorate management team supporting the application. The process is further complicated by medicines excluded from tariff. Medicines excluded from tariff are expensive medicines whose cost is not covered by the tariff income. In these cases PCTs pay for these excluded medicines separately. The mechanism varies between different health economies, but often involves recharging the cost to the patient's PCT. Therefore, an application for funding to the PCT, usually through the hospital contracting and commissioning system, has to be made for formulary applications involving these medicines. For hospitals that are tertiary referral centres, such as cancer centres, the patient's PCT may not be the local host PCT, adding a further complication to the process. Figure 11.2 illustrates the medicines management process in the author's health economy showing how complex the process can be if all stakeholders are to be involved.

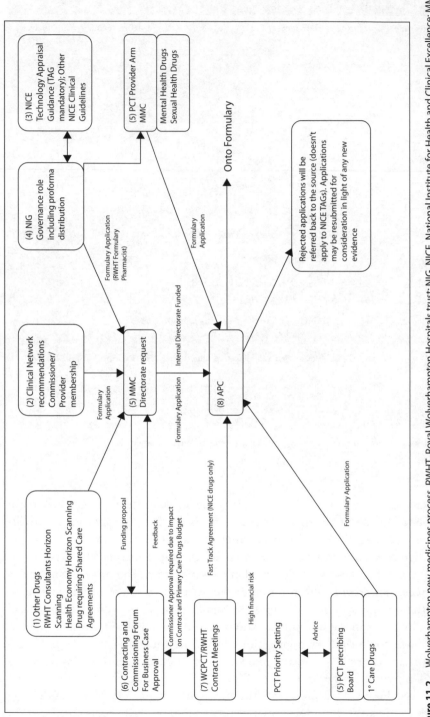

Figure 11.2 Wolverhampton new medicines process. RWHT, Royal Wolverhampton Hospitals trust; NIG, NICE, National Institute for Health and Clinical Excellence; MMC, medicines management committee; PCT, primary care trust; WCPCT, Wolverhampton City primary care trust; APC, area prescribing committee.

Prescribing policies and guidelines

National guidance

At a national level the most authoritative guidance is that issued by NICE.

Prior to 1999, hospitals had discretion as to which new medicines were prescribed there. If funding a new medicine was problematic, decisions were taken in conjunction with the district health authority. This resulted in variations in availability of new medicines across the whole NHS – so-called postcode prescribing. NICE was established in 1999 with the explicit remit of eliminating postcode prescribing.

The terms of reference for NICE were:

- to reduce inequalities in treatment
- to produce evidence-based guidance on treatments
- to identify new developments which will most improve patient care
- to help protect patients from outdated and inefficient treatments. With respect to medicines, there are two key types of NICE guidance: clinical guidelines and technology appraisals.

Clinical guidelines are recommendations by NICE on the appropriate treatment and care of people with specific disease conditions. The guidelines are based on the best available evidence but it is recognised that these are guidelines and cannot replace the health professional's knowledge and skill being applied to specific patients.

Technology appraisals are recommendations on the use of new and existing medicines and treatments within the NHS; for medicines they usually focus on one or a small group of medicines. The recommendations are based on NICE's review of clinical and economic evidence. Unlike clinical guidelines there is a statutory obligation (in England) for medicines supported by a technology appraisal to be funded via the NHS.

Whilst NICE guidelines and technology appraisals are based on critical review of clinical and economic evidence, they also take into account the views of stakeholders, including patient groups and the pharmaceutical industry.

NICE outputs are aimed at the NHS in England and Wales, though they are accessed much more widely. In Scotland, the Scottish Medicines Consortium provides guidance on medicines that may be used. Its remit is to provide advice to NHS boards and their D&T committees about the status of all newly licensed medicines, all new formulations of existing medicines and new indications for established products.[15] The All Wales Strategy Group undertakes a similar role.

There are other types of national guidelines produced by Royal Colleges and organisations such as the Scottish Intercollegiate Guidelines Network. The NHS Health Information Resources (formerly the National Library for Health) provides a single portal for accessing these guidelines through its website (www.library.nhs.uk). Searching by disease on the guidance section of the website, various guidelines can be accessed through hyperlinks to the appropriate guideline producer.

At a more local level, guidelines can take a variety of forms such as complete care pathways designed around a particular disease state and include instructions on the use of medicines. The advantage is that the prescribing message is an integral part of the care pathway the doctor will be using rather than a separate guideline.

A good example of this is the West Mercia guidelines that have been developed by a consortium of hospitals in the West Midlands and North West of England.[16] The guidelines are then individualised by each hospital (for example, to complement local formularies). These guidelines take the practitioner through the whole treatment of a particular event, including diagnostic tests and medicines to be used. Other guidelines focus mainly on the use of medicines.

The most widely used example of local guidelines focusing on the medicines is antibiotic guidelines. The emergence of resistance to antibiotics first gained national attention in the UK with the publication of the House of Lords inquiry.[17] This was followed by the Standing Medical Advisory Committee report[18] and the Department of Health document *Getting Ahead of the Curve*.[19] The latter resulted in the Department of Health allocating £12 million to establish antibiotic pharmacists within hospitals in England, as discussed in Chapter 9. The need for such posts has been further strengthened by the association of certain antibiotics with *Clostridium difficile*-associated diarrhoea (CDAD).[20] Antibiotic guidelines are a tool that is central to this area of work, which can take a variety of forms, but need to be readily accessible, and in a form that can be easily understood. Leeds teaching hospitals have developed a web-based set of antimicrobial guidelines that can be searched by body system.[21]

Monitoring and feedback on medicines use

Clearly, if senior management is to be aware of prescribing issues, there needs to be a robust system for collating and reporting information on medicines usage. All hospital pharmacies have computerised stock control systems for medicines. These systems have been designed around purchasing and stock control, and not producing prescribing reports. However, the main suppliers of these systems have built in reporting modules in newer versions, although the ease of reporting varies from system to system. Prescribing reports can be used for a variety of purposes. The most common is providing feedback to clinical directorates on medicines use and expenditure for budget management purposes. Most hospitals are managed on a directorate structure, whereby wards or clinical specialties are grouped together as a clinical directorate, with their own budget and management team. The directorate usually has a clinician as clinical director who is supported by a manager, financial accountant and human resources manager. In large hospitals, these clinical directorates may be grouped into clinical divisions (that is, medicine, surgery, and so on) that are directly accountable to and represented on trust management boards. A survey published in 1997 indicated that 77% of drug budgets were devolved to clinical directorates.[14] The Audit Commission in its review of acute hospitals medicines management systems showed that 21% of trusts managed the drug budget at directorate level, 27% at specialty level and 45% at ward/consultant level, with only 6% managing the budget at trust level.[3] In the same review 96% of budget-holders received medicines budget reports. In many hospitals these reports are supported by directorate pharmacists, a concept which was established over a decade ago.[22,23] These pharmacists are employed by the pharmacy to provide prescribing advice at clinical directorate level.

In the author's own trust directorate pharmacists present prescribing reports to their clinical directorates, usually at directorate governance meetings. These reports address not only financial issues but also clinical issues and prescribing initiatives either specific for the directorate or across the trust. More recently we have introduced a system where common prescribing errors picked up by clinical pharmacists on the wards are fed back to clinical teams as a learning exercise. This non-blame approach has resulted in a reduction in prescribing errors.[24]

Since much of the work at directorate level involves reviewing medicines usage data and producing graphical representation of prescribing trends, pharmacy technicians are now being employed to support directorate pharmacists.[25]

Medicines management reports are also produced for trust level committees. In view of the increased interest in antibiotic use, particularly as a relationship has been established that antibiotics predispose patients to develop CDAD, antibiotic-prescribing reports are presented regularly to the trust's infection prevention group.[20]

Although monitoring of medicines use has a long history in hospitals, there is no national comparison of hospital prescribing similar to the system which exists in primary care using practice detailed prescribing information data, previously called PACT data. This is detailed information on an individual primary care practice prescribing patterns, and allows PCTs to compare practice prescribing patterns to PCT and national patterns.

A project was initiated over a decade ago by the National Prescribing Centre (NPC) to undertake comparison of hospital prescribing patterns. This aimed to collect detailed prescribing information routinely from a cohort of hospitals.[26] The results of this pilot project showed some interesting trends, but it proved impossible to roll out across the whole of the NHS because there are a variety of commercial pharmacy systems being used with no common identifier for medicines. Computerised prescribing linked with electronic patient records will alleviate this problem and provide better information on hospital prescribing patterns, since usage data can be linked to individual patients and diagnosis. More importantly, where computerised prescribing has been implemented, it has delivered significant improvements in the quality of patient care.[27] However, the national information technology project to develop electronic prescribing for hospitals that was aimed to be in place by 2004 has now largely been abandoned, and individual trusts are developing their own solutions.[28] This suggests that the problems identified in the NPC project over a decade ago will still remain.

More recently the concept of comparing medicines use across hospitals has been resurrected. However, the methodology is much different from that adopted by the NPC. In this new initiative the author and colleagues have used existing data sets, such as IMS and PharmEx data, which are already collected routinely from hospital pharmacy computer systems. However, even when data are available, comparing hospitals of different size, activity and case mix is problematic.[29] We are developing tools to compensate for these variables, such as defined daily dose/finished consultant episode and proportionality.[30,31] We have shown that it is possible to support change in hospital medicines use using such comparative data.[32] For example, Figure 11.3 shows use of different formulations of lansoprazole expressed in terms of proportionality to compensate for activity variable in a group of

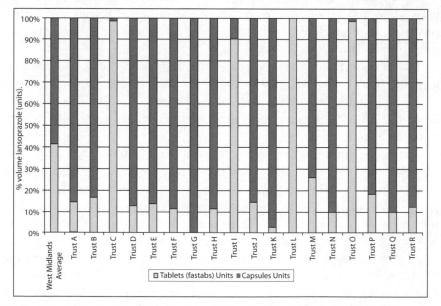

Figure 11.3 Lansoprazole usage across strategic health authority by proportion of tablets to capsules (pre data-sharing).

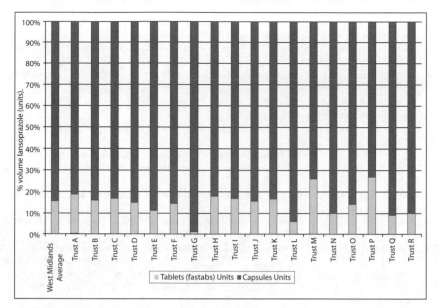

Figure 11.4 Lansoprazole usage across strategic health authority by proportion of tablets to capsules (post data-sharing).

hospitals in one English strategic health authority. Figure 11.4 shows the use in the same cohort of hospitals after an action plan to reduce the use of tablet formulation of lansoprazole was put in place.

Conclusion

Strategic medicines management is essentially about influencing prescribing at a national level, across a health economy and for secondary care at corporate level, within a hospital. There are three key elements to strategic medicines management: (1) managed entry of new medicines; (2) prescribing policies and guidelines; and (3) monitoring and feedback on medicines use. This chapter has described various ways in which these concepts can be implemented in practice. There are many examples in the literature on the various approaches, with increasing levels of sophistication, and evidence of their impact on medicines use in hospital. Medicines play an increasingly important role in all aspects of patient care, particularly in hospital. As these medicines become more complex and patients present more difficult therapeutic challenges, the involvement of the hospital pharmacist will be vital for effective strategic medicines management.

References

1. Healthcare Commission. *The Best Medicine. The Management of Medicines in Acute and Specialist Trusts.* London: Healthcare Commission, 2007.

2. National Reporting and Learning Service. *Safety in Doses. Improving the Use of Medicines in the NHS.* London: National Patient Safety Agency, 2009.
3. Audit Commission. *A Spoonful of Sugar – Medicines Management in NHS Hospitals.* London: Audit Commission, 2001.
4. NHS Information Centre. *Prescriptions Dispensed in the Community, Statistics for 1998 to 2008: England.* Leeds: Health and Social Care Information Centre, 2009.
5. NHS Information Centre. *Hospital Prescribing: England 2009.* Leeds: Health and Social Care Information Centre, 2010.
6. Tredree R. A current perspective on biopharmaceuticals. *Hosp Pharm Europe* 2008; 37: 47–49.
7. Ministry of Health Central Health Services Council, Standing Pharmaceutical Advisory Committee. *Report of the Sub-committee on Hospital Pharmaceutical Services.* London: HMSO, 1955.
8. Nuffield Commision. *Report of the Nuffield Pharmacy Inquiry Committee.* London: Nuffield Foundation, 1986.
9. Department of Health. *Health Services Management: The Way Forward for Hospital Pharmaceutical Services.* HC(88)54. London: HMSO, 1988.
10. Department of Health. *Pharmacy in the Future.* London: The Stationery Office, 2000.
11. Dornan T, Ashcroft T, Heathfield H *et al. An In Depth Investigation into Causes of Prescribing Errors by Foundation Trainees in Relation to their Medical Education.* EQUIP study. Manchester: University of Manchester Medical School Teaching Hospital, 2009.
12. Fitzpatrick RW, Mucklow JC, Fillingham D. A comprehensive system for managing medicines in secondary care. *Pharm J* 2001; 266: 585–588.
13. George C, Hands D. Drug and therapeutic committees and information pharmacy services: the United Kingdom. *World Dev* 1983; 11: 229–236.
14. Fitzpatrick RW. Is there a place for drug and therapeutics committees in the new NHS? *Eur Hosp Pharm* 1997; 3: 143–147.
15. Scottish Medicines Consortium website: http://www.scottishmedicines.org.uk/smc/CCC_FirstPage.jsp.
16. West Mercia Guidelines Partnership. Developing evidence based guidelines for general adult medicine. Presented at The NICE Clinical Excellence – Spreading Good Practice Conference, Harrogate, 1999.
17. House of Lords Science and Technology Committee. *Resistance to Antibiotics and Other Antimicrobial Agents.* London: The Stationery Office, 1998.
18. Standing Medical Advisory Committee Sub-group on Antimicrobial Resistance. *The Path of Least Resistance.* London: The Stationery Office, 1998.
19. Department of Health. *Getting Ahead of the Curve. A Strategy for Combating Infectious Diseases.* London: Department of Health, 2002.
20. Bignardi GE. Risk factors of *Clostridium difficile* infection. *J Hosp Infect* 1998; 40: 1–15.
21. Sandoe J, Howard P. Development of web-based antimicrobial guidelines. *Br J Clin Pharm* 2009; 1: 221–222.
22. Barber N. Improving quality of drug use through hospital directorates. *Qual Healthcare* 1993; 2: 3–4.
23. Ketly D, Godfrey BD. Pharmacy and clinical directorates at Leicester Royal Infirmary. *Pharm J* 1992; 248: 588–589.
24. Reynolds M, Cook N. Engaging junior doctors in patient safety: medication errors. Presented at the Eighth National Conference on Reducing Medication Errors, Manchester, 2010.
25. Edwards L. The role of the directorate liaison technician. *Hosp Pharm* 2000; 8: 115–116.
26. Walker D, Jackson C. Prescribing information in secondary care – the value of a national database? *Pharm J* 2000; 264: 263–265.
27. Ford NG, Curtis C, Paul R. The use of electronic prescribing as part of a system to provide medicines management in secondary care. *Br J Hosp Care* 2000; 17: 26–28.
28. NHS Executive. *Information for Health. An Information Strategy for the Modern NHS 1998–2005.* London: The Stationery Office, 1998.

29. Pate R, Fitzpatrick R. Why we need to compare medicines use in hospitals. *Br J Clin Pharm* 2009; 1: 179–180.
30. Fitzpatrick RW, Edwards CM. Evaluation of a tool to benchmark hospital antibiotic prescribing in the United Kingdom. *Pharmacy World Sci* 2008; 30: 73–78.
31. Fitzpatrick R, Pate R. Comparing the use of inhalational anaesthetics. *Pharm J* 2009; 283: 540–541.
32. Pate R, Fitzpatrick R. Using prescribing activity comparators to change medicines use in secondary care. *Pharm J* 2009; 283: 597–598.

Further reading

National Institute for Health and Clinical Excellence website: http://www.nice.org.uk
National Prescribing Centre website: http://www.npc.co.uk, including guidance on prescribing committees: http://www.npc.co.uk/policy/local/apc_guide.htm.
Pate R, Fitzpatrick R. Using prescribing activity comparators to change medicines use in secondary care. *Pharm J* 2009; 283: 597–598.
Stephens M. *Strategic Medicines Management*. London: Pharmaceutical Press, 2005.

12

Risks with medicines

Gillian Cavell

Pharmacists working in hospitals play a significant role in managing medicines risk. But what is medicines risk?

Risk is defined in a number of ways:

- As a noun, risk is a situation involving exposure to danger, the possibility that something unpleasant will happen and a person or thing causing a risk or regarded in relation to risk.
- As a verb, risk is to expose to danger or loss, to act in such a way as to incur the risk of, and to incur a risk by engaging in an action.[1]

Medicines risk therefore can refer to medicines themselves and to the actions of people handling medicines. Chapter 11 dealt with the financial risks relating to medicines use; this chapter will focus on the risk of harm to the patient. The principles discussed apply throughout the National Health Service (NHS) and beyond, but the organisational context is based on the NHS in England.

Medicines risk

The characteristics of medicines expose people taking those medicines to the risk of adverse drug reactions. There are a number of terms which are used to describe adverse drug reactions and these have been defined by the World Health Organization:

> An adverse drug reaction (ADR) is a response to a medicine which is noxious and unintended, and which occurs at doses normally used in man.[2]

Adverse drug reactions are associated with the way the individual patient responds to the medicine. The patient may exhibit an unexpected or exaggerated response to the medicine which is unpleasant for the patient. Adverse drug reactions may be side-effects. A side-effect is 'any unintended effect of a pharmaceutical product occurring at doses normally used by a patient which is related to the pharmacological properties of the drug'.[3] For example, a patient might experience an unexpectedly large reduction in blood pressure following administration of a licensed dose of an antihypertensive medicine. Such a reaction is related to the pharmacology of the drug.

Sometimes adverse drug reactions are not related to the pharmacology of the drug and are unpredictable. These unexpected adverse reactions are less common than side-effects but have the potential to be more serious. An unexpected adverse reaction is 'an adverse reaction, the nature or severity of which is not consistent with domestic labelling or market authorisation, or expected from characteristics of the drug'.[3] Serious adverse events are those events with the potential for permanent patient harm, including death. A serious adverse event is any event that falls into one of the following categories:

- is fatal
- is life-threatening
- is permanently/significantly disabling
- requires or prolongs hospitalisation
- causes a congenital anomaly
- requires intervention to prevent permanent impairment or damage.

Adverse drug reactions

When a medicine is first licensed and marketed there will be limited information about its side-effects and potential to cause adverse drug reactions. For a medicine to be safe the benefits to the patient of taking the medicine should be greater than the risks of harm to the patient. The marketing authorisation for the drug is granted on the basis of a balance of benefits and risks. Once a drug is used more widely and more doses are taken by patients, more side-effects will become evident, and less common and potentially more serious side-effects will emerge. Table 12.1 provides a classification of adverse drug reactions.

Table 12.1 Classification of adverse drug reactions		
Type A	Augmented	Dose-related
Type B	Bizarre	Non-dose-related
Type C	Chronic	Dose-related and time-related
Type D	Delayed	Time-related
Type E	End of use	Withdrawal
Type F	Failure	Failure of therapy

To protect patients from the risks of medicines a system must be in place to be able to collect information about, and identify trends in, the adverse drug reactions these medicines may cause. Pharmacovigilance is a process for monitoring the use of medicines once they have been licensed for use to ensure information about adverse effects not identified prior to the drug being marketed can be collected and collated. It is also a means of identifying changes in the patterns of adverse effects to drugs already widely used. By understanding these patterns and the frequency of adverse effects, risks and benefits can be assessed to determine whether action needs to be taken to improve their safety, for example, by providing additional information to prescribers and patients about cautions and contraindications. The ultimate aim of pharmacovigilance is to ensure medicines have a positive impact on patients and the risk of harm from those medicines is minimised.

In the UK, the Medicines and Healthcare Products Regulatory Agency (MHRA) is responsible for monitoring medicines safety. It does this by collecting data about the use of medicines from a wide variety of sources, including clinical studies, published medical literature, pharmaceutical companies and from individual case reports submitted to the MHRA as part of a spontaneous reporting system, the Yellow Card scheme.

The Yellow Card scheme is a mechanism by which patients and healthcare professionals can report actual and suspected adverse drug reactions to new and established medicines. The reports are evaluated alongside other information to identify whether any action needs to be taken to minimise the risk and maximise the benefits of the drug to the patient by changing product information, restricting the indications for using the medicine or, in extreme situations, removing the product from the market completely.

Risks with medicines use

In addition to the potential for harm from adverse drug reactions to medicines when used correctly, patients may be harmed as a result of incorrect medicines use.

Awareness of the risks associated with healthcare has risen over the past decade following the publication in 2000 of *To Err is Human* in the USA by the Institute of Medicine.[4] This milestone document acknowledged that healthcare is not as safe as it should be and pointed to medical errors, including medication errors, being a leading cause of death and injury. One of the events which triggered this publication was the death of a *Boston Globe* health reporter from an accidental overdose of chemotherapy.

In England, in 2000 the Department of Health published its own account of patient safety in the NHS. *An Organisation with a Memory* was written by an expert panel, chaired by the chief medical officer.[5] It recognised that serious adverse events had been allowed to recur within the NHS due to a lack of capacity to learn from infrequent but devastating events.

A specific example used to illustrate the problem was the fatal consequence of inadvertent spinal injection of vinca alkaloids intended for intravenous administration in chemotherapy regimens for the treatment of some haematological cancers. Between 1985 and publication of the report, 12 cases of maladministration of intravenous vinca alkaloids were known to have occurred, of which 10 were known to have resulted in either death or paralysis of the patient. The outcomes in the other two were unknown. Despite the known toxicity of vinca alkaloids, and warning labels on products, these preventable errors were being repeated with devastating consequences for patients, their families and the staff involved in their care.

An Organisation with a Memory recommended the establishment of an independent scheme for mandatory reporting of adverse healthcare events and near-misses to which staff could report confidentially. It recommended a single system for analysing and disseminating lessons learnt from these adverse events, making recommendations to improve patient safety and encouraging further reporting. The implementation of these recommendations was described in *Building a Safer NHS for Patients*.[6] Published in 2001, *Building a Safer NHS for Patients*: *Implementing an Organisation with a Memory* further recognised the complexity of healthcare and the risks associated with it. Patient safety was identified as a worldwide problem, and the need to improve safety in healthcare by strengthening systems through capturing data on error and learning from the analysis of incidents was described.

More specifically, the document established the National Patient Safety Agency (NPSA) and listed four key areas that should be the focus for change, two of which specifically referred to the use of medicines. The two targets for medication safety were to:

- reduce to zero the number of patients dying or being paralysed by maladministered spinal injections by the end of 2001
- reduce by 40% the number of serious errors in the use of prescribed drugs by 2005.

The way in which the NHS should work towards achieving these two targets was described in two subsequent documents, *The Prevention of Intrathecal Errors*[7] and *Building a Safer NHS for Patients: Improving Medication Safety*.[8]

The report into the prevention of intrathecal errors described two main strategies for error prevention: (1) human factors, encompassing training and education, ward and pharmacy procedures and policies; and (2) design changes. The concept of design or engineering safety was a new concept in risk management in healthcare at the time. The report highlighted the inherent risk

Table 12.2 High-risk drugs and patient groups highlighted in *Building a Safer NHS for Patients: Improving Medication Safety*[8]

High-risk drugs	Drugs in anaesthetic practice
	Anticoagulants
	Cytotoxic drugs
	Intravenous infusions
	Methotrexate
	Opiate analgesics
	Potassium chloride
High-risk patient groups	People with allergies
	Seriously ill patients
	Children

of misconnection due to the universal use of a Luer connector as a root cause of the error, compounded in some situations by human actions. The themes of root cause analysis (RCA) and design change have since become embedded into the processes for investigating serious adverse events in the NHS.

Building a Safer NHS for Patients: Improving Medication Safety addressed the target of reducing the number of serious errors in the use of prescribed medicines.[8] It described the published literature on medication safety and highlighted the processes, medicines and situations known to be associated with harm. The document recommended actions to be taken by NHS organisations to recognise and reduce these risks, although at the time these had not been accurately quantified. The publication drew attention to drugs known to be harmful and patient groups who were known to be at risk of harm from medicines: Table 12.2 lists these.

Identifying risk

Incident-reporting systems

Risks with medicines are usually identified through incident-reporting systems.

All NHS organisations are required to have incident-reporting systems in place to capture patient safety information, including information on adverse events with medicines. Review of reports submitted to local incident-reporting systems is essential to gain an understanding of the medicines and processes which are prone to error or introduce risk in individual organisations.

Incident reporting is voluntary and relies on recognition of an adverse event, understanding the need to report, knowing how and what to report and willingness to report. Because of these and other factors, such as fear of blame and disciplinary action, there is underreporting to local incident-reporting schemes. Information collected through such schemes is limited but it does provide valuable qualitative information about medication error types. Voluntary reporting schemes cannot be used for quantitative analysis of error frequency or as a measure of the safety of medicine use systems.

Medication errors that have a noticeable clinical impact on a patient and can be attributed to a particular medicine are most likely to be reported as an adverse incident. Investigation of these incidents is usually carried out locally within the organisation by a multidisciplinary team to identify root causes and predisposing factors. Steps can then be taken to raise awareness of risks or make changes to eliminate risks.

Because incident reports are completed and submitted by individuals the amount of information they contain varies widely and descriptions may lack sufficient detail to understand fully exactly what events led to the incident. Electronic reporting systems set mandatory fields to be completed but accurate supplementary information is essential to the usefulness of reports. Because of this and other limitations of voluntary incident-reporting systems, proactive methods of identifying risks are useful.

The NPSA and the National Reporting and Learning System aggregate incident reports from NHS organisations in England and Wales to identify themes and trends. Centralisation of data increases the opportunity for the NHS to recognise recurring themes and identify rare but serious untoward events and issue guidance to NHS organisations to take action to prevent patient harm.

The NPSA issues patient safety alerts, rapid response reports and signals to NHS organisations detailing these actions and giving deadlines before which recommendations should be implemented.

Trigger tools

Triggers are used as a proactive tool for identifying adverse drug events. Triggers can be changes in a patient's clinical condition, an abnormal laboratory test or a prescription for a drug which might prompt investigation into a medicine-related cause of the event. Medicines which might be triggers for adverse drug events include vitamin K to reverse overanticoagulation in patients receiving warfarin, glucagon for insulin-induced hypoglycaemia, naloxone for opioid toxicity and flumazenil for oversedation with benzodiazepines. Pharmacists should be prompted to investigate the reason why trigger drugs are prescribed and report any adverse drug reactions or medication errors identified. Similarly, abnormal laboratory results may indicate medication-related problems. Elevated serum potassium levels may indicate inappropriate use of potassium-sparing diuretics and rapid falls in haemoglobin may indicate gastrointestinal bleeding in a patient receiving non-steroidal anti-inflammatory medicines. Pharmacists can use triggers to identify risks with medicines proactively, prevent patient harm by contributing to changes in medication regimens and report adverse incidents.

Triggers are used in the Patient Safety First campaign to measure the incidence of patient safety incidents, including medication incidents.[9]

Tools for investigating and managing medicines risk

Root cause analysis

RCA is the tool that is most commonly used to identify underlying reasons for an adverse event. RCA aims to find out what happened, why it happened and what will prevent it from happening again.

Evidence provided by individuals involved in the incident allows contributory factors to be identified and used in error prevention strategies. RCA is a relatively simple process, although it may be complicated by the complexity of the issue or the number of personnel involved. Success depends on the clarity of information provided and presented, the generation of practical and feasible recommendations and ensuring that actions taken to prevent future similar events are the correct ones. Ideally RCA should remove the temptation to jump to conclusions about the reasons for failure and implement an inappropriate intervention. A variety of tools for mapping and analysing information gathered during an incident and for generating solutions are available. Some of these are listed in Table 12.3. The NPSA has published a toolkit describing these in more detail.[10]

Table 12.3 Tools for root cause analysis	
Narrative chronology	Chronological account of what happened
Timelines	Used for mapping and tracking a sequence of events in an incident
Time–person grids	Used to map the involvement and movement of multiple people involved in an incident
Tabular timelines	Used to incorporate additional information, such as good practice and care delivery problems, into the timeline
Brainstorming	Unstructured or structured way of generating ideas for analysis or generating possible solutions
Brainwriting	Similar to brainstorming, but ideas generated are written down instead of being spoken, and are therefore anonymous
Nominal group technique	A tool for building consensus within a group
Change analysis	Used to determine what changed, resulting in the failure of a previously functioning process
Barrier analysis	Used proactively or retrospectively to identify barriers which have failed or need to be put in place
Five whys	A questioning tool to ensure the root cause is identified

Failure mode and effects analysis

Whereas RCA is a tool used to analyse retrospectively incidents to identify a cause, failure modes and effects analysis (FMEA) is used to identify risks in systems before they fail and potentially result in an incident. It can be used to predict the risks associated with systems already in place and also to predict the risks associated with potential solutions while they are still in consideration, to ensure that the solution is going to have the desired outcome and not introduce new risks.

FMEA is usually conducted by a multidisciplinary group, ensuring that the views of all disciplines involved in a process are considered. The process is mapped and the potential failures at the stages of the process under scrutiny are described. The failures are scored according to the probability of occurrence (O), the severity of the outcome if the failure reached the patient (S) and the likelihood that the failure would be detected before it reached the patient (D). A failure or an error very likely to happen, unlikely to be detected and likely to harm the patient would attract a high score. The aims of risk reduction strategies are to reduce the risk score of any given stage of the process. Barriers to failure can be proposed to reduce risks. However, new risks associated with risk reduction strategies must also be scored to ensure that overall a safer system is developed.

Barriers to error

Barriers are defences and controls that are in place to increase the safety of a system. Barriers usually fall into one of four types:

1   physical barriers
2   natural barriers
3   human action barriers
4   administrative barriers.

Physical barriers are the most effective and may even be failsafe, eliminating all possibility of error. Human action barriers and administrative barriers are the least reliable. In healthcare, human and administrative barriers are heavily relied on as solutions to problems. However, these barriers are weak and, wherever possible, should only be considered alongside more robust solutions to problems. Table 12.4 gives examples of types of barriers in recommendations made by the NPSA to reduce risks with specific aspects of medicines use.

Quality improvement programmes for managing medicines risk

A number of quality improvement programmes which include medicines risk have developed within the NHS:

Table 12.4 Examples of barriers to error proposed by the National Patient Safety Agency (NPSA) to promote safe medicines use

NPSA recommendation	Barrier type	Condition
All oral anticancer medicines should be prescribed only in the context of a written protocol and treatment plan (http://www.nrls.npsa.nhs.uk/)	Administrative barrier	Relies on knowledge of the protocol and decision to follow it
Use clearly labelled epidural administration sets and catheters that distinguish them from those used for intravenous and other routes (http://www.nrls.npsa.nhs.uk/)	Human action barrier	Relies on the correct devices being used and labelled correctly
Standard ready-to-use heparin 1000 units/ml should be used (http://www.nrls.npsa.nhs.uk/)	Physical barrier	Other concentrations of heparin are not available
There should be judicious use of colour and design on the label, outer packaging and delivery bags to differentiate further minibags containing vinca alkaloids from other minibag infusions (http://www.nrls.npsa.nhs.uk/)	Natural barrier	Infusions of vinca alkaloids are separated from other cytotoxic infusions

Patient Safety First campaign

The vision of the Patient Safety First campaign is 'no avoidable death and no avoidable harm'.[9] The campaign, which, at the time of writing, is sponsored by the NPSA, the NHS Institute for Innovation and Improvement and the Health Foundation, focuses on five interventions, one of which is reducing harm from high-risk medicines: anticoagulants, opiates, injectable sedatives and insulin. Organisations signing up to Patient Safety First are expected to develop and implement improvement programmes specifically designed to reduce the risk of harm from these high-risk medicines by making changes at organisational, clinical area and patient level. The campaign provides participants with tools to support the design of improvement programmes. Suggestions are made for monitoring the outcomes of strategies implemented and organisations are invited to share their successes with other participants. It is not clear how this programme will continue following the 2010 arm's-length body review.

Never events

In 2009 the NHS published a list of never events (http://www.nrls.npsa.nhs.uk). Never events are serious, largely preventable patient safety incidents that should not occur if the available preventive measures have been implemented. At the time of writing, the core list of never events includes two that relate to medicines use:

1   wrong route administration of chemotherapy
2   intravenous administration of misselected concentrated potassium chloride

Both of these aspects of medicines use have been covered by national guidance to minimise the risk of error and incidents can be used as a marker of the quality and effectiveness of risk management systems that have been implemented within organisations. Trusts are obliged to record and report information on these incidents to commissioners, and from 2010–2011 national service contracts will include a financial penalty against organisations involved in a never event.[11] If an organisation is involved in a never event, commissioners will be entitled to recover the cost of the patient's procedure and any care subsequent to the event, introducing a financial incentive to ensure risks, including risks with medicines, are managed. Primary care trusts are also required to monitor the occurrence of never events within the services they commission and publicly report them on an annual basis. It is likely that the never event list relating to medicines will be extended.

NHS Litigation Authority risk management standards

The NHS Litigation Authority sets a risk management programme to reduce the number of negligent or preventable incidents. NHS organisations are regularly assessed against a series of standards that have been developed to reflect the types of issues that arise in claims to the NHS Litigation Authority. Trusts are given incentives to achieve compliance with the standards set in the form of reductions in the financial contributions they make to the schemes Clinical Negligence Scheme for Trusts and Risk Pooling Scheme for Trusts. Standards for hospitals are defined in the NHS Litigation Authority risk management standards for acute trusts, primary care trusts and independent sector providers of NHS care. Standards that specifically relate to medicines management are included and require organisations to have an approved documented process for managing the risks associated with medicines in all care environments that are implemented and monitored. Pharmacists make a significant contribution to the development of policies for the safe use of medicines and play a role in auditing and monitoring the impact of such policies. They therefore play a key role in supporting organisations to achieve the standards of high-quality organisations.

Conclusion

The pharmacy team has a vital role in ensuring medicines are used safely. The role of the chief pharmacist in hospitals was highlighted in the 2008 pharmacy White Paper – having a responsibility for ensuring safe medicines practice is embedded into patient care.[12] Clearly, this is in collaboration with medical, nursing and general management staff. Pharmacists must ensure they understand their role and are equipped to fulfil it.

References

1. Oxford dictionary online: http://oxforddictionaries.com/definition/risk.
2. World Health Organization. Safety of medicines. A guide to detecting and reporting adverse drug reactions. Available online at: http://whqlibdoc.who.int/hq/2002/WHO_EDM_QSM_2002.2. pdf.
3. Edwards I, Aronson J. Adverse drug reactions: definitions, diagnosis and management. *Lancet* 2000; 356: 1255–1259.
4. Institute of Medicine. *To Err is Human: Building a Safe Health System*. Washington: Institute of Medicine, 2000.
5. Department of Health. *An Organisation with a Memory*. London: The Stationery Office, 2000.
6. Department of Health. *Building a Safer NHS for Patients*. London: The Stationery Office, 2001.
7. Department of Health. *The Prevention of Intrathecal Medication Errors: A Report to the Chief Medical Officer*. London: The Stationery Office, 2001.
8. Department of Health. *Building a Safer NHS for Patients: Improving Medication Safety*. London: Department of Health, 2004.
9. Patient Safety First website: http://www.patientsafetyfirst.nhs.uk/content.aspx?path=/.
10. National Patient Safety Agency. Root cause analysis toolkit. Available online at: http://www.nrls.npsa.nhs.uk/resources/?entryid45=59901.
11. National Patient Safety Agency. *Never Events Framework – Update for 2010–11*. London: NPSA, 2010.
12. Department of Health. *Pharmacy in England. Building on Strengths – Delivering the Future*. London: Department of Health, 2008.

Further reading

Department of Health. *Building a Safer NHS for Patients: Improving Medication Safety*. London: Department of Health, 2004.

National Patient Safety Agency website: http://www.npsa.nhs.uk, including their reports on medication errors – Safety in doses – improving the use of medicines in the NHS, 2009.

Royal Pharmaceutical Society of Great Britain. The contribution of pharmacy to making Britain a safer place to take medicines. Available online at: http://eprints.pharmacy.ac.uk/1184/1/Pharmacysafer.pdf.

13

Mental health pharmacy

David Branford

Introduction

Mental illnesses are common and vary from those that have a severe impact on the person throughout his or her life to those of a more minor nature. What sets mental illnesses apart is the societal impact of these illnesses. Changing views about whether or not such illnesses should be managed within a separate setting or be seen as the same as other illnesses or diseases has affected both the development of mental health services generally and mental health pharmacy specifically. It is important to note that learning disability (LD) is different from mental illness, although there are areas of commonality. Historically, the two have been linked in that similar institutions were created to house people with LD and much of the medical care for LD is provided by psychiatrists. The pharmacy services were often the same.

Throughout the UK mental health pharmacy services vary greatly from area to area. This chapter provides an overview of mental health pharmacy and explains how such variety has occurred, including the historical perspective and the important impact of the service.

An early history of mental hospitals

This section sets out a brief historical perspective: for a more detailed account of early history of mental illness and LD, readers are referred to the mental health history timeline.[1] From ancient times both mental illness and LD were associated with evil and people suffering them were excluded from normal society. Even Socrates is reported to have stated that they should be 'put away in some mysterious place'. In England the first records of a specific place for 'lunatics' was the religious priory of St Mary of Bethlem in the 14th century. The Elizabethan *Poor Law Acts* required every parish to appoint overseers for the poor and set up parish houses for poor people who could not support themselves. After this period these remained the places where the mentally ill were housed. In the 18th century facilities for the mentally ill were generally of a very poor standard, although some were designed so that the 'lunatics' could be displayed for visitors. Many 'madhouses' were run as private facilities and housed between 50 and 400 'inmates'.

Following the attempted assassination in 1800 of George III by James Hadfield (who was deemed to be insane), the mental illness of George III himself and the passing of the *County Asylums Act* in 1808, the 19th century witnessed a large expansion of public asylums and the movement of the mentally ill from poorhouses to specific institutions. Although these institutions were originally designed to offer hope and better facilities for the mentally ill, by the late 19th century the beliefs associated with social darwinism (that insanity is the end-product of an incurable degenerative disease) saw them becoming social backwaters. Throughout this period, the powers enabled by the 1890 *Lunacy Act* led to huge expansion of the grounds for confinement of any person regarded to be 'lunatic, idiot or of unsound mind'.

By the 1930s there were 98 mental hospitals housing 110 000 patients in England and Wales. They varied in size, with the average number of patients over 1000. By the 1950s the concepts that had shaped the pre-war policy were no longer acceptable and the 1946 *Mental Health Service Act* defined a hospital as including institutions that were for 'the reception and treatment of persons suffering from illness or mental defectiveness'.

Much of the modern development of mental health services results from the 1959 *Mental Health Act*.[2] It provided for admission to mental hospitals to be on an informal basis wherever possible and made councils responsible for the social care of people who did not need inpatient treatment.

For much of the early history, people with LD suffered a similar fate to those with mental illnesses. However, by the early part of the 20th century separate institutions had been established that accommodated both children and adults with mental disabilities. The institutional model remained until the late 1960s when a series of investigations shone a light on the conditions in many 'mental handicap' hospitals. The findings of these scandals led to a policy change, later published in *Better Services for the Mentally Handicapped*, which expressed the intention to close all such institutions and move towards a community-based model.[3]

Early mental health and learning disability pharmacy

It is unclear at what stage the mental hospitals and LD institutions began to employ pharmacists. Although treatments such as insulin shock and medicines such as paraldehyde, barbiturates and bromides were popular before the 1950s, it is likely that any requirements for medicines were managed, in the main, by nurses. The therapeutic revolution following the introduction of chlorpromazine in the late 1940s increased the requirements for a wide range of medicines. However, the isolated nature of the institutions and social attitudes towards mental illness and LD resulted in such employment being unappealing. Typically, such dispensaries were situated between the segregated male and female parts of the institutions and the medicines passed through separate hatches so as to minimise the requirements for crossing sectors or for contact between patients and dispensary staff. Despite these problems there were examples of well-developed pharmacy services, for example, Central Hospital, Warwick.

Changes in the approach to mental illness

The fundamental underpinning themes of the Royal Commission[4] that led to the 1959 *Mental Health Act* were:

- that mental disorders should be regarded in much the same way as physical illness and disability
- that hospitals for mental illness should be run as nearly as possible like those for physical disorders.

These themes were further developed in the 1960s with the development of 'community care'. The main features of the policy were:

- that hospital treatment should be in psychiatric units in district general hospitals
- that as much care and treatment as possible should be provided outside hospitals.

The development of mental health wards in the middle of general medical wards proved problematic, and the approach is now to situate such wards on the periphery of the district general hospital site or on a dedicated site. This last theme has been the focus of much recent policy development, firstly with the development of community mental health teams to support patients in the community and, more recently, with the publication of the *National Service Framework for Mental Health*, the establishment of crisis intervention and home treatment teams.[5] These teams are designed to obviate, wherever possible, the need to admit people in crisis and, if admission if required, to expedite their discharge from hospital.

Mental health law

One key difference between mental health and other aspects of healthcare is the ability to detain patients against their will using the *Mental Health Act*.

The 1959 *Mental Health Act* provided for patients to be treated informally but did not provide clarity about the powers to impose medical treatment against a person's wish. The 1983 *Mental Health Act*[6] did place legal controls on the applications of treatments, particularly psychosurgery, electroconvulsive therapy and mood-altering drugs. It also moved the responsibility for formal admission to hospital into the hands of approved social workers and psychiatrists.

The 1983 *Act* provides for people to be detained for treatment using a variety of schedules:

- to be detained for assessment (schedule 2)
- to be detained for treatment (schedule 3)
- to be transferred from prison to hospital for treatment (section 37).

The 1983 *Act* also provided the first opportunity for patients detained under the *Act* to have a say in their drug treatment. Section 57, more commonly called the *'Consent to Treatment' regulations*, provides an opportunity to review the continuing requirement for the medicines after 3 months of detention.[6]

Inevitably any mental health *Act* is a compromise between the tensions identified in Table 13.1.

Table 13.1 Philosophical tensions associated with treatments in mental health

Philosophical tension 1

General freedoms	General restrictions
People with mental health problems should have the same opportunities as everybody else to live a normal life: • Normal relationships • Normal domestic life • Normal employment	People with mental health problems need to be protected from self-harm and the persecution of others Society needs to be protected from people with insane and antisocial behaviour

Philosophical tension 2

Freedoms associated with medicines	Restrictions associated with medicines
Patients have the right to stop taking their medicines once discharged if they do not feel they are necessary Safeguards need to be in place to ensure that patients only receive necessary medicines Safeguards need to be in place to ensure that treatments that cause them harm are not imposed Medicines are prescribed within agreed guidelines Patients and their representatives have a choice about whether to receive medicines and the medicines chosen Medicines are not used as a form of social control	Prescribers need to have the freedom to prescribe medicines that they feel may benefit the patient, even if the patient does not agree Medicine administration should be enforced when the patient is deemed as mentally unwell and meets the criteria for detention Society has the right to insist that mentally ill people who pose a danger to themselves or others if they stop taking their medicines can be recalled to hospital care and treatment implemented without their consent

Between 1999 and 2006 there was an extensive review of the *Mental Health Act 1983* and attempts to develop a new *Act*. One major change in the 2007 *Amendment Act*[7] was the power to detain and treat patients while discharged into the community; this is via the community treatment order.[8, 9]

Mental capacity and deprivation of liberty

During the 2000s, in addition to the changes to the *Mental Health Act 1983* to form the *Mental Health Act Amendment Act 2007*, there were two other pieces of legislation of key importance to both mental health and LD: the *Mental Capacity Act* and the *Deprivation of Liberty Safeguards*. Both have an impact on the authority to give medicines.[10–12]

The *Mental Capacity Act 2005*, covering England and Wales, provides a statutory framework for people who lack the capacity to make decisions, or who have capacity and want to make preparations for a time when they may lack capacity in the future.[12] It sets out who can take decisions, in which situations and how they should go about this.

The underlying philosophy of the *Act* is to ensure that any decision made, or action taken, on behalf of someone who lacks the capacity to make the decision or act for themselves is made in their best interests.

The five statutory principles of the Act are:

1   A person must be assumed to have capacity unless it is established that they lack capacity.
2   A person is not to be treated as unable to make a decision unless all practicable steps to help them to do so have been taken without success.
3   A person is not to be treated as unable to make a decision merely because they make an unwise decision.
4   An act done, or decision made, under this *Act* for or on behalf of a person who lacks capacity must be done, or made, in their best interests.
5   Before the act is done, or the decision is made, regard must be given to whether the purpose for which it is needed can be as effectively achieved in a way that is less restrictive of the person's rights and freedom of action.

The deprivation of liberty safeguards were introduced into the *Mental Capacity Act 2005* by the *Mental Health Act 2007*.[8] The safeguards provide a framework for approving the deprivation of liberty for people who lack the capacity to consent to treatment or care in either a hospital or care home that, in their own best interests, can only be provided in circumstances that amount to a deprivation of liberty. The safeguards legislation contains detailed requirements about when and how deprivation of liberty may be authorised. It provides for an assessment process that must be undertaken before deprivation of liberty may be authorised and detailed arrangements for renewing and challenging the authorisation of deprivation of liberty.

Medicines for mental illness

Medicines are commonly prescribed for people with mental health problems. These comprise the medicines for the mental health problems and, with the greater recognition of associated physical illness, medicines for physical illness. For those with severe mental health problems most will be prescribed mental health medicines for extended periods of time. This long-term, possibly lifelong, need means extended periods under the care of mental health professionals alone, jointly with shared care with a general practitioner (GP) or as discharged solely to the care of a GP. Many mental health medicines take weeks, if not months, to achieve a satisfactory response, although the short-term sedative effects may prove sufficient to allow early discharge of a still largely unwell person back into the community.

Most mental health medicines are associated with an array of side-effects that many patients find unpleasant and possibly unacceptable. In addition, many have only partial effectiveness or are only effective against some aspects of the illness. These factors make choice of medicine a key issue for pharmacists and psychiatrists, with frequent trials of alternatives. This adds to the difficulty in determining the usefulness of the medicines, as assessments are often based on subjective responses and subject to a large number of variables.

The pivotal discoveries in the late 1940s and 1950s that changed mental health medicines were those of the phenothiazine antipsychotics, the tricyclic and monoamine oxidase inhibitor antidepressants and lithium for bipolar illness. Following shortly after was the arrival of the benzodiazepines both as sedatives and hypnotics. For the first time there was an array of medicines truly effective in managing psychosis, mania and depression.

The discovery of chlorpromazine is regarded as the key event that led to the fall in population of the asylums (then almost 150 000) but others claim that the decline had started earlier, following the changes to the 1959 *Mental Health Act*. Whichever explanation, the arrival in the 1970s of the long-acting formulations of antipsychotic drugs showed the development of community psychiatry was well under way.

Throughout the 1970s and 1980s there were few novel medicines in mental health, with most introductions being chemical variations or new formulations of those already available. Many were attempts to reduce the side-effects of the original drugs, make them work quicker or enhance their efficacy. However, the movement disorders (called extrapyramidal side-effects) associated with the antipsychotics and the toxicity of lithium and the antidepressants remained sources of concern. The 1990s saw another wave of developments as research into the mode of action of clozapine caused a change of attention of antipsychotic drug research to the mesolimbic system in the brain and to different receptors. Clozapine does not chronically alter striatal D_2 receptors but does appear to affect them. It also appears to have more effect on the limbic system and on serotonin ($5HT_2$) receptors, which may explain its reduced risk of extrapyramidal symptoms. The term 'atypical' is used to categorise those antipsychotic drugs that, like clozapine, rarely produce extrapyramidal side-effects.

Although the reason for the superiority of clozapine in schizophrenia treatment remains an enigma, a variety of theories have led to the development of a new family of antipsychotic drugs. Some mimic the impact of clozapine on a wide range of dopamine and serotonin receptors, for example olanzapine; others mimic the impact on particular receptors, for example $5HT_2/D_2$ receptor antagonists such as risperidone; others focus on limited occupancy of D_2 receptors, for example quetiapine; while others focus on alternative theories such as partial agonism, for example aripiprazole.

The other revolution to occur in the 1990s was fluoxetine. Although not the first selective serotonin reuptake inhibitor, this antidepressant became the medicine for the masses in the 1990s and rivalled the 1960s' use of the benzodiazepine diazepam in popularity. Throughout the 1990s and 2000s mental health practice saw a wide range of new medicines introduced for bipolar (antiepileptic drugs and antipsychotics), attention deficit hyperactivity disorder (wider use of methylphenidate), Alzheimer's disease (cholinesterase inhibitors), schizophrenia (atypical antipsychotics) and depression (noradrenaline (norepinephrine) and serotonin reuptake inhibitors)

Medicines in learning disabilities

LD is not an illness. It requires the presence of three criteria based on the definition derived from extensive consultation in the USA:[13]

1   a significant developmental intellectual impairment
2   concurrent deficits in social functioning or adaptive behaviour
3   the condition is manifest before the age of 18 years.

Significant LD is usually defined as an intelligence quotient (IQ) more than two standard deviations below the general population mean (originally fixed at 100). This is an IQ below 70 on recognised IQ tests. Two per cent of the population have an IQ below this level. Significant deficits in social functioning are in communication, daily living skills, socialisation and motor skills.[13]

The term 'intellectual disability' is used synonymously with 'learning disability' (the common terminology used in clinical practice in the UK), mental retardation (used in the *International Classification of Illnesses*[14]) and mental handicap (used in the UK until 1994).

People with LD have significantly more health problems than the rest of the population. Around 50% have a major psychiatric or behaviour problem requiring specialist help; 25% have active epilepsy; at least 30% have a sensory impairment; and around 40% have associated major physical disabilities of mobility and incontinence. Most people with LD have communication difficulties and a lack of supported communication may compound their problems in receiving the healthcare that they need. The substantial health needs of this population are often overlooked and unmet.

Biological, environmental and social factors may contribute to the development of LD. Biological factors are present in about 67–75% of people with LD, the majority operating before birth. The two most common genetic causes of LD are Down syndrome and fragile X syndrome. In a third of people with LD, no primary diagnosis can be made.

Medicines are widely prescribed for people with LD. The medicines are broadly prescribed for four problem areas:

1 epilepsy
2 challenging behaviours
3 physical problems
4 mental illness.

In line with the government intention to close all LD institutions and to discourage the development of grouped housing, the management of people with LD has largely been devolved to the private and voluntary sectors. However, many mental health trusts (MHTs) remain responsible for the mental health aspects of care and, in some places, retain treatment beds as well as having community team roles, although such responsibilities are being transferred to local authority care.

Mental health pharmacy changes

By the 1970s the landscape of mental health services was dominated by institutional care. A report undertaken in the late 1970s showed that most mental health pharmacy departments were situated within institutions and much of the workload was associated with providing ward stock to in excess of 1000 beds.[15] The pattern of LD institutions being supplied for by the same mental health pharmacy was common, as was the model of one mental health pharmacy supplying another nearby institution. Such pharmacies were usually poorly staffed (usually just one pharmacist) with high vacancy of posts.

The Noel Hall report for pharmacy recommended that hospital pharmaceutical services be organised on an area basis and for many mental health pharmacies this provided for the first time a managerial link to the rest of hospital pharmacy.[16] However, whilst this managerial change did at first bring great benefits in the reduction of isolation, it resulted in the priorities for the now area pharmaceutical service becoming acute hospital pharmacy rather than focused on mental health and LD. As the model for mental health services changed to that of fewer beds, moving acute wards to district general hospital settings and developing community services, from a hospital pharmacy viewpoint where only bed numbers mattered this was an opportunity to cut and redeploy the available staff.[17]

Throughout the 1980s and much of the 1990s there were few new medicines in mental health and compared to other medical specialties it remained an area of low cost. In an environment of staff shortages of hospital pharmacists, poor understanding of mental health within an acute hospital environment and a continued thrust towards community care, the specialty struggled to survive. Periodic surveys of staffing indicated poor levels of service, provided by staff of low grades, very poor knowledge within hospital pharmacy of mental health and limited development of mental health clinical pharmacy. Finally, with the trend for contracting out it became common for services to mental health hospitals to be put out to tender and to be provided by others, usually via a service level agreement.[18]

By the 1990s the significance of medicines in mental health care and the attitude towards mental health pharmacy began to change. The reintroduction of the antipsychotic drug clozapine (now requiring pharmacy oversight of the necessary monitoring) and other new medicines, as described earlier, focused attention on the escalating costs and demands for pharmacy services. The development of clinical pharmacy training specifically in mental health by the UK Psychiatric Pharmacy Group (UKPPG) and the development, in England, of specialist MHTs all contributed to an awareness of the need to develop specialist mental health pharmacy services. These historical factors in general determine the nature and size of the pharmacy service now available to any MHT.

During the 2000s this focus on mental health pharmacy services led to a number of initiatives, the most significant of which are described below.

The New Ways of Working programme

The Spread Programme demonstrated a wide range of potential impacts on patient care and treatment in mental health that can be achieved by the various grades of pharmacy staff.[19]

Fundamental findings were:

- Schemes that resulted in better access to pharmacy staff for wards/community teams resulted in improved medicines management.
- Any project that placed a pharmacy staff member as a member of the clinical/ward/community team was likely to improve relationships, improve medicines management and lead to better outcomes for service users.

In addition to the Spread programme, a wide range of initiatives were undertaken to improve medicines management in MHTs. The New Ways of Working initiative included a specific programme for pharmacy, with documents developed to support frontline teams.[20]

The mental health pharmacy workforce survey

In 2005 help was enlisted of Bath University and the UKPPG to undertake a mental health pharmacy workforce survey.[21-23] The results showed that MHT pharmacy services vary significantly in size, that most are dependent on other providers for their pharmacy service (only 17% did not use another trust to provide pharmacy services) and that the number of pharmacists employed did not appear to have any rationale, with some very large MHTs employing only one or two per million population served and others employing 15–20.

The Healthcare Commission review of mental health pharmacy

The management of medicines in general hospitals had been a subject of growing interest to the Audit Commission with its publication of the document *A Spoonful of Sugar – Medicines Management in NHS Hospitals*.[24] Much of the learning from the workforce survey highlighted to the Healthcare Commission (now replaced by the Care Quality Commission) the extent to which medicines management and pharmacy had been neglected in mental health care and contributed to its 2007 report *Let's Talk About Medicines*.[25] The document made 46 recommendations relating to how MHTs can maximise the benefits from medicines across 11 broad areas. It placed leadership by a chief pharmacist as a central role.

Other aspects of the New Ways of Working programme

Following publication of the Healthcare Commission document, the Department of Health commissioned a number of follow-up projects to assist MHTs to develop their management of medicines.[26-31]

The UK Psychiatric Pharmacy Group and the College of Mental Health Pharmacy

In 1970, a psychiatric pharmacists association was established. The primary achievements of the association were to carry out a survey of pharmacy in psychiatric hospitals and to establish an annual psychiatric conference. Although the association replaced an informal group of psychiatric pharmacists, it became the organising committee for the annual conference, then later formed the Psychiatric Pharmacy Group, evolving still later into the UKPPG.

In 1989 clozapine was marketed by Sandoz (now Novartis), with a revolutionary pharmacy-managed monitoring scheme. As a part of the agreement Sandoz agreed to fund three or four training courses per year for 100 mental health pharmacists. This training framework proved pivotal in helping to revolutionise the practice of psychiatric pharmacy in the UK.

In March 1993 a joint postgraduate clinical diploma course in mental health was established with De Montfort University and the UKPPG and this then led to the programme of postgraduate courses in mental health pharmacy, now with Aston University. These educational programmes, together with leadership from the UKPPG, changed the landscape for mental health pharmacy, taking it from a clinical backwater to one of the most progressive specialties. In 1999 the UKPPG established the College of Mental Health Pharmacy, one of the first specialties to develop an accreditation scheme for its members.

Pharmacy's contribution

The New Ways of Working initiative is, of course, evidence of pharmacy's contribution to the care and use of medicines of those with mental illness and LD. As described in other chapters, pharmacy focuses on the safe and effective use of medicines and the importance of tailoring regimens to the individual. The evidence base from across pharmacy can be drawn upon, for example for reconciliation on admission, but there are also examples specific to mental illness and LD. Maidment *et al.* identified the errors that occur in mental healthcare.[31] The literature also contains a number of examples of how pharmacists can contribute, but evidence of impact is less common. Finley *et al.*[32] reported a systematic review of pharmacists' impact in mental health in 2003, noting: 'most of the investigations were small, and significant limitations in study design limited further comparison', though they went on to acknowledge the many anecdotal reports of success and urged further trials. Pharmacists working in mental illness and LD do need to help develop the evidence base to ensure pharmacy's contribution with regard to safety and improved outcomes is understood. Consultant pharmacists working in mental illness and LD may have a particularly important role to play in ensuring this happens since, alongside their leadership role, the posts should contain significant elements of research and development. Chapter 18 discusses this in more detail.

Future models for mental health pharmacy

Increasingly, secondary care mental health services are moving towards a brief intervention model with expectation of follow-up in the community by any one of an assortment of community-based teams. For those admitted to crisis teams or acute wards discharge back to more homely settings will be at the first opportunity and with only partial treatment.

As described earlier, full response to treatment may take some time but the sedative effective of medicines may allow early discharge of a still largely unwell person back into the community. Except for the period as an inpatient, the supply of medicines will almost exclusively come from the community pharmacy. Traditionally this supply of medicines has provided a demarcation of responsibility for the pharmacy profession.

However, with the development of clinical pharmacy, the expectation is that the community pharmacist will have a greater clinical responsibility for the medicines provided and the patient with mental health problems may access four services that relate to medicines and where enhanced pharmacy services could have a direct impact on the medicines prescribed. These are:

1   the community pharmacy
2   the GP
3. the community mental health team
4   the acute/crisis services of the MHT or equivalent.

In addition to the current hospital-based services, what might work better is dedicated mental health specialist pharmacists or technicians using one of the following models:

- employed by community pharmacy chains whose role is to achieve the above in liaison with secondary care
- employed by GP practices who, in addition to undertaking roles relating to mental health within the GP practice, develop the role of the community pharmacies that service the practice
- employed by MHT community teams who, in addition to undertaking roles relating to mental health within the community team, develop the role of the community pharmacies that service the team's catchment area.

Whatever model develops, the requirement for well-trained mental health pharmacists and technicians to ensure medicines are used well in mental health and LD and to provide support for patients with their medicines will remain.

References

1. Roberts A. A mental health history timeline. Available online at: http://www.studymore.org.uk/mhhtim.htm.
2. *Mental Health Act 1959*. Available online at: http://www.legislation.gov.uk/ukpga/Eliz2/7-8/72.
3. Department of Health and Social Security. *Better Services for the Mentally Handicapped*. Command paper 010146830X. London: HMSO, 1971.
4. Royal Commission on the law relating to mental illness and mental deficiency. *Modern Law Rev* 1958; 21: 63–68.

5. Department of Health. *National Service Framework for Mental Health: Modern Standards and Service Models.* London: The Stationery Office, 1999.
6. *Mental Health Act 1983.* Available online at: http://www.dh.gov.uk/en/Publicationsandstatistics/Legislation/Actsandbills/DH_4002034.
7. *Amendment Act 2007.* Available online at: http://www.legislation.gov.uk/ukpga/2007/12/contents.
8. Department of Health. *Mental Health Act 2007.* Available online at: http://www.opsi.gov.uk/acts/acts2007/pdf/ukpga_20070012_en.pdf.
9. Department of Health. Code of practice: Mental Health Act 1983. Available online at: http://www.dh.gov.uk/dr_consum_dh/groups/dh_digitalassets/@dh/@en/documents/digitalasset/dh_087073.pdf.
10. Department of Health. Mental Capacity Act 2005: deprivation of liberty safeguards – code of practice to supplement the main Mental Capacity Act 2005 code of practice. Available online at: http://www.tsoshop.co.uk.
11. Department of Health. Code of practice Mental Health Act 1983. Available online at: http://www.tsoshop.co.uk.
12. Public Guardianship Office. The Mental Capacity Act 2005 code of practice. Available online at: http://www.guardianshiop.gsi.gov.uk.
13. American Association on Mental Retardation. *Mental Retardation: Definition, Classification and Systems of Support.* Washington, DC: American Association on Mental Retardation, 1992.
14. World Health Organization. International classification of illnesses. Available online at: http://www.who.int/classifications/icd/en/.
15. Benfield M, Griffiths G, Preskey D. *Pharmacy in Psychiatric Hospitals.* Hampshire: Sandoz Publications, 1981.
16. Hall N, chair. *Report of the Working Party Investigating the Hospital Pharmaceutical Service.* London, HMSO, 1970.
17. Branford D. Pharmacy services to psychiatric hospitals. *Pharm J* 1988; 240: HS 24.
18. Branford D. Hospital pharmaceutical services to people with mental health problems or learning disabilities. *Hosp Pharmacist* 1998; 5: 49–51.
19. Pratt P, Branford D. Learning lessons from the Spread Programme – analysis of key themes. NWW/National Institute for Mental Health for England. Available online at: http://www.newwaysofworking.org.uk.
20. New Ways of Working website: http://www.newwaysofworking.org.uk/content/view/54/465/ (accessed 14 June 2010).
21. Taylor DA, Sutton J. Report on the mental health and learning disabilities pharmacy workforce survey May 2006. University of Bath. Available online at: http://www.newwaysofworking.org.uk.
22. Branford D, Parton G, Taylor D *et al.* Summary and key findings of the report on the mental health and learning disabilities secondary care pharmacy workforce survey. National Institute for Mental Health for England. Available online at: http://www.newwaysofworking.org.uk.
23. Branford D, Parton G, Taylor D *et al.* The UKPPG and CMHP report on the mental health and learning disabilities secondary care pharmacy workforce survey (phase 2). NWW/National Institute for Mental Health for England. Available online at: http://www.newwaysofworking.org.uk.
24. Audit Commission. *A Spoonful of Sugar – Medicines Management in NHS Hospitals.* London: Audit Commission, 2001.
25. Healthcare Commission. Let's talk about medicines – a report on the management of medicines in trusts providing mental health services. London: Healthcare Commission, 2007.
26. Branford D. New ways of working for mental health pharmacists and other pharmacy staff. Available online at: http://www.newwaysofworking.org.uk/content/view/54/465.
27. Improving medicines management by extending the roles of pharmacy technicians in mental health – a briefing document. Available online at: http://www.newwaysofworking.org.uk/content/view/54/465.

28. Guidance on mental health pharmacy service level agreements and contracts, with examples of SLAs and a self assessment framework. Available online at: http://www.newwaysofworking. org.uk/content/view/54/465.
29. Medicines management: everybody's business. A guide for service users, carers and health and social care practitioners. Available online at: http://www.newwaysofworking.org.uk/ content/view/55/466.
30. Mental health medicines management self assessment toolkit. Available online at: http:// www.newwaysofworking.org.uk/content/view/55/466.
31. Maidment I, Lelliot P, Paton C. A systematic review of medication errors in mental health-care. *Qual Safe Healthcare* 2006; 15: 409–413.
32. Finley P, Crismon M, Rush A. Evaluating the impact of pharmacists in mental health: a systematic review. *Pharmacotherapy* 2003; 23: 1634–1644.

Further reading

Healthcare Commission. Let's talk about medicines – a report on the management of medicines in trusts providing mental health services. London: Healthcare Commission, 2007.
Mental health medicines management self-assessment toolkit. Available online at: http://www. newwaysofworking.org.uk/content/view/55/466.
National Institute for Health and Clinical Excellence website for treatment guidelines in mental health: http://www.nice.org.uk.

14

Community health services

Theresa Rutter

Introduction

Understandably, many hospital pharmacy staff are unfamiliar with community health services (CHS), though access to CHS is essential to keep the population healthy (immunisation programmes), to maintain vulnerable people in their own homes and prevent unnecessary admissions to hospital ('virtual wards', community nursing).

Many departments provide services to the community via a contract or service level agreement (SLA) with a local CHS provider; this can include supply, advice and specialist clinical service elements. They may also employ staff who specialise in CHS or the CHS provider organisation may be integrated into a hospital or mental health trust.

Since the first edition of this book there has been divergence in the policies of the UK governments and in the organisation of health services in England, Northern Ireland, Scotland and Wales, as discussed in Chapter 1. However, the national health strategies have much in common, including:

- improving the population's health and preventing ill health
- providing patient-centred care as close to the patient as possible
- moving care outside hospital into community settings.

Examples of this third element are anticoagulant services delivered by general practitioners (GPs) and pharmacists with a special interest and musculoskeletal services delivered by physiotherapists. Each of these developments increases the volume and often the complexity of the care delivered in CHS settings. Alongside this is an increasing emphasis on the quality and safety of services, including optimal use of medicines and better communications across interfaces of care.

This chapter describes CHS and the role of the healthcare professionals who work in CHS. It also describes the support that is provided by pharmacists and pharmacy technicians specialising in this area of practice.

Community health services

These diverse and locally variable services are provided from clinics, health centres, community hospitals, care homes and in patients' own homes. They are an important element in the healthcare of many older people, of people living with disabilities, of families with young children and of people living with long-term conditions. The recipients of CHS are often among the most vulnerable members of the community.

Regardless of the care setting, all patients are entitled to services appropriate to their needs, that are safe, of high quality and operating within legal and clinical governance frameworks.

CHS can broadly be described as:

- services generally delivered outwith GP practices and secondary care by CHS professionals such as community nurses and therapists working from and in community clinics, community hospitals and other community sites
- services that reach across the population such as district nursing, school health, podiatry, sexual health services and specialist nurses
- services that help people back into their own homes from hospital and prevent unnecessary admissions, for example intermediate care, rehabilitation, 'virtual wards' (provision of a ward level of care that supports earlier discharge from or prevents admission to hospital)
- services that help individuals and their carers to maintain and manage ill health or long-term conditions that require support outside GP practices, for example respite care for children with complex medical conditions, end-of-life care
- services provided by specialist services and practitioners, for example, tuberculosis clinics, community dental services and tissue viability nurses
- services that interface with social care, for example, services supporting those with learning disability are often provided via joint health and social care teams.

Table 14.1 provides an example of the range of CHS provided in an urban area.

CHS professionals and their roles

Pharmacy support for CHS staff needs to include access to advice and information, input to the development of policies, procedures, and associated

Table 14.1 Examples of community health services provided in an urban area

Core services usually aligned to GP practices	Services usually provided on a wider, e.g. borough/local authority, basis	Specialist services which are often provided across a larger population
Health visiting	Teams caring for those with a physical disability	Rehabilitation services
District nursing	Consultant community paediatricians	Continence service
Podiatry/chiropody (routine)	Immunisation and vaccination	Homeless and refugee team
Physiotherapy (routine)	Care of the elderly, including community hospitals, outreach teams	Home enteral nutrition team
	Sexual health services, e.g. family planning, community HIV/AIDs	Diabetes resource team
	Specialist community teams, e.g. for learning disability	Tissue viability nurse
	Palliative care and end-of-life care	Interpreting service
	Child protection, working closely with social services	Respite care
	School health	Podiatric surgery
	Speech and language therapy	Infection control

GP, general practitioner; HIV, human immunodeficiency virus; AIDS, acquired immunodeficiency syndrome.

education and training. Information on the medicines that the different professionals can prescribe, supply and/or administer can be found in *Medicines, Ethics and Practice*.[1] A document on the National electronic Library for Medicines explains more fully the training, qualifications and roles of these CHS professionals.[2]

District nurses (also called community nurses)

District nurses (DN) are registered general nurses with a postregistration specialist qualification who provide skilled nursing care to patients, generally within their own homes. DN are located in community clinics or in GP practices. DN are community practitioner nurse prescribers who prescribe from a limited list of medicines providing they have fulfilled the educational requirements. The majority of pharmaceutical items that they use should be obtained on FP10 or private prescription. However, the local policy may be to have a stock supply system for dressings. At the back of the *British National Formulary* there is a list of the medicines they can prescribe. As DN prescribe and administer medicines they need to be able to access pharmacy advice about, for example, product information, stability, routes of administration and support for compliance.

Health visitors

Health visitors (HV) are registered general nurses with a postregistration qualification. Their roles mainly involve health promotion and development of the family, particularly relating to children less than 5 years of age. Some HV specialise in providing services to older people, well-woman groups, smoking cessation and so on. HV are also community practitioner nurse prescribers but as their roles are advisory and educational they tend to prescribe less than DN and have a minimal need for pharmaceutical supplies. HV need to be able to access pharmaceutical advice on topics such as drugs in breast milk, medicines in pregnancy, immunisation, treatment of head lice infection and use of medicines in children and in the elderly.

School nurses

School nurses (SN) are responsible for the health of children in primary and secondary school, both in providing medical checks at key stages of development and in implementing the school vaccination programme that includes school-leaver boosters. The support they need from pharmacy is mainly information about, for example, maintaining the cold chain for vaccines, working under patient group directions (PGDs) and specific vaccine queries. They may also need to access advice about the management of prescribed medicines in schools. SN also work in special schools to support children with severe learning and physical disabilities. These SN need access to more specific advice relating to the safe management of prescribed medicines, for example, for treatment of epilepsy.

Specialist nurses

Some nurses develop specialist expertise in defined areas such as stoma care, diabetes, paediatrics, continence and palliative care, and need pharmaceutical advice such as on policies and procedures. Many of these nurses will be nurse independent prescribers.

Many nurses now work in 'walk-in' centres and other first contact care facilities. These services are often nurse-led, although some have sessional medical input. These nurses will supply and administer an agreed range of medicines, either under PGDs or they may be qualified as nurse independent prescribers.

With care moving closer to the patient's home the role of the community matron has developed in England, their role including to assess and support patients, and thus prevent unnecessary admission to hospital. Many of these nurses will also be non-medical prescribers.

Employed dentists

Community dental officers are generally based in community clinics (these are those employed rather than the contractor dentists who provide general dental services). They provide dental care for the community with particular emphasis on schoolchildren, antenatal and postnatal women and people with physical or learning disabilities. They may also provide domiciliary care to patients who are unable to attend a clinic, including those living in care homes. Most individual patient treatment is provided on FP10 prescription. Local anaesthetics and other pharmaceuticals routinely needed in dental sessions will generally be supplied by the pharmacy service. General anaesthesia is now almost exclusively performed in a hospital setting but some community dental services may provide conscious sedation. Dentists need to comply with current guidelines for dental emergencies such as anaphylactic shock and cardiac arrest.

Podiatrists

Podiatrists (registered as chiropodists) who work within CHS are registered with the Health Professions Council and provide services to older people, diabetics and to the same groups of patients as dentists. Podiatrists who hold a certificate of competence in the use of medicines may sell or supply certain medicines in the course of their professional practice. It is important to ensure that proper labelling requirements are being met. Podiatrists who hold a certificate of competence in the use of analgesics may administer certain local anaesthetics parenterally. Podiatrists are also included in the list of health professionals who can administer and supply medicines under a PGD. Podiatrists who have additional training can offer surgical foot services. Many podiatrists now provide services within GP practices.

Other healthcare professionals

Other healthcare professionals who work in CHS include dieticians, speech and language therapists, physiotherapists and occupational therapists.

Although use of medicines may not be a major component of the roles of these professionals, they may need access to pharmacy advice and support. Examples include: dieticians involved in advising on/initiating sip feeds or recommending the use of fortified recipes; speech and language therapists involved in poststroke support and treating swallowing difficulties; physiotherapists providing musculoskeletal services who may be injecting intra-articular steroids; and occupational therapists in rehabilitation services who assess activities of daily living, including ability to open containers.

Pharmacy support for medicines management in CHS

Medicines management issues that arise in CHS have much in common with those in the hospital pharmacy service. The pharmacy support required by CHS therefore has some similarities with hospital pharmacy. For example:

- strategic advice – to inform planning of new services and redesign of existing services
- support for clinical governance – policies, procedures, audit, monitoring safe practices with medicines and reducing medication-related risks
- advice on safe appropriate use and handling of medicines
- medicines information and query answering
- education and training for other healthcare professionals
- supply and dispensing
- clinical pharmacy services – to community hospitals and to specialist teams
- medication reviews in care homes.

However, significant differences and factors need to be considered by the CHS pharmacy team. For example, in the CHS environment healthcare professionals work more autonomously and may work in isolation from colleagues, such as when caring for someone in his/her own home. The pharmacy staff supporting CHS need to understand the range of environments where medicines are used and who will be using them, as well as having a good understanding of the legal framework so that they can risk-assess practice and provide advice accordingly.

Strategic advice

National Health Service (NHS) (and non-NHS) organisations providing CHS need to have access to advice from a suitably experienced senior pharmacist (typically at band 8b or above) with competency in CHS. They may be directly employed or support the organisation via a contract or SLA. The role of the senior pharmacist will include responsibility for safe systems for managing medicines across the organisation. This includes ensuring that controlled drugs are managed within the legal framework and providing support to the accountable officer (see Chapter 5).

An ability to access strategic pharmacy advice is particularly important at a time of rapid change with services moving from hospital into community settings and redesigned to be closer to the patient. These changes may bring additional risks that need to be assessed and managed.

Response to emergencies may need review, as basic life support only will be available in community settings, along with dialling 999 when necessary.

There may be additional issues relating to safe disposal, for example, when cytotoxics are being administered in a patient's home. There may be a need for new policies and procedures to support safe practice. There may be a need for the development of PGDs for supply and/or administration of medicines within a new service or for training of new non-medical prescribers. There may need to be advice on the legal route for the supply of appropriately labelled medicines, especially for supply under PGD.

Support for clinical governance

There should be pharmacy input to the clinical governance structure and to the committees and groups responsible for managing any aspect of care involving use of medicines across the organisation, such as the drugs and therapeutics committee and the patient safety group. There also needs to be pharmacy input to the clinical audit programme. Each CHS organisation needs to have an overarching medicines policy that links to other relevant policies and procedures on specific topics.[3] There must be policies and procedures in place to support all aspects of the safe, appropriate use of medicines, as detailed below. These policies and procedures must be accessible, perhaps via an intranet, and any associated training needs must be identified and met. Knowledge of the working practices of community health staff is essential in formulating policies for safe use of medicines. It must not be assumed that the medicines policy from an acute setting would fit CHS as there are distinct differences in practice that need to be taken into account, as referred to previously. CHS pharmacists are often required to utilise their knowledge and expertise on legal issues relating to medicines and to apply this to address the complex circumstances that community-based health staff may encounter.

Pharmacy input is also needed for any aspect of new and established services that involve the prescription, supply and/or administration of medicines such as the need to develop PGDs.

Patient group directions

The use of PGDs for the administration and/or supply of appropriate prescription-only medicines is common within CHS, for example in family planning or walk-in centres. The devolved governments have provided their own guidance about the use of PGDs so it is important to refer to the correct advice.[4]

Table 14.2 Examples of patient group directions (PGDs) in use within community health services

Service	PGD
Family planning	Supply and administration of oral contraceptives
District nursing	Administration of flu vaccine
School nurses	Administration of childhood vaccines given at school
Musculoskeletal services	Administration of intra-articular steroid injections
First-contact care services	Supply of medicines, for example, oral analgesics

It is a legal requirement that a pharmacist has involvement in writing and signing PGDs. Pharmacists may also be involved in the approval process. CHS pharmacists must have the legal knowledge to be able to advise a service of the appropriate route for prescription, supply and/or administration of medicines. Table 14.2 provides some examples of PGDs from a CHS setting. Knowledge of the environment in which CHS staff operate, for instance the way in which school vaccination sessions are organised, is essential in order that PGDs are legal, workable and appropriate to the working practices of the health professionals concerned.

Advice on the safe, appropriate use and handling of medicines

All CHS staff need access to appropriate professional pharmaceutical support for their practice in relation to the following range of issues:

- safe and secure handling and storage of medicines in all areas of use, including the transportation of medicines[5]
- handling and use of cytotoxics
- treatment of anaphylactic shock (vaccines are administered in schools and patients' own homes as well as in clinics, and staff need regular training and access to kits containing adrenaline (epinephrine))
- safe disposal of unwanted medicines (DN may find patients who have a stockpile of medicines that have expired or are no longer prescribed)
- use of pharmaceutical samples
- control of infection
- handling, use and transport of vaccines within the 'cold chain'
- public health issues such as treatment of head lice infection
- patient safety incident and adverse reaction reporting
- hazard recall
- implementation of National Patient Safety Agency and other alerts

- Control of Substances Hazardous to Health
- medicines information and query answering.

The provision of information and advice on medicine-related issues to CHS staff and, where appropriate, to the public is a key role for pharmacists working with CHS. The same standards of checking content and logging and documenting queries apply as in medicines information departments in hospitals (see Chapter 8). There should also be access to a medicines information department (via an SLA or contract) and clear lines of communication should be agreed so that urgent queries can be answered quickly. CHS pharmacists may also produce active information such as regular bulletins on appropriate topics and single-subject newsletters on specific issues.

Education and training

It is often the role of CHS pharmacists to identify relevant training needs of healthcare staff in the community. As individual staff often work in isolation they may find it difficult to maintain professional development. Training may be needed across a range of topics; Table 14.3 provides some examples. Training sessions are often developed and provided with colleagues from other disciplines.

Supply and dispensing of medicines

The supply of medicines to staff in CHS has usually been provided by an acute or mental health hospital/trust under a contract or SLA. This route is also used for dispensed medicines for patients in community hospitals. In some areas these services are now obtained from a local community pharmacy under a contract or SLA. Any services obtained must meet required standards and ensure cost-effective use of pharmaceuticals. Contracts, SLAs and so on should be monitored by the lead CHS pharmacist. There should be written policies that comply with the safe and secure handling of medicines.[5] Procedures for the ordering, supply and safe delivery of pharmaceuticals to community premises must be in place. Stock lists and levels need to be agreed between the health professionals and the pharmacy team. They must be available, as a basis for ordering and stock control in every clinic and

Table 14.3 Examples of training sessions provided
Core induction for all staff who handle medicines
Managing emergencies such as anaphylaxis for staff who do immunisations
For staff who work under patient group directions
To maintain and develop the competencies of non-medical prescribers
To support changes in practice in new/redesigned services

community site, and safe and secure storage must be provided. There may be a trend to seek independent providers for supply services in a similar way to the provision to mental health trusts and for outpatient dispensing.

Clinical pharmacy services in CHS

Clinical pharmacy services are needed for patients in community hospitals, respite and rehabilitation units and by specialist teams providing end-of-life care. These are similar to those in acute hospitals but often involve visiting sites that do not have a pharmacy department. The pharmacists and pharmacy technicians providing the service need to work with the multidisciplinary team to assess ability to manage medicines after discharge and to encourage self-administration to support independence. As in acute settings, medicines reconciliation and communications across interfaces are essential for consistency of care. The pharmacy team needs to be aware of the different ways in which community hospitals may receive medical cover, for example by GPs, hospital doctors or a mix of both.

Specialist knowledge for CHS pharmacy staff

Below are some of the areas where CHS pharmacy staff need specialist knowledge and expertise.

Vaccines and immunisation

The UK has a childhood immunisation schedule to protect infants and children from illnesses that can cause morbidity and mortality. The range and timing of vaccines are subject to regular revision as new vaccines become available: a recent example is the addition of human papilloma-virus vaccine to the schedule in 2008. There are other regular vaccination campaigns such as against seasonal flu as well as additional campaigns in response to public health concerns. The latter is well illustrated by the flu pandemic response in 2009. Immunisation against infectious disease is set out in what is known as the *Green Book*.[6] Updates to the *Green Book* can only be found online.

Vaccine supplies for GPs are provided via a national contract. Deliveries using refrigerated lorries may be direct to GP practices (where most childhood immunisations are given) and to community clinics and health centres (for the school nursing service) or to nominated distribution centres. It is essential that the 'cold chain' is maintained and monitored, from supplier to clinic fridge, up to the point of administration, with an audit trail covering each stage. Advice on appropriate and verified cool boxes and monitoring of temperatures is an essential part of the pharmacy team's involvement.

Sexual health services

The reduction of unwanted pregnancies and sexually transmitted diseases is an important part of the UK government's sexual health strategies. Family planning clinics provide free birth control advice and contraceptives to any person needing them. Sexual health services, for example, diagnosis and treatment of *Chlamydia*, are increasingly being provided in community settings; of course, this includes the important role of community pharmacists, but goes beyond the remit of this text.

The provision of family planning items such as oral contraceptives and other medicines used in sexual health clinics needs to be within an agreed stock list and/or formulary. The appropriate and cost-effective use of medicines within these services needs to be monitored. There also needs to be appropriate pharmacy input to ensure that legal requirements such as appropriate labelling of oral and emergency contraceptives are in place.

Intermediate care, rehabilitation services, admissions avoidance teams, respite care

Many services and care pathways are now designed to keep people out of hospital and/or to promote independence so that they can return home more quickly with support from a multidisciplinary team. Intermediate care is defined as rehabilitation programmes of usually not more than 6 weeks and can be provided in community hospitals, by rehabilitation teams, in 'step-down' units and by other nurse-led services. CHS pharmacy staff are involved in providing advice about medicines for an individual, assessing the needs of an individual patient for support to take his or her medicines safely and advice on support for concordance (compliance).

Vulnerable patients may need help with self-administration of their medication, for example using memory aids. They may also require information in a more accessible form such as instructions in simple English (or translated into their spoken language), large print labels or a pictorial reminder. Many will be supported by family and other carers who may also require advice and support. Effective communication is particularly important when patients move across interfaces of care. Pharmacists have a key role in ensuring this is achieved.

Support for people with learning disabilities

Learning disability services are discussed in Chapter 13: services may be provided by CHS staff because people with learning disabilities are now integrated as far as possible within local communities. They often live in group homes and hostels with a multidisciplinary community learning disability team coordinating any specialist healthcare required. Pharmacy staff may contribute to this team along with therapists, specialist nurses and consultants. In addition, they may work with organisations providing health and social care to ensure that there are safe systems for the management of medicines in these settings.

Working with other agencies

Social services

Historically, in parallel with health authorities, local authorities have been responsible for commissioning the social care needed by their residents, particularly children and vulnerable groups such as older people. These needs include access to care homes, domiciliary care, 'meals on wheels', fostering services, adoption, social care assessments and occupational therapy. Successive governments have encouraged local authorities to outsource these services from the private or voluntary sector and this has led to an expansion of private home care agencies.

Nurses are employed by care homes that provide nursing care. In most other social care environments social care workers are involved with medication in the course of their duties. In residential care homes, social care workers administer medication to their service users unable to manage their own medicines. Domiciliary home care workers support service users living in their own homes with their medicines in line with their employer's policy. Both groups need to access training, professional advice and medicines information from pharmacists. While community pharmacists will provide support to individual service users and carers, CHS pharmacists often work with social care organisations to support safe practices with medication, including local policies, training programmes and advice on documentation.

Local education authorities

Education authorities should work with health professionals such as SN, specialist SN, community paediatricians and CHS pharmacists to ensure that there are proper policies for the control and use of medicines both within mainstream and special schools and in early-years settings. Procedures need to be in place so that children can access their medicines and medicines are handled and stored responsibly. All staff involved with medicines need appropriate in-service training so that they, other staff and parents are clear about their roles.

Voluntary agencies

Many of the voluntary agencies such as Age UK and the Parkinson's Disease Society have concerns around the proper use of medicines by their service users. They may access help from their local CHS pharmacist to give talks to individual self-help groups such as stroke clubs or to give advice to agencies in formulating information leaflets on the use of medicines.

The Primary and Community Care Pharmacy Network (PCCPN)

PCCPN is a UK-wide special-interest group established to provide peer support, networking and education opportunities to those working in this field. There is an uneven spread of CHS posts across the UK along with a great variation in the size and organisation of CHS pharmacy services. Some posts are part-time or sometimes linked to other duties within hospital pharmacy. There is also a range of seniority, with chief pharmacists of large CHS providers at band 8c or 8d. Most CHS posts are band 8a or 8b, reflecting the autonomy and scope of these posts and the competencies needed. There are also band 7 posts for pharmacists with less experience of CHS. CHS pharmacy technician posts tend to be graded at band 5 or 6. A competency framework has been developed for pharmacy staff working in CHS; this is under review at the time of writing.[7]

Organisation of pharmacy support to CHS

England

As explained in Chapter 1, the NHS is undergoing a significant organisational change as the text is compiled. Prior to this, CHS were recently reorganised as primary care trust provider services, separated from commissioning. Some CHS providers may develop into independent organisations as foundation trust or social enterprises; others may vertically integrate with an acute or mental health trust. As the White Paper 2010 changes are implemented[8] it is essential that the skills and competencies of CHS specialist pharmacy staff are maintained in order to support other CHS professionals and vulnerable patients who may have complex needs in relation to their medication.

The emerging models for pharmacy services include:

- a team of pharmacists, technicians and support staff directly employed by the larger CHS providers with SLAs in place with an acute or mental health trust for supply and dispensing
- a lead pharmacist directly employed by the CHS provider with responsibility for advising the organisation on medicines management and coordinating and monitoring pharmacy services provided in contracts or SLAs

- integration of the CHS provider functions into an acute or mental health trust such that CHS pharmacy staff are employed by and are part of the hospital pharmacy team independent provider provision.

Scotland

NHS trusts for acute, mental health and primary care were disbanded in Scotland in 2006 when the concept of single-system NHS boards was created. These boards are re-empowered with the delivery of healthcare (previously devolved to trusts) as well as responsibility for the planning and assessment of health needs. The NHS boards also paved the way for more integrated health and social care under joint management arrangements. Although some support for CHS is provided by primary care-based pharmacists, the majority of it is integrated into the roles of acute and mental health pharmacy teams. The CHS work is likely to be part of an individual's role rather than there being a specialist post.

Wales

The reorganisation of NHS Wales means that health boards are responsible for planning and providing healthcare to all their population. This includes primary, secondary, tertiary and community care. At the time of writing, individual health boards are still determining their structure but locality working is becoming common. Health board pharmacy teams are responsible for providing support across the area and will need to become more involved with CHS.

Nationally, a strategic delivery group has been charged with delivering pharmacy services, including contractual services, and a director for medicines management in Wales has been appointed.

Northern Ireland

The Health and Social Care Board in Northern Ireland works with the Public Health Agency to address the health needs of the population. As in Scotland, the majority of support for CHS is integrated into the roles of acute and mental health pharmacy teams and is likely to be part of an individual's role rather than there being a specialist post.

The future

CHS pharmacy is an interesting and rewarding area of practice, particularly with the opportunities it offers for multidisciplinary and multiagency working. With the trend to move care closer to the patient as well as delivery of services in community rather than acute settings, the need for pharmacy support for CHS is likely to increase rather than diminish.

References

1. Royal Pharmaceutical Society of Great Britain. *Medicines, Ethics and Practice: A Guide for Pharmacists and Pharmacy Technicians*, vol. 33. London: RPSGB, 2010.
2. Health and social care staff working in the community: a briefing for pharmacists. Available online at: http://www.nelm.nhs.uk/en/NeLM-Area/Community-Areas/Primary–Community-Care/.
3. Developing medicines management arrangements in provider organisations. Available online at: http://www.nelm.nhs.uk/en/NeLM-Area/Community-Areas/Primary–Community-Care/.
4. Patient group directions in the NHS. Available online at: http://www.nelm.nhs.uk/en/Communities/NeLM/PGDs/.
5. Royal Pharmaceutical Society of Great Britain. *The Safe and Secure Handling of Medicines: A Team Approach. Revision of the Duthie Report (1988)*. London: RPSGB, 2005.
6. Immunisation against infectious disease. Available online at: http://www.immunisation.nhs.uk.
7. PCCPN competency framework. Available online at: http://www.pccpnetwork.nhs.uk.
8. Department of Health. *Equity and Excellence: Liberating the NHS*. London: Department of Health, 2010.

Further reading

Health and social care staff working in the community: a briefing for pharmacists. Available online at: http://www.nelm.nhs.uk/en/NeLM-Area/Community-Areas/Primary–Community-Care/.

Primary and Community Care Pharmacy Network website: http://www.pccpnetwork.nhs.uk.

Refer to the current issue of *Medicines, Ethics and Practice* for information on the prescription and supply of medicines by community health services professionals.

15

Information technology

Ann Slee

The Audit Commission's 2001 review of medicines management in hospitals set out a vision of the use of information technology (IT) in hospital pharmacy that largely remains unchanged today.[1] It stated that:

> New medication is agreed between members of the clinical team and ordered at the bedside through a radio-computer link to an automated dispensary, where robotic systems pick the new medicines and dispatch them to the patient's ward via a pneumatic tube.

Ten years later, this vision remains a long way off for many, though in a small number of hospitals it is tantalisingly close to full implementation, yet after 10 years still not there. This chapter will examine the developments in IT as they apply to hospital pharmacy practice and how the vision set out has been modified in some areas, as the national programme for IT has evolved and pharmacy practice moved on. It will describe the main developments in IT relating to hospital pharmacy, the use of stock control systems, electronic prescribing and medicines administration and electronic patient records (EPRs).

The definition that is assumed for e-prescribing is that utilised by NHS Connecting for Health, namely:

> the utilisation of electronic systems to facilitate and enhance the communication of a prescription or medicine order, aiding the choice, administration and supply of a medicine through knowledge and decision support and providing a robust audit trail for the entire medicines use process.[2]

History

Pharmacy has a long history of using IT to support service development. Computerised stock control systems were introduced to pharmacy during the 1980s to provide machine-generated labels.[3, 4] Some of these systems also provided limited management information about which drugs had been used and by whom. Systems were further developed to provide automatic stock control, patient medication records and drug interaction warnings. Despite these advances, many systems are still not used to their full potential and have developed at a slower pace over the past few years as the supplier focus has moved towards e-prescribing and medicines administration.

The introduction of automation and automated drug cabinets, as discussed in Chapter 4, as well as advances in e-commerce, has further evolved the supply model. Full systems integration has remained a challenge, with many of these developments operating as stand-alone systems. A key element of integration has been the development and use of key information standards, many of which are starting to go through the formal NHS standards route but to date still remain unused in key systems.

E-prescribing and the EPR were introduced into a number of hospitals in the USA in the 1970s and first introduced into the UK in the early 1990s. The publication of *Information for Health* in 1998 set out an ambitious timetable for the introduction of the EPR, including electronic prescribing.[5] It proved to be too ambitious and was superseded in June 2002 with *Delivery of 21st Century IT Support for the NHS: National Strategic Programme*.[6] This introduced the national programme for IT that aimed to speed up the delivery of systems by centrally procuring systems via local service providers (LSPs). Replacing the National Health Service (NHS) Information Authority, it also aimed to develop key NHS information standards, working in collaboration with the Information Standards Board for Health and Social Care to underpin system development.

Delivery of the national programme has not been without controversy or delay, resulting in a further Department of Health informatics review in July 2008.[7] This focused the national programme towards five key deliverables ('the clinical 5' – see Table 15.1) identified by the NHS as supporting the *Next Stage Review*.[8] It also reintroduced the opportunity for local system

Table 15.1 The five key elements for secondary care – 'the clinical five'	
	Functional requirements
1	A patient administration system with integration with other systems and sophisticated reporting
2	Order communications and diagnostics reporting (including all pathology and radiology tests and tests ordered in primary care)
3	Letters with coding (discharge summaries, clinic and Accident and Emergency letters)
4	Scheduling (for beds, tests, theatres)
5	E-prescribing (including 'to take out' medicines)

development with the advent of local programmes for IT and a more service-led delivery model. It is clear that the 'replace all' policy from 2003 is being superseded by a 'connect all' philosophy. Whilst this may seem to be a step forward it leaves doubt as to how this is to be managed and how delivery of systems into secondary care is to proceed. At the time of writing, the change of government and the review of IT systems has now been outlined with a consultation document issued by the Department of Health in October 2010 – *Liberating the NHS: An Information Revolution.*[9] This reiterates the connection and joining up of systems whilst also signalling more of a focus on meeting individual and local needs. It also outlines that the government will move away from being the main provider of systems, with a greater range of organisations offering services. In essence it looks at information and not systems, leaving further doubt as to what will happen to the existing national contracts for the delivery of systems. It is clear that the strategy of delivering systems via connecting for health is now superseded; what remain to be clarified are how the remaining contracts will be delivered and the impact on local system delivery; given the current financial climate this gives cause for concern.

Stock control systems

Perhaps the earliest IT to be introduced into pharmacy practice, stock control systems allowed the production of a clear printed label, often with information support about interaction checking and materials management for medicine procurement. Many systems produced limited management information allowing pharmacists to review the use of medicines – by specialty, for example. This drug use review was particularly helpful to the financial side of medicines management and it has been extensively used in the USA. There the use of systems for billing purposes has ensured good-quality data capture and reporting.

In the UK the provision of drug expenditure information showing month-on-month comparisons and top 50 expenditure items on a trust or specialty level is common practice. We underestimate the ease with which such information becomes available due to its routine collection during the supply and dispensing process. The advent of payment by results and exclusions, as well as service line reporting to support foundation trust status and hospital at-home services, has forced the development of more detailed reporting. This has created a number of challenges as the information may be required at patient level, necessitating the development of often manual data collection/reporting, as stock control and other IT systems are not always sufficiently developed.

The use of patient medication records, common in community pharmacies, has had relatively limited application in hospital practice but has potential advantages in operational terms which are beginning to be realised.

Information is being used to reduce unnecessary redispensing, facilitate one-stop dispensing and also to track individual patient costs to support, for example, payment by results.

Sadly, systems are still not as developed or utilised as they might be. This has been particularly challenging as the national programme for IT did not include pharmacy stock control systems for hospitals. Thus there has been no national standard defined for system functionality or development; drug files largely continue to be maintained at each site, interfaces with third-party databases are in their relative infancy and there is no requirement for an up-to-date system to be in place.

The Dictionary of Medicines and Devices (dm+d)

One of the barriers to the seamless electronic transfer of information has been the lack of a common drug dictionary. The use of such a dictionary is a key requirement to support the delivery of systems that aim to facilitate reduction in clinical risk, for example, e-prescribing. Its use will facilitate the use of standard descriptions for all medicines, as well as the use of a common coding system and structure. The lack of use of such a dictionary was further highlighted in 2009 as the main barrier for the development of the pharmacy supply chain and key for addressing problems with pharmacy computer systems in hospitals.[10] Driving existing systems towards the use of dm+d (see below) has remained problematic.[11]

The Department of Health and the National Health Service Information Authority started working to produce a common drug dictionary for secondary care via the UK Standard Clinical Products Reference Source Project, which worked to produce three component parts – (1) the primary care drug dictionary; (2) the secondary care drug dictionary; and (3) the medical devices dictionary. This project is now better known as dm+d and has developed to become a partnership between the Business Services Authority (BSA) and NHS Connecting for Health (NHS CFH), amalgamating the three components outlined above.

The BSA and NHS CFH have produced a drug dictionary which contains all items prescribed more than three times a year in primary care as well as an extended range of products to meet secondary care needs. Information on the content can be accessed via a browser available on the internet, from which users can register to receive regular downloads of the content.[12] The medicines content is largely complete, and additional items are added as they are marketed or become known.

The dictionary is not simply a list of medicines that are utilised within the NHS; it also contains a number of other items of information which include, but are not limited to, controlled drug status, product availability and flags identifying whether brand prescribing is required.

The dictionary has continued to develop since its initial release to meet secondary care prescribing requirements. It has now been incorporated into Snomed CT, the key clinical data standard that is being rolled out across the NHS.

Details about the editorial policy, the structure and content of dm+d and implementation guidance for primary and secondary care can be found on the dm+d website. It is hoped that future work will extend the content to link with the Profile database of NHS-manufactured specials and to incorporate medical devices. This latter project is complex and is likely to take some time to deliver fully.

We can see that one of the key building blocks required to support the development of IT systems is now largely in place and has started to proceed through the information standards route. It was accepted at the requirement stage as a fundamental standard in March 2009 and looks set to become the NHS standard for describing and coding medicines by around 2015 in primary care. Secondary care will miss this first standard requirement and will likely take a little longer to move through the process. This will require that NHS trusts use the standard within their systems, thus helping to drive its use forward. Incorporation into pharmacy stock control systems, e-prescribing systems and any other systems used to support NHS medicines management is going to be key to supporting integrated patient care moving forward.

Electronic patient record

The advancement of computer systems in the USA has demonstrated the potential advantages of the introduction of EPRs, with many of the benefits related to the introduction of electronic prescribing systems within them. Whilst introduction of these systems into the UK is still very limited, the previous government's stated ambition was to have EPR systems, including electronic prescribing systems, in place in all acute hospitals. The report from the Treasury, the Wanless report, underlined the importance of investment in IT, which could be taken as supporting the development of the national programme for IT.[13] It identified that:

> one of the major benefits to accrue from such systems arises from physician order entry which requires the doctor to input requests for new medicines, X-rays or other investigations into the system directly. This physician order entry has been a feature of most UK applications whereas the health system in the USA, delivered as it is by independent private physicians, does not lend itself to mandatory requirements for physician order entry. As a consequence, despite having advanced computer systems, many of the advantages of an electronic record are missed due to lack of physician involvement with the system.

The use of EPR systems has shown a number of benefits in terms of improving communication and reducing risks to patients. A patient safety internet site estimated that computerised physician order entry could lead to the avoidance of 522 000 serious medication errors each year in the USA.[14] This has been demonstrated in terms of improved legibility and completeness of prescriptions and dramatic improvements in patient care, with reduction in risks associated with inappropriate dosing or drug choice.[15, 16] Advanced systems that include clinical decision support with dose and interaction checking or checks of the appropriateness of the prescription allow review of the prescription at the point of decision-making.[17–19]

The sentinel paper that highlighted the potential of e-prescribing to reduce errors was published by Bates *et al.* in 1998.[20] A more recent systematic review reports a relative risk reduction in medication error rates in 23 out of 25 systems of between 13% and 99%. Six of the nine studies reviewed looking at the effects on potential adverse drug events showed a relative risk reduction of between 35% and 98%.[21]

Thus there are a number of different ways in which e-prescribing systems can reduce the incidence of medication-related error. However, caution is required: many of the studies published that describe the benefits can be criticised for poor methodology and outcome measures. Also, it should not be forgotten that there are also ways in which systems can introduce new errors or increase error rates. These must be taken into consideration during design and implementation.

The main areas of benefit for a well designed e-prescribing system include:

- Legibility and completeness – prescriptions are legible and complete. Structured pathways for ordering medicines ensure that full descriptions are used, doses use appropriate units of measure and frequencies are selected for individual medicines. For example, the word 'unit' can be forced for insulin doses, micrograms can be forced in place of μg, addressing known errors with hand-written scripts.
- Decision support – this can be utilised in a number of different ways:
  - Passive decision support: systems can be configured to ensure that prescribers are guided to select the most appropriate prescription content, namely route, unit of measure, frequency and other supporting requirements, such as appropriate rates of administration or diluents. Routes of administration can be limited; for example, the intrathecal route can be excluded for selection for all vinca alkaloids. Much of the reduction in error rates reported by Brigham and Women's Hospital has been due to this type of support.[22]
  - Active decision support: active checking of prescriptions can be undertaken using prebuilt third-party or local rules. When a rule is 'broken' an active alert will fire a warning to the prescriber. Areas that

can be supported include allergy checking, drug–drug interaction checking, dose range checking, therapeutic duplication and local rules to support, for example, meticillin-resistant *Staphylococcus aureus* prophylaxis and antibiotic course length review.

- Formulary management – this can be used in a number of ways. It can be used to ensure that medicines prescribed are available, thus potentially reducing delays in administration. It may also be used to limit access to specific medicines on safety or clinical grounds, supporting compliance with local policy.[23] For example, improvements in the use of antibiotics have been reported, including a reduction in misselection and excessive doses.[24] It may also be used to support improvements in prescribing appropriate prophylaxis such as for heparins.[25]

- Communication – prescriptions are available where and when they are required as they can be accessed via many terminals or locations at the same time. Current paper processes require prescriptions to be moved around, meaning that they may not be in the correct place or are lost. E-prescribing promises much in terms of improving communication between different care sectors in the future and supporting medicines reconciliation.

- Administration: the introduction of bar code checking to support the correct identification and recording of medicines administered has been reported to have reduced the incidence of error by up to 80%.[26]

- Introduction of new errors: there have been a series of reports outlining problems with e-prescribing systems. Many of these have been due to poor implementation or configuration decisions, often where clinical input has been weak or planning inadequate. A case in point is the implementation of a paediatric system in the USA that initially increased mortality rates.[27] Other problems vary but include: (1) poor system design, particularly relating to decision support; (2) the process flow used within systems; (3) poor screen design; and (4) a lack of decision support.[28–30] In particular, if alerts are not relevant or fire off late in the prescribing process, it is more likely that they will be ignored and important warnings missed. There is a fine balance to be achieved to ensure that overalerting is avoided.

Poor screen design may repeat many of the problems seen with poor handwriting, for example, the use of abbreviations, truncated descriptions and inappropriately wrapped text. Many basic system errors that can be mitigated via system design or configuration are outlined in the hazard frameworks published by the e-prescribing programme at NHS CFH and in user interface guidance for medicines which can be found at the common user interface program.[31, 32] The NPSA has also published guidance on the safe on-screen display of medication information which illustrates some of the basic design elements that can be used to reduce risk in this area.[33]

The Leapfrog Group in the USA has continued to champion the introduction of e-prescribing (or computerised physician order entry (CPOE), as it is known in the USA) into hospitals. Over the past 10 years it has developed a tool to review individual system implementation of CPOE at hospitals to see whether key patient safety benefits are met.[14] This is being used by various accreditation bodies in the USA to support patient safety benefits at hospital level and has been funded by the Agency for Healthcare Research and Quality. At the time of writing, summary results of the initial use of this tool have yet to be published. Personal communication with the author has suggested that implementation of CPOE (and thus the benefits) can be very variable between sites using the same system; this highlights that local configuration decisions and ongoing development are key to supporting system benefits realisation. Work is under way to see whether the tool might be used in the UK to support ongoing system review and development at trust level. Initial results have been promising and have demonstrated that Anglicisation is entirely possible.

The benefits of e-prescribing are increasingly being sought by UK hospitals to support the quality and safety agenda of which improvement in the use of, and the management of, medicines forms a large part. Communication between different care providers by facilitating medicines reconciliation and transfer of information are areas that are being highlighted as being particularly beneficial to patient safety. The Care Quality Commission report identifying the challenges with managing patients' medicines after discharge from hospital highlights that IT could be used to facilitate improved information transfer between care settings.[34]

A significant number of medication-related errors due to poor hand-writing and incomplete information are likely to be reduced with the introduction of e-prescribing. The 2009 General Medical Council report highlighting the number and type of errors in prescribing adds further weight to organisations' need to introduce systems to facilitate improvements in prescribing practice.[35]

E-prescribing is one of the most, if not the most, complex areas of health IT to develop and implement – both technically and culturally. One of the significant challenges for the introduction of IT is the cultural change required for the successful implementation of these systems.[36] There are a number of difficulties in getting buy-in from a range of different professional groups. Successful implementation requires strong clinical champions, a commitment from the highest level in the organisation and a clear expression of the clinical benefits that patients will gain from its introduction.

Prescribing is an activity that affects almost every patient admitted to hospital and requires the active participation of the majority of hospital staff. It is also an area that must be failsafe and there is no leeway for mistakes to be made. It is an area that, to many, seems too complicated to implement and often most enthusiasm for implementation comes from pharmacy. Given these challenges with the introduction of e-prescribing, NHS CFH commissioned a report to identify the lessons learnt from successful and unsuccessful UK implementation of e-prescribing.[37] This highlights the main lessons and areas that must be addressed to facilitate clinical buy-in and successful system rollout. The publication also contains six briefing documents aimed at the various groups and clinical professions that must be involved, demonstrating the size of the engagement challenge.

It should not be forgotten that, although e-prescribing is generally one, if not the main, focus for delivery within an EPR, support for clinical pharmacy and medicines management services should also be incorporated. Work has started to define the core standard requirements laying the foundation for a pharmaceutical care record that can be shared across and beyond the pharmacy profession within an overall individual patient record. The profession must develop its requirements to support developments and advances in practice called for in the 2008 pharmacy White Paper.[38] It needs to ensure that information is included within the overall patient record and input is visible to the wider healthcare team. Whilst EPRs offer many opportunities to develop pharmacy practice by freeing time to focus on clinical input, they may also represent a threat if the automated elements are seen as staff-saving.[39] Systems are not a panacea for all medication-related problems and this is not always understood. Failure to understand the opportunities and threats from the introduction of systems may create challenges in terms of staffing and service development, of which the profession must be aware if a reversal in clinical input is to be avoided.

Delivery of e-prescribing into UK hospitals

There are real clinical benefits to accrue from the implementation of e-prescribing which have quite rightly meant its inclusion as one of the five key clinical elements of health-related IT that form the current strategy for delivery of systems into hospitals. Support has continued to grow nationally over the past few years to underpin this. The 2009 patient safety Health Select Committee report[40] highlighted e-prescribing as being key, as did the National Audit Office recommendations in its report on reducing healthcare-acquired infections.[41] The increased awareness of the need to manage medication errors, as demonstrated by National Patient Safety Agency alerts and the Patient Safety First initiative, continues to add pressure for delivery.[42]

As outlined earlier, delays in the delivery of the national programme for IT have created a number of challenges for trusts. A planning blight has effectively stalled the implementation of systems pending delivery of the national strategic solutions, meaning that e-prescribing rollout has moved on little over the past 10 years. The exception to this is in oncology, where pressure from the national clinical director for cancer brought about government support for bringing forward the e-prescribing system delivery in 2005. Work by the e-prescribing programme at NHS CFH and the Cancer Action Team at the Department of Health identified system requirements at that time and bench-marked existing systems to determine whether they met current need. Trusts were then invited to bid for monies to support local procurement and imple-mentation of interim systems. Nineteen bids were successful, resulting in a key number of cancer services having systems in place or being implemented.

There have also been a number of discharge systems implemented throughout hospitals to support the target of providing legible discharge information to general practitioners within 24 hours. Many of these systems have been home-grown and lack any form of sophisticated decision support. Implementation has been largely pharmacy-driven, particularly as medical staff see little benefit to themselves in using the system. Errors in transcription are not uncommon and create pressure within pharmacy departments which have to correct them.

More recent national pressure has resulted in a systems of choice approach being adopted for the southern strategic health authority areas following the loss of the southern LSP and stringent deadlines for delivery being set for the remaining two LSPs. Computer Services Corporation is contracted to deliver iSoft's Lorenzo system in the north, midlands and east and BT is contracted to deliver Cerner's Millennium system for London. These developments, as well as the need to deliver safer services, should allow us to see progress in the next few years.

Trusts that have implemented systems have been key in supporting system development and in highlighting where benefits may be accrued. Sites that have well-developed systems include Burton, Doncaster, Heart of England, Salford, Sheffield mental health, Sunderland, University Hospital Birmingham, Winchester, Wirral and the first specialist paediatric trust implementation at Great Ormond Street.

The e-prescribing programme at NHS CFH has developed a number of resources that are available to facilitate and support the development and delivery of e-prescribing.[43] Resources are available to support four key areas: (1) system selection and evaluation; (2) clinical safety; (3) implementation; and (4) decision support. Information available includes the functional requirements for systems, hazard frameworks, dose range checking, lessons learnt and challenges with implementing hospital e-prescribing, frequently asked questions, system evaluation methodology and results.

One of the barriers to the rollout of EPR is undoubtedly the perceived cost of introducing an integrated information system. Most hospitals have some degree of IT implementation at the department level, with systems such as patient administration, outpatient scheduling and often laboratory ordering and results reporting available at ward level. As a consequence the IT budget for most hospitals is probably sufficient to support the introduction of an integrated system if spread over the lifetime of the system. However, the perceived procurement and implementation costs are still the biggest barrier to implementation in this area. For those who have introduced such systems, these have tended to be imported from the USA and have required extensive local work to anglicise the existing system or to build it from scratch. There are now systems that have been developed specifically for and implemented in the UK market – whilst these have mostly (but not all) been developed from pharmacy stock control systems, they do offer some of the benefits that e-prescribing systems would be expected to deliver and will certainly support the development of a culture that utilises electronic systems. In the medium to long term those that are stand-alone will require development to integrate with other hospital systems such as pathology, to use NHS IT standards and to deliver sophisticated decision support.

The features of an ideal system are that it should be fast, reliable, locally adaptable to meet user preferences, easy to learn and intuitive in its use, fully integrated or allowing easy interfacing with other systems (such as departmental systems or medical devices and automated systems), and allowing easy access to patient data for audit purposes (as well as patient care) – with speed being of prime importance to users. The debate between fully integrated hospital information systems or interfaced 'best-of-breed' systems is fiercely contested amongst the varying proponents. The author's preference is for a fully integrated system that allows users to view relevant data from other applications such as pathology when prescribing medicines such as warfarin, insulin or drugs with a narrow therapeutic index. Whichever option you choose, it is imperative to be able to see the system in operation at a working site and not just accept the impressive demonstration that the vendors offer.

Conclusion

IT offers significant advantages to both patient care and pharmacy practice. Electronic prescribing systems, with integrated knowledge-based checks for dose and drug and other interactions, that interface directly with automated dispensing systems will allow pharmacy staff to spend their time where it is of most value – with the patient. The growing support for such systems suggests that these will indeed be introduced into clinical practice within the next 5–10 years, providing that current budgetary constraints do not prevent this. However, implementation of IT requires a significant effort on behalf of organisations. The cultural change required to ensure effective implementation is a much greater challenge than finding the right technology and, without the support of staff, systems are just expensive, and possibly dangerous, toys.

References

1. Audit Commission. *A Spoonful of Sugar – Medicines Management in NHS Hospitals.* London: Audit Commission, 2001.

2. Connecting for Health definition of e-prescribing. Available online at: http://www.connecting-forhealth.nhs.uk/systemsandservices/eprescribing/news/eprescribing.pdf (accessed 14 August 2010).

3. Anonymous. Hospital computer package from Pharmed. *Pharm J* 1980; 225: 329.

4. Hughes IR. Computer systems in pharmacy: II. *Br J Pharm Pract* 1982; 4: 15–24.

5. NHS Executive. *Information for Health. An Information Strategy for the Modern NHS 1998–2005.* London: The Stationery Office, 1998.

6. Department of Health. *Delivering 21st Century IT Support for the NHS: National Strategic Programme.* London: Department of Health, 2002.

7. Department of Health. *Health Informatics Review Report.* London: Department of Health, 2008.

8. Department of Health. *High Quality Care for All: NHS Next Stage Review, Final Report.* London: Department of Health, 2008.

9. Department of Health. *Liberating the NHS: An Information Revolution.* London: Department of Health, 2010.

10. Anonymous. Steps identified to improve supply chain in secondary care. *Pharm J* 2009; 283: 88.

11. Davies A, Finesilver J, Stokoe H. Addressing pharmacy computer system issues within NHS hospitals. *Pharm J* 2009; 282: 280.

12. Dictionary of Medicines and Devices: http://www.dmd.nhs.uk/dictionary.

13. Wanless D. *Securing Our Future Health: Taking a Long-term View. Final Report.* London: HM Treasury, 2002.

14. Leapfrog Group patient site re errors: http://www.leapfroggroup.org.

15. Hughes DK, Farrar KT, Slee AL. The trials and tribulations of electronic prescribing. *Hosp Presc Eur* 2001; 1: 74–76.

16. Evans RS, Pestotnik SL, Classen DC *et al.* A computer-assisted management program for antibiotics and other antiinfective agents. *N Engl J Med* 1998; 338: 232–238.

17. Bates DW, Leape LL, Cullen DJ *et al.* Effect of computerized physician order entry and a team intervention on prevention of serious medication errors. *JAMA* 1998; 280: 1311–1316.

18. Raschke RA, Gollihare B, Wunderlich TA *et al.* A computer alert system to prevent injury from adverse drug events. *JAMA* 1998; 280: 1317–1320.

19. Hunt DL, Haynes RB, Hanna SE *et al.* Effects of computer-based clinical decision support systems on physician performance and patient outcomes: a systematic review. *JAMA* 1998; 280: 1339–1346.

20. Bates DW, Leape LL, Cullen DJ *et al.* Effect of computerized physician order entry and a team intervention on prevention of serious medication errors. *JAMA* 1998; 280: 1311–1316.

21. Ammenwerth E, Schnell-Inderst P, Machan C *et al.* The effect of electronic prescribing on medication errors and adverse drug events: a systematic review. *J Am Med Inform Assoc* 2008; 15: 585–600.

22. Bates DW, Teich JM, Lee J *et al.* The impact of computerized physician order entry on medication error prevention. *J Am Med Inform Assoc* 1999; 6: 313–321.

23. Slee A, Farrar K. Formulary management – effective computer systems. *Pharm J* 1999; 262: 363–365.

24. Evans RS, Pestotnik SL, Classen DC *et al.* A computer-assisted management program for antibiotics and other antiinfective agents. *N Engl J Med* 1998; 338: 232–238.

25. Teich JM, Merchia PR, Schmiz JL *et al.* Effects of computerized physician order entry on prescribing practices. *Arch Intern Med* 2000; 160: 2741–2747.

26. Cescon D, Etchells E. Barcoded medication administration: a last line of defense. *JAMA* 2008; 299: 2200–2202.

27. Han Y, Carcillo J, Venkataraman S *et al*. Unexpected increased mortality after implementation of a commercially sold computerised physician order entry system. *Pediatrics* 2005; 116: 1506–1512.
28. Koppel R, Metlay JP, Cohen A *et al*. Role of computerised physician order entry systems in facilitating medication errors. *JAMA* 2005; 293: 1197–1203.
29. Ash J, Berg M, Coiera E. Some unintended consequences of information technology in healthcare: the nature of patient care information system-related errors. *J Am Med Inform Assoc* 2004; 11: 104–112.
30. Nebeker JR, Hoffman JM, Weir CR *et al*. High rates of adverse drug events in a highly computerised hospital. *Arch Intern Med* 2005; 165: 1111–1116.
31. Connecting for health system design: http://www.connectingforhealth.nhs.net/systemsandservices/eprescribing.
32. Connecting for health, common user interface: http://www.cui.nhs.uk/Pages/NHSCommonUserInterface.aspx.
33. National Patient Safety Agency. Design for patient safety: guidelines for the safe on-screen display of medication information 2010 v1. Available online at: http://www.nrls.npsa.nhs.uk/resources/?entryid45=66713&q=0%c2%acdesign+for+patient+safety%c2%ac.
34. Care Quality Commission. *Managing Patients' Medicines after Discharge from Hospital*. London: Care Quality Commission, 2009.
35. Dornan T, Ashcroft D, Heathfield H *et al*. *Final Report. An In Depth Investigation into Causes of Prescribing Errors by Foundation Trainees in Relation to their Medical Education*. EQUIP study. Manchester: University of Manchester Medical School Teaching Hospital, 2009.
36. Lively BT, Shrader KR. High tech and the human condition: impact on employees. *Am Pharm* 1986; 26: 24.
37. Cornford T. Electronic prescribing in hospitals: challenges and lessons learnt. Available online at: http://www.connectingforhealth.nhs.uk/systemsandservices/eprescribing/challenges (accessed 30 December 2009).
38. Department of Health. *Pharmacy in England. Building on Strengths – Delivering the Future*. London: Department of Health, 2008.
39. Slee A, Farvar K, Hughes D *et al*. Electronic prescribing – implications for hospital pharmacy. *Hosp Pharm* 2007; 14 217.
40. Health Select Committee report. Available online at: http://www.publications.parliament.uk/pa/cm200809/cmselect/cmhealth/151/151i.pdf (accessed 30 January 2009).
41. National Audit Office report. Available online at: http://www.nao.org.uk/publications/0809/reducing_healthcare_associated.aspx (accessed 30 January 2009).
42. Patient Safety First website: http://www.patientsafetyfirst.nhs.uk/content.aspx?path=/.
43. Connecting for Health website: nww.connectingforhealth.nhs.uk/systemsandservices/eprescribing (access via NHS net required).

Further reading

Dictionary of Medicines and Devices: http://www.dmd.nhs.uk/.
Information Standards Board for Health and Social Care: http://www.isb.nhs.uk/.
NHS Connecting for Health: http://www.connectingforhealth.nhs.uk.
NHS Connecting for Health ePrescribing Programme: http://www.connectingforhealth.nhs.uk/systemsandservices/eprescribing.
Oscheroff J (ed.) *Improving Medicines Use and Outcomes with Clinical Decision Support: a Step-by-Step Guide*. Chicago: HIMSS, 2009.

16

Research and development

Alison Blenkinsopp and Moira Kinnear

This chapter aims to explain key principles of research and development (R&D) from a practitioner perspective, providing an introduction for pharmacists who are, or want to become, involved as research users, research practitioners and research leaders. It will describe what is meant by research, development, service evaluation and audit followed by an overview of each stage from planning through resourcing, conducting and disseminating research.

Research, audit and service evaluation

Evidence is both needed and expected to underpin clinical and commissioning decisions about the way services are organised and delivered. The Department of Health's White Paper *Pharmacy in England* highlighted the need for the profession to strengthen further the evidence base for pharmacy.[1] However, not all evidence is created by research and understanding the differences between research, audit and service evaluation is important in deciding how to answer a particular question that may guide future practice. The National Research Ethics Service for the National Health Service (NHS) states:

> the primary aim of research is to derive generalisable new knowledge, whereas the aim of audit and service evaluation projects is to measure standards of care. Research is to find out what you should be doing; audit is to find out if you are doing planned activity and assesses whether it is working.[2]

Table 16.1 summarises the differences between these activities, all of which make a valuable contribution to the evidence base.

Research in the NHS is needed to support the key goal of providing high-quality care, care with effective health outcomes, delivered safely.

Table 16.1 National Research Ethics Service – differentiating clinical audit, service evaluation, research and usual practice/surveillance work in public health

Research	Service evaluation	Clinical audit	Surveillance	Usual practice in public health
Seeking generalisable new knowledge, including studies where hypotheses are tested	Seeking to define or assess current care	Assessing current care against a set of defined standards, then taking action to improve that care	Assessing the level and risks of an outbreak	Investigating an outbreak or incident to help control disease or for prevention
Quantitative – hypothesis testing Qualitative – exploring themes using established methodology	Asks: what does the service achieve?	Asks: are the standards met? and seeks improvement	Asks: what caused this outbreak?	Asks: what caused this outbreak? and treats
A defined question with aims and objectives	Describing or measuring current service	Assessing current care against a set of defined standards, then taking action to improve that care	Systematic, statistical methods to allow timely public health action	Systematic, may use statistical methods
Quantitative – may involve a new intervention and includes comparison with alternatives Qualitative – explores how interventions and relationships are experienced	Looks at current practice	Looks at current practice	May involve data and sample collection for purpose of managing incident	Treatments based on current evidence
Data collection beyond routine care required	Usually requires analysis of existing data but may require additional collection such as by questionnaire	Review of clinical data against standards may require additional collection such as by questionnaire	May involve analysis of existing data or administration of questionnaire or interviews	May involve administration of questionnaire or interviews
Quantitative – study design may require allocation to specific intervention groups Qualitative – uses a clearly defined sampling framework that is supported by conceptual or theoretical justifications	No allocation – looks at current practice	No allocation – looks at current practice	No intervention	May include a control group – but these are from those not exposed to the risk

Table 16.1 (*continued*)				
Research	Service evaluation	Clinical audit	Surveillance	Usual practice in public health
Randomisation to a particular treatment or course of action may be required	No randomisation	Cases might be sampled randomly but no randomisation of treatment or other intervention	No randomisation	Randomisation not used to decide treatment
Ethical opinion required – research ethics committee	No ethical opinion required from research ethics committee (sensitive issues may arise and require consideration, or even referral to a clinical ethics group, but this is not the norm)	No ethical opinion required from research ethics committee (sensitive issues may arise and require consideration, or even referral to a clinical ethics group, but this is not the norm)	No ethical opinion required from research ethics committee	No ethical opinion required from research ethics committee

Adapted from www.nres.npsa.nhs.uk/rec-community/guidance/#researchoraudit.

Pharmacy practice research

Pharmacy practice research, as a discipline, has been developing since the 1970s; a summit involving key stakeholders in 2008 concluded:

> pharmacy practice research has come some way over the last 10 years and some highly influential research has been undertaken in all four nations. However, in general the research is largely small-scale and exploratory in nature, due in part to a comparatively small research workforce and a shortage of academic and research pharmacists with PhDs.[3]

The Pharmacy Practice Research Trust identified five priorities:

1   long-term conditions
2   public health
3   minor ailments/self-care
4   integrating research into practice
5   integrating evidence into practice.[3]

NHS organisations have identified clinical priorities such as cancer, coronary heart disease, stroke and mental health that usually form the basis of local

NHS R&D strategies. Some NHS organisations will have well-established research programmes and some may have health services research programmes into which pharmacy practice research fits. Some organisations may have their own pharmacy practice R&D detailing service priorities. Practitioners will also have local questions arising in their organisation and areas of personal interest that they will want to pursue. However, because there are capacity constraints, R&D activity is more likely to be supported if it addresses identified local and/or national priorities or organisational issues.

This chapter will go on to discuss how to plan a research or development project, looking at research questions and outcome measures, literature-searching, study design, necessary approvals (research ethics and governance), resources needed and how to disseminate findings. Finally some thoughts on collaborations between practice and academia for the future are discussed. There are many useful books and articles that can help. Here we provide a summary of key points and there is a list of resources at the end of the chapter.

Project design and planning

Who needs to be involved?

Collaborating with others is important at every stage in R&D, finding people who are interested in the topic you want to study and also who are experts in research methods. Talking with colleagues and with other healthcare professionals can help to develop a broader perspective from initial ideas and allows input from those with a track record in R&D. Collaborators might include academics at a school of pharmacy or other health or social sciences discipline. Advice can also be sought from an organisation's local NHS R&D office that can also provide contact with a local forum for input from patients and the public. Depending on whether the idea is research or service development, a local clinical governance office can also be helpful.

As others become involved, it is useful to establish early in the planning of the project the extent of collaboration and the contribution they will provide; this is particularly true for academic colleagues in terms of expectations around co-authorship of published output.

What question am I trying to answer?

Designing a robust study is dependent on having a clear question to answer. The starting point may be from interest in a particular area of research; this will need to be channelled into a general, and then more specific, research question. The aim is to arrive at a single question that is specific and as unambiguous as possible. Then work to break down the question further and to develop objectives for the study is required. For example, a team of researchers aiming to reduce medication problems after discharge from hospital asked: 'What is the impact of a pharmacist-facilitated hospital discharge programme?' and defined their objectives as: 'to characterise medication discrepancies at hospital discharge and test the effects of a pharmacist intervention on healthcare utilisation following discharge'.[4] This example does not explicitly state the outcomes that will be used other than the broad term 'healthcare utilisation'. Pharmacy practice research is now strengthening its use of outcomes and there are still areas where existing research is particularly sparse, for example for clinical and economic outcomes.

Two issues are raised for pharmacy because many of its interventions are as part of care provided by a team: firstly, the need for multidisciplinary research to take this into account and, secondly, not choosing outcomes where it would be unlikely or even impossible for a pharmacy intervention alone to lead to improved health outcomes. The Medical Research Council has produced guidance for evaluating complex interventions that include conducting feasibility studies to define interventions and outcomes.[5] This framework could be followed if the research asks complex questions comparing pharmacist-led services with usual care.

It is perhaps helpful to consider an example. If the service were a hypertension clinic, a feasibility study would define the processes in care and facilitate power calculations to be undertaken to determine an appropriate sample size for a randomised controlled trial that would demonstrate any likely impact on the health outcome, in this case, blood pressure control. Process outcomes such as patient satisfaction and acceptability of the service by other healthcare professionals may provide positive outcomes but there may be no difference in blood pressure control. Economic evaluation may be appropriate in such a study to demonstrate that a change in service delivery is more efficient with no detriment to patient care.

If the question is more about why and how, then the outcomes will be more descriptive and qualitative methods may provide the answers. If the question is what, then a questionnaire may provide the answer. The challenge is to generate a question that is not too ambitious and can clearly be answered. Once the question is developed, before proceeding any further, there is a need to know if the work has been done before.

Has someone already answered my question?

Searching and reviewing relevant literature will prevent reinventing the wheel and is a key element in study design. Summarising what is known and not known from previous work will help give a better understanding of both the context and issues in the chosen topic. It is then possible to build upon existing published evidence and make a useful and relevant contribution. Depending on the strength of the researcher's skills in constructing an electronic literature search, assistance from the medicines information team or from a medical librarian can be key at this stage. As for clinical evidence, the principles of information mastery apply, drilling down through a hierarchy of sources beginning with systematic reviews and moving through to individual studies.[6] A useful starting point might be the Cochrane Collaboration on effective professional practice. Learning resources available through the UK Medicines Information website (www.ukmi.nhs.uk) may help with your search strategy and provide examples of research in medicines information. It is important to remember that there are many published abstracts from pharmacy conferences, such as the British Pharmaceutical Conference, Health Services Research and Pharmacy Practice Research Conference and UK Clinical Pharmacy Association (UKCPA) conference. These can usually found at the relevant website and are a valuable source because not all of these make their way into the wider literature if they are not subsequently written up as full papers. Local NHS R&D and clinical governance offices may also hold local and national databases of R&D projects. An advanced Google search can also be useful. Accessing full copies of published papers may be possible through the organisation's clinical library or medicines information team.

The literature review must go beyond being descriptive to being critical, showing an understanding of the strengths and limitations of the studies being appraised. Results and conclusions need to be assessed in the light of the research design used and the appropriateness of the methods to answer the question posed.

Finding out whether key authors in the relevant field have ongoing studies that are due to be published is another important step. Most researchers are happy to be contacted and there may even be the possibility for collaboration. Papers in peer-review journals almost always have address and e-mail contact details for the corresponding author; otherwise 'googling' by name and organisation is usually fruitful.

Which methods?

Depending on the question and the outcomes to be measured, an experimental or descriptive approach or a mixture of the two may be selected; quantitative or qualitative methods, or both, may be appropriate. Experimental studies are used to test the effects of an intervention and they aim to investigate causes and associations. Experimental research designs include 'true' experiments (randomised trials) and quasiexperimental studies. Their aim can be 'proof of concept' or 'proof of generalisability'. Choosing the appropriate method/s is a balance between selecting the ideal design (highest validity) with the most practical (highest feasibility).

Both quantitative and qualitative methods are used in pharmacy practice research. In the former the data are numbers and measurements, and in the latter narrative descriptions and observations. Qualitative methods are valuable in stand-alone studies and also have an important role in setting content for quantitative methods, including surveys. Survey studies are commonly used; they collect information in a standardised form from groups of people and are useful providing the questions have been framed. They usually employ questionnaires or highly structured interviews to obtain a small amount of data from a large population. Self-completed questionnaires are efficient in terms of researchers' time and effort. Closed questions will provide more concise replies, but wording needs to be carefully developed and tested. Rating scales are often used to collect data in questionnaires, for example, strength of agreement or disagreement about statements. Open questions generate qualitative data that can be subjected to a content analysis. Coding of content can be used to produce a quantitative profile of responses that can be supplemented by illustrative quotations; this is a time-consuming process requiring considerable skill. Semistructured interviews are a key tool in qualitative research and enable rich and in-depth information to be collected. Focus groups use a topic guide and facilitated discussion to cover the topics. The Delphi and nominal group techniques are used in specialist areas of practice to obtain consensus, but again can be time-consuming. To choose the best methodology or tool, other research in the topic can be examined as a guide; there may even be a validated tool that would be ideal for the planned research.

Consideration must be given to the study population, how many subjects are required and how they will be recruited. The inclusion and exclusion criteria will need to be established to help arrive at participants who will help answer the question posed. For a quantitative study a sample size or power calculation will be necessary, checking to see the study has sufficient participants to give an answer that is not merely down to chance. If there is no statistical expertise in the team, the NHS R&D office should be able to help. It is also a good idea to consider how the data will be analysed and to obtain statistical advice at an early stage. This may also help design the data collection tools. A decision on who will measure the outcomes will need to be made. Depending on the intervention, it may be more appropriate to engage an independent researcher such as a research nurse to administer questionnaires or take clinical measurements. The local R&D office or clinical research facility may be able to help.

It is a good idea at this stage to develop a study protocol outlining the project as this provides a focus for collaborators to provide feedback and it will be required for approval processes. It will also help to clarify whether or not they will be part of the project team. A more detailed protocol will need to be developed as plans progress. There is no set outline for a research protocol and funding bodies may specify their own template, but the following headings would usually be expected

- title of the study
- study team and contribution of individual members
- summary of aims, objectives, methods and outcomes to be measured
- background: this section justifies the need to undertake the research based on the literature review and any pilot work done
- aims and objectives
- study design and methods:
  - setting where the research will take place
  - subjects/patients, including how they will be identified and recruited, and inclusion and exclusion criteria. The sample size must be justified and, for a quantitative study, say whether a sample size calculation has been used
  - methods of assessment or measurement: explain what data will be collected, data collection instruments to be used and why they were chosen. If equipment needs to be used, describe it, and how its measures will be used
  - outcome measures need to be stated for both quantitative and qualitative studies
  - interventions (if applicable): if the study involves an intervention, it should be described. If giving a treatment or investigation, the dose, timing, method of providing, administering and receiving the treatment should be detailed. All necessary safeguards and potential risks should be made clear, including the methods by which intervention will be monitored
- data collection, management and analysis, including how data will be collected, method of data entry, plan of analysis, and any data analysis packages
- ethical considerations
- benefits of the research to patients and the NHS
- costs, including staff salaries, equipment, running costs (for example stationery, telephone, postage, travel) and any overheads (such as costs for office space, lighting, heating)
- timescales
- references
- appendices (draft or actual data collection forms, questionnaires, interview schedules)
- which approvals are needed for my study?

The main aim of research governance is to ensure all NHS researchers comply with a framework of activities and minimum standards and to be able to demonstrate their research quality through defined audit trails. There are two main types of NHS approval for research studies: (1) research ethics; and (2) R&D management approval. If the study is going to involve patients or staff working within the NHS, advice must be sought on whether ethical and local R&D approval is needed. This hinges on whether the project is considered to be 'research', hence the importance of the earlier definitions. The local R&D office will be able to advise on this as well as on local procedures that may be required for audit or service evaluation, which are sometimes overseen by clinical effectiveness teams. The electronic Integrated Research Application System ethics form (www. myresearchproject.org.uk/) gives an idea of the issues for consideration. Projects which are not 'research' will probably require approval through clinical governance structures. Irrespective of whether the study is deemed 'research' or 'audit', Caldicott principles, patient consent and data protection should be considered, though the project design will determine if particular actions are required. Training programmes may be available through the local NHS R&D office or through partner academic institution.

What resources will I need?

Regardless of whether the study is self funded or an application for funding is to be made, it is important to understand the resources that will be needed, including time, equipment, consumables, travel and dissemination costs. These need to be clear on all approval forms and the local NHS R&D office may be able to help with templates for estimating and costing resources. The National Institute for Health Research is a major funder of health research (www.rdinfo.org.uk; http//rdfunding.org.uk) and has several funding streams, some of which are commissioned on specific topics and some are responsive and intended to meet needs identified within the service. There are many other possible sources of funding, such as www. cso.scot.nhs.uk (in NHS Scotland) and many clinical specialist charities. Any bid needs to be targeted appropriately to the relevant body. Some pharmacy organisations have awards to support pilot or development work and small projects, and these are valuable to test out ideas if you are thinking of applying for funding for a larger study. It is important that the proposal has been well reviewed by all members of the project team before it is submitted for funding or approval.

Bringing it all together

An example of how a research programme was developed from the starting point of an audit of care is shown in Text box 16.1.

Box 16.1 Developing a research programme in pharmaceutical care in secondary prevention of stroke

Starting from audits of care in patients who had had a stroke, an application was made for a research grant to:

- explore beliefs and concerns about medicines
- identify the difficulties experienced taking medicines
- design documentation incorporating the evidence base and pharmaceutical needs as identified by patients and carers.

The application was successful and the study was conducted with 30 patients who were purposively sampled and had been discharged after stroke or transient ischaemic attack within the past 12 months. Semistructured interviews covered self-reported adherence with prescribed medication and patients were asked to complete the Beliefs about Medicines questionnaire. The medicine-related problems identified were then addressed. The draft document produced as a result was reviewed by patients, general practitioners, community pharmacists and the local stroke managed clinical network.

Using the results from the study a further grant application was made to conduct a randomised exploratory trial of a pharmacist-led home-based clinical medication review in people after stroke. The purpose of this study was to conduct an exploratory trial to define the intervention, outcome measures and sample size. Pharmacist-led home-based clinical medication review at 1 and 3 months after discharge ($n = 20$) is being compared with 'usual care' ($n = 20$), and 6-month follow-up which ended in May 2010. Further grant application has been made to test the feasibility of recruitment from primary care and to include telephone interview.

The research is a collaboration between pharmacy, geriatric medicine, community health sciences, psychology and the Stroke Research Group.[7–9]

How should I disseminate my findings?

Much greater emphasis is now placed on dissemination than used to be the case. Effective dissemination of results to those who need to take action is now widely recognised as an essential part of the research process. In the past there has been more emphasis on academic methods of dissemination so that information is publicly available and open to peer review. This has changed to incorporate dissemination to key stakeholders because ultimately R&D activities are done with a view to change and improvement. This can only happen if the findings are acted upon. Research can be disseminated in many ways, including full original peer-reviewed journal publications, articles in professional journals, oral and poster conference presentations, newsletters, reports, briefings and entries in research databases. A dissemination plan should be agreed by the project team at the outset of the study, as there may be differences in opinion as to where research should be published. Guidance on preparing and presenting research is available from various pharmacy organisations. For example the UKCPA, UK Medicines Information and European Society of Clinical Pharmacy include guidance on preparation of abstracts and posters on their websites (http://www.ukcpa.org.uk; www.ukmi.nhs.uk; www.escpweb.org). Abstracts from posters and presentations at previous pharmacy conferences (for example, British Pharmaceutical Conference, Health Services Research and Pharmacy Practice Research Conference and UKCPA conference) can usually be found on their websites. It may be possible to present findings at both pharmacy conferences and at multidisciplinary specialist conferences such as Diabetes UK.

Publications are rewarding for researchers and raise not only their individual profile but also the profile of the profession in a multidisciplinary environment. Proactive dissemination to stakeholders is an important part of the overall strategy and requires creative thinking. A strategy might include targeted presentations to relevant boards or committees, written briefings sent to a targeted audience and multi-stakeholder workshops at which findings can be discussed and actions needed prioritised. Again collaboration is helpful, whether it is academic support for writing for peer-review journals and conferences, or review of briefings and articles by some of the intended audience.

The future

Pharmacy practice research next needs to develop to become a more integral part of the wider health services research effort, represented in more of the existing and future large successful multidisciplinary groups. Not all of the studies that result will be of pharmacy and pharmacists but there will be greater opportunities to include pharmacy interventions as an arm in more trials than is currently the case, supported by infrastructure and expertise in experimental study design. Pharmacists are taking the lead in service redesign within their clinical specialities and these changes in service delivery should be evidence-based. There are opportunities to work in collaboration with clinical teams to evaluate new models of care in a scientific way with full economic evaluation. As pharmacists recognise the need to research their core practice and demonstrate equal or better alternatives to service delivery, the culture will change from R&D being an add-on to it being integral to practice.

Acknowledgement

This chapter is based on work by Sarah Hiom for the previous edition of this book.

References

1. Department of Health. *Pharmacy in England: Building on Strengths – Delivering the Future.* London: Department of Health, 2008.
2. National Research Ethics Service. *Defining Research.* London: National Research Ethics Service, 2009.
3. Pharmacy Practice Research Trust. *A Strategic Direction for Pharmacy Practice Research.* London: Pharmacy Practice Research Trust, 2009.
4. Walker PC, Bernstein SJ, Jones JN *et al.* Impact of a pharmacist-facilitated hospital discharge program: a quasi-experimental study. *Arch Intern Med* 2009; 23: 2003–2010.
5. Craig P, Dieppe P, Macintyre S *et al.* Developing and evaluating complex interventions: the new Medical Research Council guidance. *Br Med J* 2008; 337: a1655.
6. Slawson DC, Shaughnessy AF. Teaching evidence-based medicine: should we be teaching information management instead? *Acad Med* 2005; 80: 685–689.
7. Palenzuela E, Kinnear A, Kinnear M. Adherence to prescribing guidelines and design of a pharmaceutical care plan for stroke patients. *Pharm World Sci* 2009; 31: 54.
8. Souter C, Kinnear A, Kinnear M. Optimisation of pharmaceutical care for secondary prevention of stroke. *Int J Pharm Pract* 2009; 17(Suppl 1): A34.
9. Souter C, Kinnear A, Kinnear M *et al.* Optimisation of secondary prevention of stroke: qualitative study of patients' beliefs, concerns and difficulties with their medicines. *Int J Pharm Pract* 2010; 18(Suppl 1): 62.

Further reading

Department of Health. *Research Governance Framework for Health and Social Care*, 2nd edn. London: Department of Health, 2005.

Greenhalgh T. *How to Read a Paper*. London: BMJ Publishing, 1997.

Hart C. *Doing a Literature Review*. London: Sage, 2000.

http://www.knowledge.scot.nhs.uk/home.aspx: a range of resources including electronic databases for literature searching.

International Committee of Medical Journal Editors. Uniform requirements for manuscripts submitted to biomedical journals: ethical considerations in the conduct and reporting of research: authorship and contributorship: http://www.icmje.org/ethical_1author.html.

Oppenheim AN. *Questionnaire Design, Interviewing and Attitude Measurement*. London: Cassell, 1992.

Robson C. *Real World Research*, 2nd edn. Oxford: Blackwell, 2002.

Royal Pharmaceutical Society of Great Britain library: https://my.rpsgb.org/login/index.asp.

Scottish Executive Health Department. *Research Governance Framework for Health and Community Care*, 2nd edn. Edinburgh: Scottish Government, 2006.

Smith F. *Conducting your Pharmacy Practice Research Project*, 2nd edn. London: Pharmaceutical Press, 2010.

17

Workforce development

Trevor Beswick and Lyn Hanning

It would not be unreasonable to suggest that, over the past 20 years or so, hospital pharmacy in the UK has been the most innovative area of pharmacy practice. In large part this has been possible because of the steps taken to develop the hospital pharmacy workforce in delivering advances in patient care. Role development and accreditation, adoption and delegation of authority and skill mix have all been successfully used within the hospital pharmacy sector. These issues are recognised in the 2008 Department of Health White Paper *Pharmacy in England: Building on Strengths – Delivering the Future.*[1]

This chapter will briefly review the recent approaches taken to the development of the hospital pharmacy workforce. It will also address a number of factors that will have an impact on those developments in the future. These factors include:

- changes in the regulation of the profession
- health service reform and government policy
- new approaches to workforce planning
- continued development of the clinical roles of pharmacy staff
- development of advanced and specialist practice.

Recent developments

Clinical pharmacy became well established in UK hospital pharmacy practice during the 1980s as a result of both the profession's aspirations and government policy. The role of pharmacists and support staff in managing medicines, both at organisational and individual levels, was seen as being crucial to delivering clinical and cost-effective treatment.[2] This led to a drive to improve the training of pharmacists in clinical knowledge and skills at undergraduate, preregistration and, predominantly, at postregistration levels.

As a result of the change in role of hospital pharmacists, pharmacy technicians, supported by additional post-basic qualification training and accreditation, took on wider roles and more delegated authority.

Hospital pharmacy services are still underpinned by the traditional specialist roles such as those in technical services, quality assurance and medicines information. There is, however, an increasing emphasis on the development of clinical specialities, a change driven by a variety of professional pharmacy organisations, such as UK Clinical Pharmacy Association and the College of Mental Health Pharmacy, as well as by the inclusion of advanced and specialist practice by the Department of Health in the framework for consultant pharmacists.[3]

Alongside these significant developments in practice there have been a number of changes in teaching, learning and assessment. The Competency Development and Evaluation Group describes a set of competency frameworks, based on qualitative and quantitative research findings that can be applied to both general and advanced practice.[4] It has provided a tool to define and measure performance standards of practice.

Factors that will influence workforce development in the coming years

Health service reform

In common with many countries, the National Health Service (NHS) has undertaken major reviews of how it meets society's health needs. Changing demographics, advances in healthcare and increased patient involvement and expectation mean that the NHS, in common with health systems in other countries, is now entering another phase of major reform.

Economic pressures

The financial pressure on public services caused in large part by international problems in financial sectors has brought renewed urgency to the need to reform the NHS. It has been necessary to identify how to manage reduced budgets and still meet a range of growing and competing demands.

Changes in professional regulation

Following on from the Kennedy report into the problems in Bristol Heart Surgery Services, the Council for Healthcare Regulatory Excellence was established to oversee the roles of the individual professional regulatory bodies.[5, 6] For pharmacy, this led to a change in the role of the Royal Pharmaceutical Society of Great Britain (RPSGB), with all of its statutory professional regulatory functions being transferred during 2010 to the General Pharmaceutical Council.[7] Amongst these functions are the professional standards and codes of conduct that govern the education, training and CPD of pharmacists and pharmacy technicians.

Workforce planning

Whilst the NHS has always undertaken workforce planning in an attempt to match the workforce demands of the service with the commissioned numbers of professionals in training, it has recently been severely criticised for not being fit for purpose.[8] This is a difficult task that needs to make informed assumptions about the factors affecting both the demand and the supply side of this system. The Centre for Workforce Intelligence has been established to improve this process.[9] One of the key approaches that it is hoped will improve workforce planning is the transition to a focus on care pathways: by determining how key groups of patients will be managed, a workforce model can then be built to estimate more accurately the numbers and types of staff required. One of the challenges with this approach will be to ensure that this planning has sufficient granularity to estimate smaller professional groups such as the pharmacy workforce, and in particular the very specialised roles that may not be obvious when considering a pathway but that make an important contribution to healthcare as a whole.

Advanced and specialist practice

Advanced practice has been defined as when a new role is so significantly different from the original registered qualification that members of the profession and public need to be able to identify the new practitioner and understand the education, training and assessment associated with the new role. This is a complex area that has to achieve a balance between providing services that are fit for purpose and affordable, meet collective and individual professional aspirations and protect the public interest.

Currently, apart from pharmacists with extended prescribing responsibilities, there is no statutory recognition of advanced and specialist practice; registrants are either pharmacists (with or without prescribing responsibilities) or they are pharmacy technicians.

Medical Education England and the Modernising Pharmacy Careers Project Board

Medical Education England was set up in 2009 to align professional training, education and workforce needs with the needs of the service and patients following on from the Lord Darzi *NHS Next Stage Review: A High Quality*

Workforce.[10, 11] Medical Education England will provide independent expert advice on education and training and workforce planning for doctors, dentists, healthcare scientists and pharmacists. The pharmacy agenda is being taken forward by the Modernising Pharmacy Careers Project Board. At the time of writing, their work programme covers the following areas that, clearly, will lead to change in the education and training of the hospital pharmacy workforce:

* the development and implementation of a new approach to pharmacist undergraduate education and preregistration training
* enabling the registered pharmacy workforce to acquire the additional skills needed to deliver a wider range of clinical services
* building on current arrangements for advanced pharmacy practice
* determining and facilitating changes in the training of key pharmacy support staff to improve pharmacy skill mix, making the best use of all those working in pharmacy.

Undergraduate and preregistration education and training

Since 1997, pharmacy has been a 4-year undergraduate course, leading to the MPharm degree. National initiatives to increase NHS staffing numbers have led to recognition of the need for greater numbers of pharmacists to undertake new roles and provide a greater range of pharmacy services. Most universities have increased their intake of students, and in recent years a number of new sites have become accredited. There are now a total of 25 Schools of Pharmacy across the UK. Two universities offer sandwich courses delivered over 5 years, incorporating the preregistration year.

To become a pharmacist in the UK, all graduates must complete a 1-year period of preregistration training under the supervision of a registered pharmacist. In addition, all trainees must pass a registration assessment. The General Pharmaceutical Council sets the standards for the training, and monitors the quality to ensure that it is acceptably high across all sites.

A full revision of the preregistration training programme was undertaken by the RPSGB in preparation for the intake of the first graduates from the new 4-year degree in August 2001. The aim of the new training programme was to develop pharmacists who had patients as their primary focus and who were fit for practice in any sector of the profession. Putting patients at the centre of care was a clear theme within *Pharmacy in the Future*, the document dealing with pharmacy's part in delivering NHS change agenda in the late 1990s, so the change in focus was timely.[12] Cross-sector experience was introduced at this time, although logistically it has not been possible to implement this across all sectors. The work of the Modernising Pharmacy Careers Board looking at developments in undergraduate and preregistration education may suggest a new approach to this in the coming years.[13] This will address a range of issues including the context for theoretical learning; late exposure to pharmacy practice; the large variation in quality of preregistration training and tutors; and a need for greater coooperation between higher education institutes and employers.

The current training programme comprises performance standards which state what a newly qualified pharmacist is expected to be able to do. These were devised in consultation with members of all sectors of the profession and describe generic skills required of all pharmacists. The examination syllabus was revised and updated at that time, and now has a strong emphasis on the ability of pharmacists to perform calculations.

The shift to a more outcome-focused programme enables preregistration trainees to assess themselves against the performance standards and so identify what their learning needs are, hence reinforcing the culture of CPD that is being developed throughout the profession. In tandem with the trainee, preregistration tutors also have to demonstrate a commitment to CPD and maintain a portfolio in which they document how they have identified and met their learning needs.

The vast majority of hospital trainees undergo an in-house training programme that typically consists of a planned rotation through the main sections within the pharmacy department. This will often include periods in the dispensary, wards and clinical services, medicines information, technical services and quality assurance. Depending on the size of the hospital and the scope of services offered, there may well be a period of training at a neighbouring hospital for specialist experience. Most in-house training programmes are supplemented by a programme of regionally taught courses, which may be delivered either as 1-day courses or as residential blocks.

Trainees undergo formal assessments with their tutor during the year, and the results of these are sent to the registration body. In addition, the registration body requests copies of the in-house and taught course programmes, and may sample the tutor portfolios to enable closer monitoring of the quality of training.

Postregistration education and training

The current provision of structured postregistration training for pharmacists is varied but includes a number of common elements. After qualification most newly qualified pharmacists in the NHS take up a band 6 position, many of which include an opportunity to study on a clinical diploma. This is the standard route for most hospital pharmacists and many universities provide clinical diploma courses – these courses are not formally accredited by the current pharmacy regulator and vary across the country in their design and delivery. Opportunity to study a clinical diploma may be an aid to recruitment and retention for employers as well as a means of developing its employees.

The clinical diploma is usually a 2-year postgraduate diploma-level qualification which teaches pharmacists much of the clinical application of their knowledge with an emphasis on applying their knowledge to practice-based situations. The course is usually funded by the individual trust or, at time of writing, via the relevant strategic health authority.

Recent developments have seen a number of institutions, for example the University of Bath, launching a range of learning opportunities to meet the needs of mid-career pharmacists.[14] These have been mapped to the Advanced and Consultant Level Framework and support pharmacists in developing in areas such as teaching and learning, research methods, management and leadership.

Technician training

Student technician training has evolved significantly over recent years since the introduction of the National Vocational Qualification (NVQ) level 3 in pharmacy services in 1997. This is a competency-based training programme, consisting of a total of nine (seven core and two optional) units that the student undertakes in the workplace. The student must demonstrate consistent competence in a range of activities and undergoes assessment by local work-based tutors. The tutors must gain formal qualifications that help to ensure that they are able to judge evidence fairly and consistently.

In addition to the work-based units, students must also gain evidence of their underpinning knowledge. This may be achieved in several ways – some hospitals use distance-learning packages, such as those provided by the National Pharmaceutical Association or the Buttercups scheme. Others attend Further Education Colleges to undertake specific Business and Technology Council (BTEC) courses in order to attain the required underpinning knowledge.

After qualification, many hospital pharmacy technicians take up further structured postqualification training in order to develop new roles within and take on additional responsibilities. The need for formal training and accreditation to perform these new roles is well developed.

The first major development for technician training was the introduction of technician checking schemes, which have allowed technicians to perform the final accuracy check of dispensed items. Most NHS regions have now developed accredited schemes that specify the training that an individual must undergo, and the mechanisms for assessment. Upon completion of all stages they gain formal accreditation, which can be recognised by other NHS employers.

Pharmacy technicians also develop other roles working more closely with patients to improve medicines management. A range of schemes to enable accreditation of technicians in medicines management, technical services and medicines information is available.

Support staff

In tandem with the developing roles of pharmacists and pharmacy technicians, pharmacy assistants are offered appropriate support to underpin the roles that they are now performing within the pharmacy. This staff group undertake training relevant to their roles and to meet the requirements of the RPSGB for training of support staff,

Management and leadership

In 2001, the Audit Commission made it clear that excellent pharmacy services require good leadership.[15] This theme was restated in the broader sense for all clinical services in the *Next Stage Review*.[11] Development of management and leadership skills in pharmacy is therefore an important aspect of CPD. Chapter 19 deals with the key aspects of management; this chapter will briefly mention some important training initiatives. Often the first aspects of management training will be taught in the local hospital on a multiprofessional basis – personnel management, understanding the organisation, budget control, for example. Access to external training may be provided, such as to the Open University health management courses or to Masters in Business Administration, for those taking on full-time management roles. The national development scheme for senior pharmacists, and the more recently introduced national course for technicians, is an invaluable opportunity to gain insight and develop skills in a uniprofessional setting.[16]

Postgraduate pharmacy education centres

Access to materials and programmes from the Centre for Pharmacy Postgraduate Education is open to pharmacists and pharmacy technicians in England. Their products include the learning@lunch portfolio aimed at hospital pharmacy teams and including modules on topics such as medicines reconciliation and venous thromboembolism.[17] NHS Education for Scotland (Pharmacy) is the Centre for Continuing Pharmaceutical Education in Scotland and it provides an education and training programme, including face-to-face courses, distance learning and other flexible methods for hospital pharmacists working within the NHS in Scotland. Wales has a similar centre.

The future

The NHS will continue to modernise and change. This will bring new demands on the profession that will need to be underpinned with well-educated, trained and competent staff. Among these factors will be:

- revised General Pharmaceutical Council standards for education, training and CPD for pharmacists and pharmacy technicians
- training, often delivered by employers on a mandatory basis, to support medicines governance, for example, to ensure competence for prescribing, prescription screening and dispensing chemotherapy
- greater uptake of new ways to support learning and assessment, for example, greater use of e-portfolios, e-learning and e-assessment
- the further definition of advanced and specialist practice and the specification of the learning needs of those practitioners
- the incorporation of new elements of practice into undergraduate and preregistration training, for example, elements of prescribing competencies and supply through patient group directions
- CPD and revalidation to practice
- new systems for workforce planning.

References

1. Department of Health. *Pharmacy in England. Building on Strengths – Delivering the Future.* London: Department of Health, 2008.
2. Department of Health. *The Way Forward for Hospital Pharmaceutical Services.* HC88(54). London: HMSO, 1988.
3. Department of Health. *Guidance for the Development of Consultant Pharmacist Posts.* London: Department of Health, 2005.
4. Competency Development and Evaluation Group (CoDEG) website: http://www.codeg.org/.
5. Learning from Bristol: the report of the public inquiry into children's heart surgery at the Bristol Royal Infirmary 1984–1995. Available online at: http://www.bristol-inquiry.org.uk/final_report/Summary.pdf.
6. Council for Healthcare Regulatory Excellence website: http://www.chre.org.uk/.
7. General Pharmaceutical Council website: http://www.pharmacyregulation.org/.
8. House of Commons Health Committee Workforce Planning 2007. Available online at: http://www.publications.parliament.uk/pa/cm200607/cmselect/cmhealth/171/171i.pdf.
9. Centre for Workforce Intelligence website: http://www.dh.gov.uk/en/MediaCentre/Pressreleasesarchive/DH_114870.
10. NHS Medical Education England website: http://www.mee.nhs.uk/.
11. Department of Health. *Next Stage Review, Final Report.* London: Department of Health, 2008.
12. Department of Health. *Pharmacy in the Future – Implementing the NHS Plan.* London: The Stationery Office, 2000.
13. MEE press release. Stakeholders welcome cross-sector discussion of pharmacist undergraduate education and pre-registration training. Available online at: http://www.mee.nhs.uk/latest_news/news_releases/mpc_stakeholder_event_report.aspx.
14. University of Bath website: http://www.bath.ac.uk/pharmacy/pg_ap3t/AdvCPD_Overview.html.

15. Audit Commission. *A Spoonful of Sugar – Medicines Management in NHS Hospitals.* London: Audit Commission, 2001.
16. National Development Schemes for Senior Pharmacists and Pharmacy Technicians website: http://www.waypointers.co.uk/.
17. CPPE learning@lunch portfolio. Available online at: http://www.cppe.ac.uk/learning/ programmes.asp?ByTheme=false&format=h&ID=52 (accessed 27 August 2010).

Further reading

Centre for Pharmacy Postgraduate Education website: http://www.cppe.ac.uk/default.asp.
Modernising Pharmacy Careers Board website: http://www.mee.nhs.uk/programme_boards/ modernising_pharmacy_careers_p.aspx.
National Health Service Education for Scotland, pharmacy: http://www.nes.scot.nhs.uk/pharmacy/.

18

Consultant pharmacists

Nina Barnett and Mark Tomlin

Introduction

Whatever the sector of practice, pharmacists are experts on medicines. This may be in their discovery, manufacture, preparation, dispensing, provision of medicines information, clinical usage, dealing with adverse events, costs, medicines management or general safety. The question is: what distinguishes an advanced or consultant-level practitioner? Chapter 17 touched on the issue of advanced practice and its regulation, including the role of the Modernising Pharmacy Careers Board. This chapter will focus on developments in the UK hospital sector, detailing the history that led to the development of the consultant pharmacist role, key characteristics of the post-holders and the way forward, including non-hospital-based developments. It is worth noting here that the term 'consultant pharmacist' is used in the context of the Department of Health guidance, developed for use in England.[1]

Leaders in hospital pharmacy have traditionally been chief pharmacists, as professional leaders and strategic thinkers, in addition to managing a department. The new and emerging role of the consultant pharmacists differs from the chief pharmacist role, and is based on the provision of clinical leadership as part of the pharmacy team, working with chief pharmacists to deliver improvements in practice. Consultant pharmacists will have developed their expert practice area to an advanced level and have significant demonstrable experience in pharmacy leadership, education and research.

There has been some confusion in the use of the terms 'advanced', 'higher-level', 'specialist' and 'expert' in the context of the consultant pharmacist. In reality, consultant pharmacists may be any or all of these: they will be 'advanced' in their knowledge of their area of practice and may be working at a 'higher' clinical or technical level, they may have a specific clinical or technical area in which they have expertise, or may be 'expert' in a general area of practice. However, in National Health Service (NHS) hospitals in

England, pharmacists may only use the title consultant if they are employed in an organisation where their post has been approved by the strategic health authority in accordance with Department of Health guidance. This guidance makes provision for an experienced practitioner to remain in a practice-based post for the benefit of patients.

How did these roles emerge?

Career pathways in hospital pharmacy

Prior to the 1970s hospital pharmacy was a medicines supply role and the developments over the following 20 years saw a move towards ward-based pharmacy and then into the more proactive clinical pharmacy role, as discussed in Chapters 9 and 13.

Just as medical practice moved into specialisation according to clinical areas, pharmacy practice and the specialist pharmacist role emerged, together with advances in pharmaceutical, clinically based expertise in these areas. The 1990s saw the emergence of directorate pharmacists, giving clinical pharmacists the opportunity to develop business skills and roles in budgeting and formulary development. Career paths continued to move from clinical practitioner to dispensary manager to chief pharmacist, leaving the 'clinical specialist' pharmacist with no other route to progress. In the 1990s it became more accepted that highly skilled clinical pharmacists might work in a generalist role, providing cover across several specialties from their senior clinical pharmacy or clinical pharmacy manager posts. Nevertheless, progression to chief pharmacist from both specialist and generalist higher-level roles required practitioners to reduce the time spent in clinical work and spend time in management and supervisory functions. Thus promotion was linked to the loss of the direct clinical contribution to patients.

Developments in education and training

As discussed in Chapter 17, the development of clinical pharmacy was underpinned by education and training. In 1982 the UK Clinical Pharmacy Association (UKCPA) was formed as a broad umbrella for all clinical areas of pharmacy. This has provided an opportunity for pharmacists to share best clinical practice through conference workshops and case study discussions, as well as through clinical networks where ideas and strategic developments are shared. Some specialists formed their own groups, such as oncology, paediatric and mental health pharmacist, and became faculties of the College of Pharmacy Practice, developing their specialisms through individual study days, conferences and postgraduate courses.

Use of practice frameworks

Early years

Despite the exciting advances in hospital pharmacy practice, recruitment to junior posts remained challenging, not helped by the salary differential between hospital and community pharmacy. This was addressed by the introduction of work-based formal clinical training programmes to attract and then retain junior pharmacists. In the south-east, this was known as the Structured Training and Experience for Pharmacists (STEPS) project – a focused development programme with staged objectives.[2] This was a London-based project, with Southampton as a control site. Junior pharmacists were given a structured rotation through London hospitals with defined achievements at each clinical rotation. The project showed that pharmacists developed competencies that could be defined and assessed in order to achieve performance targets. This progression was achieved more rapidly when the targets were described at the beginning of the programme and the Competency Development and Education Group (CoDEG) used this to produce the evidence-based, validated general-level competency framework, which emerged in 2003.[3]

Higher-level and advanced practice

Senior clinical pharmacists who had not moved into a management position, including those who had taught on postgraduate or training programmes, expressed their desire for recognition of their higher-level/advanced practice. At the time, there was no method of defining higher-level/advanced practice in pharmacy and reputation relied on recognition by peers and medical colleagues. Some practitioners working at higher-level specialist practice aligned themselves more closely with the medical team than the pharmacy team, making it difficult to identify the pharmacy level at which they practised.

Hospital-based practice

In the late 1980s US pharmacy practice began to move away from the traditional pyramid structure of hospital pharmacy where promotion to a higher level relied on managerial responsibility. The parallel career ladders describe a more rectangular model where those with relevant clinical competencies can be promoted to the same level as their manager, who deals with human resources issues – akin to models in business. Promotion was linked to a review board considering a variety of documentation (evidence) and portfolios now included self-evaluation against competencies, peer evaluations, letters of recommendation, records of teaching and supervision of juniors.

This was a way of rewarding mentorship and supervision of junior pharmacists and allowed practice to develop where supply activities were delegated to technicians. Promotion might require delivery of a practice development project or new service such as pharmacokinetic support or nutrition.

The Americans struggled with the classification of young pharmacists. Their pathway was the generation of evidence, which consisted of intervention log, descriptions of projects, research published papers, case reviews, contributions to hospital committees and mentor recommendations – much like portfolios of practice today.

The top of these parallel career ladders was occupied by an associate director who was managed by the pharmacy director. The pharmacy director was generally supported by a top-level team, each contributing to the external perception of the pharmacy contribution to hospital care. There might be an operational manager below the director, mirrored by a clinical pharmacy manager in the UK.

In the UK, many clinical pharmacists had developed in the single ladder of clinical practice with the additional skill of building strong working relationships with other clinical specialities and good communication skills. Pharmacy was lacking capacity in practice research. The question that followed was: could multidimensional practitioners be created with not just the ladder of expert practice and education but also research and leadership capabilities?

Consultant pharmacists

The answer to clinical leadership for patient-facing clinical roles came in the late 1990s with the emergence of the consultant nurse role, as Project 2000 moved nursing into a degree-based profession. Later the consultant allied health professional (AHP) role was developed, paving the way for consultant pharmacists, for which Department of Health guidance was published in 2005.[1]

Suggestions of the consultant pharmacist role had been developed in the UK in the early 2000s.[4]

Following the success of the general-level competency framework, CoDEG set up a PhD project to look at a framework for advanced practice. The College of Pharmacy Practice faculty groups and UKCPA were asked to nominate 'experts' to participate in the research, which would attempt to determine competencies of advanced practice and the levels of practice. This research demonstrated that there were at least 50 practitioners in the UK working at a very high ('consultant') level and led to the development of the advanced-level framework. This information contributed to the Department of Health working party on consultant pharmacists, with a wider reference group as part of the Department of Health consultant pharmacist project in 2004. The

Department of Health utilised the framework in its 2005 guidance, renamed as the advanced and consultant level framework (ACLF).[5]

Contribution of the critical care model

In 2000, the modernisation agency produced a document entitled *Comprehensive Critical Care*, which outlined how critical care should be provided over at least the following decade.[6] Crucially, it facilitated the set-up of clinical networks that focused multidisciplinary collaboration across a geographical area, creating the opportunity for consultant nurses, AHPs and pharmacists to influence the development of practice outside their base hospital.

In 2002 the Modernisation Agency followed up this report with a description of the functions of healthcare professionals who supported doctors and nurses, including the roles of AHPs and healthcare scientists.[7] This was the first document to describe the activities of clinical pharmacists and provide a benchmark of staffing levels (0.1 whole-time-equivalent posts (WTE) per level 3 bed and 0.05 WTE per level 2 bed). The publication of this document triggered the UKCPA critical care pharmacists group, many of whom were leading in local critical care networks, to form an expert panel and convert the description of these roles into a list of competencies that were required to support critical care. The work was supported by the Department of Health lead for critical care and described what networks and trusts needed to commission from pharmacy. It also gave pharmacists a career development plan for working in critical care from new practitioner to higher levels of practice and a syllabus of knowledge that needed to be acquired. The competencies were described in a way that matched the ACLF and in the same format.

Consultant posts and post-holders

Requirements for the consultant pharmacist post

The guidance clearly sets out the functions of the post:

- Expert practice (up to 50% of role) (the guidance took note of the issue from nurse consultants where patient-facing roles varied from as little as 20% clinical practice to over 80%, and stated that about 50% of the consultant pharmacist role should be in expert practice): delivering high-level expertise, recognised as an expert in their area of practice, having professional autonomy and driving professional and strategic development.
- Research, evaluation and service development: contributing to audit, service evaluation, research, education and training, supporting clinical governance and strengthening links between research and practice.

- Education, mentoring and overview of practice: working with higher-education institutions at a strategic level, teaching and enhancing links between pharmacy bodies and practice.
- Professional leadership: communicating across sectors and organisations, developing services strategies and leading introduction of best practice, working in partnership with managers, advanced practitioners and other healthcare leaders to achieve successful outcomes.

The guidance was unique in that it encouraged creation of these posts across localities, which could span acute, primary care and/or mental health trusts together with higher-education institutions.

Establishing local posts

The publication of the Department of Health guidance in 2005[1] heralded a new way of establishing posts in the NHS, hitherto unseen. Local organisations were required to identify the service need and produce a submission/ business plan to their local organisation as usual. However, the proposal then had to be presented to a specially convened panel at their strategic health authority, which determined whether the post met the requirement of the Department of Health guidance. The panel members were specified in the guidance as:

- chief pharmacist or director of pharmaceutical services
- lay member or patient representative
- pharmacist with appropriate expertise in the practice area under consideration
- strategic health authority representative
- higher education institution representative

The business plan/submission is required to contain the service need for patient benefit and outline of the appointment process as well as the job description, person specification and competency requirements for potential post-holders with details of time allocated for each of the four main post functions. Competencies were measured against the ACLF, as documented in the Department of Health guidance.

Applying for a post

Pharmacists wishing to apply for a consultant pharmacist post were required to demonstrate competence according to the Department of Health guidance. The framework provided was divided into six 'clusters' and practitioners were required to submit evidence of highest-level practice (mastery) in a minimum of three clusters: (1) expert practice; (2) building working relationships; and

(3) leadership, with a minimum of the middle level, 'excellence', in management, education and training, and research and evaluation. This would form part of an interview submission for new applicants.

In order to facilitate the establishment of the posts, the first 2 years after the consultant post establishment allowed for 'transitional' arrangements. Organisations with posts matching the consultant profile could submit an application for strategic health authority approval of these posts and practitioners, who were already in the post, operating at consultant level, were permitted to submit evidence of their suitability for the post, using the ACLF to facilitate demonstration of competence.

However, NHS reorganisation in 2005 made it difficult for the process of appointment to become established. The process was the same as for nurse and AHP consultants, with more constraints, as the nurse consultants had in some cases become a rebadging of advanced practitioners. Academic links were particularly difficult to establish as schools of pharmacy were not experienced with work-based learning and practitioner teaching to the same level as seen in schools of nursing. In addition universities were being challenged by new financial constraints.

The result of this has been that, at the time of writing, there are about 40 consultant pharmacist posts established.

Current posts/where we are now

While the majority of consultant pharmacist posts are in the hospital sector and specific clinical specialties, the importance of primary care contribution is increasingly clear and new roles recognise this. In addition, the guidance is flexible enough to allow a number of different models of consultant role.

The models include:

- Specialist hospital consultant pharmacist: for example in critical care, human immunodeficiency virus, where the pharmacist provides on-site expertise to a specific cohort of patients in a ward and/or clinic-based setting. In the latter example, there are strong connections with primary care.
- Generalist hospital consultant pharmacists: this model can include a consultancy role where pharmacists have a number of areas of expertise (two or three, rather than one) and their caseload is through referral from other pharmacists and healthcare professionals. They may also have ward-based commitment. Another version of this model is seen within the acute admissions unit in hospitals where consultant pharmacists are the lead pharmacy practitioners for these units that admit general medicine and/or surgery patients.

- Specialist primary care consultant pharmacist: this role is less common but includes practitioners leading general practice services and/or running their own clinics, such as cardiology or substance abuse.
- Generalist primary care consultant pharmacist: this is a developing role and currently only exists for care of older people; however, there is great potential for support of community pharmacists and pharmacists with a special interest (see Department of Health guidance[8]).

At present there are no established consultant pharmacist posts in service-led pharmacy, for example medicines information, technical services, although there are many recognised pharmacy experts in these areas. In the current financial climate, establishment of consultant posts must demonstrate clear outcomes for patient benefit that maximise use of resources in a difficult health economy.

Next steps

The introduction of a clinically based leadership role in pharmacy is greatly welcomed and supports the establishment of a flexible career pathway for pharmacists, benefiting patients by providing access to experts across localities and ensuring that good practice and expertise are disseminated. However, at present there is no formal mechanism for career development from the general level/early years of practice to higher-level practice. While these developments are much needed, it is crucial that they take account of the need for a flexible workforce and avoid the overspecialisation seen in the medical model.

The Department of Health guidance for consultant pharmacists has the key to flexible service development through use of the ACLF, which describes a majority of practice areas that are applicable to all pharmacists wishing to develop their practice. This is particularly relevant as most patients are supported by community-based pharmacists, whether in retail outlets or primary care, and there is a need for advanced generalists to fulfil these roles for more complex patients.

While the medical model of registrar development is well established, it suffers from the 'silo effect', where practitioners are required to undertake a complete registrar programme again if they wish to change specialities. A more flexible approach would be to engage the networks of expert pharmacy practitioners, whether general or specialist, in producing a curriculum of practice for advancing practitioners, up to consultant level, allowing those practitioners who wish to progress to complete the curriculum, however they choose to (which may be self-directed learning and/or through courses). If the practitioners also submitted evidence of achievement in the five non-expert clusters of the ACLF, this could then be assessed by the experts and contribute to the establishment of professional designations as nationally recognised levels of practice, reflecting these achievements. The Royal Pharmaceutical Society (the professional leadership body for pharmacy) has adopted this approach and is working with networks of expert practitioners to achieve this.

This discussion has focused on the NHS hospital sector. However, it has been shown that this can apply to primary and community pharmacy practitioners. The concept of higher-level practice also exists in industry, as the qualified person, and in academia through postgraduate Masters and Doctorate-level qualification, and it is not known whether there is benefit to establishing consultant-level practice outside the NHS.

Already those using the restricted title 'consultant pharmacist' are showing leadership in non-medical prescribing, where there is an external perception that all consultant pharmacists are prescribers (which is not the case). Leadership in risk management initiatives and managing antimicrobials has achieved outcomes for patient benefit. Consultant pharmacists are engaging in research into specific drugs such as melatonin, disease states such as delirium, broad therapeutic areas such as gene therapy and participating in technology appraisals for national bodies.

Conclusion

This chapter has outlined how the role of the consultant pharmacist has developed. Consultant pharmacists are working together, through regular meetings and e-mail networking, gathering data on their outputs and achievements. In 2010 there are around 40 of these posts but the question of how advanced practitioners or preconsultant ('registrar') posts will be developed is, as yet, unanswered.[9]

References

1. Department of Health. *Guidance for the Development of Consultant Pharmacist Posts*. London: Department of Health, 2005.
2. Antoniou S, Webb DG, McRobbie D *et al*. A controlled study of the general level framework: results of the south of England competency study. *Pharm Educ* 2005; 5: 201–207.
3. Competency Development and Education Group general-level framework. Available online at: http://www.codeg.org/fileadmin/codeg/pdf/glf/GLF_October_2007_Edition.pdf (accessed 27 August 2010).
4. Hebron B, Graham-Clarke E, Bleasdale J. The consultant clinical pharmacist's role. *Pharm J* 2003; 270: 261.
5. Competency Development and Education Group advanced-level framework. Available online at: http://www.codeg.org/fileadmin/codeg/pdf/ACLF.pdf (accessed 27 August 2010).
6. Department of Health. Comprehensive critical care. Available online at: http://www.dh.gov.uk/prod_consum_dh/groups/dh_digitalassets/@dh/@en/documents/digitalasset/dh_4082872.pdf 2000 (accessed 27 August 2010).

7. National AHP and HCS Critical Care Advisory Group. Critical care staffing guidance: a guideline for AHP and HCS staffing levels. Critical Care Programme Modernisation Agency. Available online at: http://www.ukcpa.org/ukcpadocuments/2.pdf (accessed 27 August 2010).

8. Department of Health. *Implementing Care Closer to Home – Providing Convenient Quality Care for Patients: A National Framework for Pharmacists with a Special Interest*. London: Department of Health, 2006.

9. Barnett NL, Mason J, Stephens M. Meeting the needs of our patients – the case for pharmacist 'registrars'. *Pharm J* 2009; 283: 71–72.

Further reading

CoDEG website: http://www.codeg.org/.

Department of Health. *Guidance for the Development of Consultant Pharmacist Posts*. London: Department of Health, 2005.

19

Managing services

Pippa Roberts

Introduction

Preregistration trainees and newly registered pharmacists entering hospital pharmacy may have given little consideration to their potential future roles as managers. At this early stage of a hospital pharmacist's career, attention will usually be focused on gaining experience in a broad range of pharmacy services and having the opportunity to apply knowledge to practical situations. Many pharmacists will have aspirations to work in a clinical setting where they are able to operate as part of a clinical team, directly contributing to the management and care of patients.

Junior pharmacists look to their managers to provide them with training opportunities, guidance and support. There will be a reasonable expectation that their managers will be experienced, knowledgeable and accessible, and able to provide a continuous and dependable source of ready-made solutions to problems they encounter. Junior pharmacists will probably have little appreciation of the wide range of leadership and management skills that their managers have acquired and are using for their benefit.

So what is the difference between leadership and management and are both skills required when you are responsible for the whole or part of the pharmacy service? There has been much written on this subject and this short chapter cannot, and is not intended to, do it justice. In summary, leadership is more concerned with finding direction and purpose in the face of critical challenges, whereas managing is about organising to achieve desired purposes efficiently, effectively and creatively. Leaders ensure vision is developed and conveyed to the whole team. A good manager will require leadership skills, but leadership must be displayed by staff at all levels if they are to navigate local circumstances and deliver the best care possible for an individual or group of patients.

Progression up the career ladder, beyond the rotational training grades, will lead to appointment to posts, with an increasing management component within them that may involve staff management and/or responsibility for a section of the service. Indeed, it is rare to find jobs from *Agenda for Change* band 7 upwards[1] that do not have certain elements of managerial tasks within them, with management and clinical practice becoming increasingly entwined as clinical pharmacists need to align their practice to organisational objectives. This is the stage of a pharmacist's career pathway when he or she must acquire the ability to balance managerial responsibility with the stimulation of working in a clinical setting, as pharmacists are expected to deliver change to the way pharmaceutical care is provided to large groups of patients rather than simply those under their direct care on a ward or in a clinic. Some of the skills needed for a role in management are listed in Table 19.1.

Table 19.1 Attributes for managers

Personal qualities
  Strong leader
  Self-motivated
  Proactive
  Copes with conflicting pressures
  Team player
  Able to work in multidisciplinary environment

Skills and abilities
  Presentation skills
  Communication skills – oral and written
  Personal time management
  Analytical skills
  Project management
  Devise, plan and manage complex work programme
  Numeracy and computer-literacy skills

Managing staff
  Individual performance review
  Personal development plans
  Continuing professional development
  Disciplinary procedures
  Workforce planning
  Recruitment and retention

Business planning
  Writing business cases
  Project management
  Budget-setting and management
  Financial skills

Experience
  Evidence of working in relevant settings
  Knowledge of National Health Service

This chapter is intended to provide an appreciation of the roles pharmacy managers undertake within the pharmacy department and how they interact with other managers and clinicians in the wider hospital environment. It also provides some insights into the recruitment process and provides some advice to support newly qualified and junior pharmacists when applying and being interviewed for new posts.

Pharmacy management

The National Health Service (NHS) is sometimes criticised for employing excessive numbers of managers whose existence diverts resources away from front-line clinical services. In reality, hospitals are extremely complex organisations that depend on experienced, well-trained managers and clinicians with good management skills for the development and delivery of high-quality, efficient and patient-centred services. Hospital pharmacy departments, albeit on a much smaller scale, are also complex, offering a wide selection of services provided by professional, technical and support staff often over a number of different hospital sites and in community clinics. Pharmacy managers, working at different levels in the department, make a critical contribution to patient care by applying a wide variety of skills, expertise and experience to the delivery and development of clinical and support services that are compatible with the overall aims of the hospital.

Overall managerial responsibility for the pharmacy service will rest with the NHS trust's chief pharmacist who will be accountable to a senior manager, often one of the executive directors. The chief pharmacist will also be accountable to the trust's board of directors for all aspects of medicines management, including the safe procurement, storage, handling, distribution and use of all medicines throughout the hospital. This responsibility encompasses the need to ensure that all practice involving medicines complies with current legislation, NHS rules and regulations, and nationally accepted statutory clinical protocols and good practice guidelines. This includes the regulatory standards for medicines management introduced by the Care Quality Commission in 2010.[2] Also included are corporate governance requirements that necessitate probity and financial control within all aspects of the organisation's day-to-day business. Additionally, the chief pharmacist will be responsible for pharmacy's contribution to the clinical governance agenda. This requires that all patients receive the highest possible standard of care, that practice is evidence-based, delivered by appropriately trained and qualified staff and that risks to patients during their treatment are minimised. Chief pharmacists are expected to take action if any aspect of the medicines-handling process in their organisation is not congruent with the aims of clinical governance and to escalate issues of concern within the organisation as required.

Effective management of pharmacy services demands high levels of leadership and team work. The chief pharmacist is not only required to lead the pharmacy service but also to act as an advocate for and representative of the service within the organisation as a whole. This will often mean that the chief pharmacist will spend considerable periods of time contributing to the wider trust agenda, becoming a respected part of the trust senior management team.

The two broad types of management that occur are generally referred to as strategic and operational management. As staff progress up the management ladder there should be an increasing shift away from substantially operational management to a significant element of strategic management. Hence, the strategic management role performed by the chief pharmacist should receive far more emphasis and time, and much of the operational workload should be delegated to deputies or department team leaders. Delegation is not only important to the chief pharmacist, but also ensures that the team can develop their own managerial capabilities. It is critical that the chief pharmacist has a vision about the future direction of the overall pharmacy service and can draw up plans for changing methods of service delivery. However, the entire management team must be developed to be able to contribute to the vision for the whole department and their own areas of responsibility if the vision is to be based on specialist practice, owned by those who will be charged with delivering the vision. In practice, the split between strategic and operational management undertaken by the chief pharmacist will be a balancing act, because, as the responsible person for medicines management, the chief pharmacist will be held to account if something goes wrong. As a result, the chief pharmacist must be confident that the systems and processes governing medicines in their trust are robust and applied in practice. This will require the development of leadership and management skills in members of the pharmacy team. A strong management team is essential if the chief pharmacist is to free up time to develop and market pharmacy services at a corporate level.

Operational management focuses on the wide range of functions which underpin the day-to-day smooth running of the pharmacy department; thus the chief pharmacist's leadership role will be supported by a team of senior pharmacists and technicians. These staff will take responsibility for major sections of the department, such as patient services, clinical pharmacy services, medicines information, aseptic dispensing, non-sterile and sterile production, quality assurance, procurement and stores. Such managers need to acquire a wide range of skills and expertise and will have the opportunity to attend training courses in order to develop and refine their management skills, but there is no substitute for gaining experience and developing expertise through performing the job, being given new tasks and experiences, and being supported to develop through constructive feedback and open two-way communication with a line manager.

A particularly positive development in the management of pharmacy services during the past decade has been the increasing number of pharmacy technicians and support staff who hold senior management positions within the pharmacy department. This recognises the significant contribution that these staff groups can make to managing key sections of the department, such as the dispensary, procurement, stores and distribution, or having overall site management responsibilities, and is an important means of providing support staff with improved prospects for career progression. This development also allows pharmacists to concentrate on clinical pharmacy services.

In summary, chief pharmacists and their senior management team hold considerable power, insofar as they can determine, negotiate and implement the future direction of the pharmacy service. Not only will a strong management team be able to make the best use of staff and resources, it will also be able to exert a strong influence beyond the confines of the pharmacy department in achieving a high profile for the service.

Business planning

An NHS trust is essentially a non-profit-making business whose chief executive and board are accountable for delivering high, safe standards of care for its patients through the effective and efficient use of resources within an agreed annual budget. Each year trusts undertake a business-planning exercise. Within each NHS trust the business-planning process is intended to align trust services with national priorities and local priorities. National priorities are described each year by the Department of Health in a document called the NHS operating framework, and primary and secondary care organisations must plan their services with this in mind. Local priorities will be dictated by the additional requirements of those commissioning the services (primary care trusts at the time of writing but soon to be general practitioner consortia) and these will depend on demographics and epidemiology in the local health economy as well as the specialist services that the trust provides.

For an NHS trust the primary objective of the business-planning process is to describe its vision and to develop organisational objectives that will support the delivery of that vision. Chapter 1 described the organisational arrangements of trusts – divisions or directorates making up the whole. Divisional and directorate objectives will be developed which then support the trust objectives, and the pharmacy objectives should be derived from these and other documents which relate to the quality, safety and the professional pharmacy agenda. It is important that all staff have an annual appraisal and have their own objectives agreed which are derived from the pharmacy business plans so that staff are clear what they are required to deliver during the year and how their work supports the trust's plan.

Preparing a business case

The business-planning process is often underpinned by a requirement to prepare a detailed business case that provides a thorough analysis of the implications for changing or developing services. Not only will a business case be used to judge the merits of the specific proposal and how it contributes to the delivery of trust objectives and performance targets, it may also be compared with business cases from other departments or directorates as part of a prioritisation exercise. Pharmacy managers need, therefore, to muster all their skills, knowledge and expertise to produce a well-reasoned, robust case which can withstand detailed scrutiny and then market the benefits of the changes that any funding will bring. Understanding the intended recipient of the case is vital – what are their priorities and objectives?

In most business cases it is expected that a range of options will be described. These may range from the 'do nothing' approach to an option that requires the highest level of funding in terms of capital investment and revenue consequences. The business case will need to be well argued, show a detailed financial analysis and, perhaps most importantly, set out the benefits to the organisation and to patients.

Financial management

The total annual budget for a hospital trust will vary greatly depending on the size of the organisation. About 70% of a trust's expenditure will be taken up in staff costs. Medicines expenditure will account for about 15–50% of the remaining non-staff expenditure depending upon the nature of the services provided (for example, the provision of human immunodeficiency virus services can increase the proportion of medicine costs). Not surprisingly, managing and controlling medicines expenditure is often given high priority by hospital management teams; Chapter 11 addresses this issue.

Trust managers will expect the chief pharmacist to take responsibility for all aspects of financial management relating to pharmacy services and the organisation's medicines budget. This requires the ability to obtain sufficient resources to maintain and develop services and to respond to the introduction of new services arising from changing trust priorities. It means working with the pharmacy team to ensure that pharmacy services are as efficient as they can be, that they deliver value for money and that the contributions made are recognised at trust level. With the increasing emphasis on efficiency savings in the NHS, budgetary management cannot be solely the responsibility of the chief pharmacist, and specialist pharmacists in particular will be essential to the delivery of savings in drugs budgets.

Budgets are set on an annual basis, although some changes may be incorporated during the financial year, particularly where changes to staffing levels have been agreed or cost improvements have been delivered. The chief pharmacist, as the budget-holder, will be expected to ensure that expenditure does not exceed the agreed budget. Income and expenditure used for pay and non-pay costs during the year are described in financial terms as revenue. Capital is used for the construction of new or refurbished facilities or the purchase of new equipment. Availability of capital depends on the organisation delivering a surplus – income exceeding costs – unless specific funds are made available for the NHS or from charities.

In many trusts, the chief pharmacist will be expected to be involved in the contracting process that occurs between the commissioner (primary care trusts at the time of writing, but soon to be general practitioner consortia) and the hospital (the provider) to ensure that sufficient money (income) is gained to cover the full cost of providing services (expenditure). The chief pharmacist can, with the support of his or her team of specialists, bring valuable expertise to the contracting negotiations in relation to the predicted medicines expenditure for the year ahead.

Within the organisation, an NHS hospital trust will normally devolve the budget to the individual clinical and non-clinical directorates or divisions. Directorate/divisional managers will have responsibility for managing their budgets and for developing their own business plans and constructing budgets with their finance advisers to cover their services. The crucial role of the chief pharmacist, supported by the rest of the pharmacy management team, is to act as an advocate for the pharmacy service and ensure that sufficient resources are available to maintain and develop services in line with the overall direction and objectives of the directorates and the trust. This will invariably require the application of considerable negotiating skills to secure an appropriate share of limited resources. As new hospital services are identified and developed, the chief pharmacist will need to ensure that their impact on the pharmacy service has been properly assessed and, where appropriate, additional resources are allocated. This requires the chief pharmacist to be well connected and informed at a corporate level to avoid overlooking pharmacy service costs.

Within the current financial climate, with the quality–productivity challenge, chief pharmacists are expected, with their teams, to think differently about the way services are delivered so that pharmacy services deliver more in terms of quality and breadth of service for less expenditure. Although a proactive approach to service development may not always be successful, a positive outcome is more likely to be achieved when pharmacy managers recognise that strategic planning aligned to the trust objectives is essential. Requesting realistic funding for new services or managing to deliver a change in service provision without the need for additional funding will also enhance the pharmacy team's reputation and increase success in these negotiations.

Staffing budgets

Staffing levels vary greatly between trusts. The staffing establishment will comprise professional, technical, ancillary, administrative and clerical staff, as well as pharmacist and technician trainees. As often staff work on a part-time basis, the number of people employed, known as the head count, will generally exceed the number of established whole-time-equivalent posts (WTEs). A ratio of 1:1:1 (pharmacist : technicians : others) has been suggested as an appropriate balance.[3]

The final staffing budget will be calculated on the agreed staffing establishment for the department, measured as WTEs. The budget will reflect the grades, salaries and allowances, such as emergency duty commitments, for each staff member and will also include the employer's overhead costs, such as national insurance and superannuation (pension) payments. A hospital pharmacy with a staff of 160 WTEs will have an annual budget of about £4.5 million.

When managers experience difficulty in filling vacant posts on a long-term permanent basis they may rely on the availability of temporary staff supplied by locum agencies. Such staff are more expensive than permanent staff and present a particular challenge for budgetary management and for maintaining the morale of the permanent staff members. The financial position in the NHS currently means that in many trusts agency staff are not employed and existing staff resources have to cover services or discussions occur about service reductions.

Medicines budgets

As part of a trust's annual business-planning process, pharmacy managers, in collaboration with their directorate pharmacists, should be involved in the estimation of medicines budgets for the forthcoming year. The primary purpose of this exercise will be to set budgets that have been adjusted for the impact of a variety of critical factors and influences. These may include anticipated changes in clinical activity and case mix, the potential impact of new – invariably more expensive – recently licensed drugs, changes in drug treatment preferences, savings from negotiated purchasing contracts and, conversely, increases in the acquisition costs of medicines. Although it would be extremely difficult to achieve total accuracy in the budget-setting process, it is important to achieve a level of confidence in the budgets so that a greater commitment to effective expenditure control can be maintained during the financial year. This is also important for the ex-tariff medicines (see Chapter 1 for an explanation of ex-tariff medicines).

Benchmarking

Managers working at all levels of the organisation have an obligation to ensure that their services are continually reviewed and adapted to meet the changing needs of patients and staff. In the current NHS climate where productivity and efficiency need to be maximised, benchmarking has become increasingly recognised as a valuable management tool for assessing the performance of a service and identifying opportunities for developing better services and using staff more effectively and efficiently.[4, 5] An important feature of benchmarking is the comparison with other similar-sized hospitals or services, as this allows managers to consider alternative ways of planning and delivering their services based on the wider experience of others.

The primary aim of a benchmarking exercise is to use and collect data to provide quantitative and, preferably, qualitative means of measuring performance through the production of a range of indicators, which can be compared with other similar organisations. Benchmarks for pharmacy are produced by combining, for example, clinical activity, workload data and staffing information to produce indicators such as the number of staff per 1000 inpatient bed days or 1000 outpatient attendances. These indicators can then be used both to compare different hospitals and to produce annual trend data for an individual hospital.

As previously described, the hospital pharmacy service is characterised by the number of posts in the staffing establishment, measured as WTEs. The establishment will comprise professional, technical, administrative and clerical staff, as well as pharmacist and technician trainees. The numbers, grades and types of staff employed are commonly referred to as the skill mix. The process of reviewing the composition and size of the staffing establishment is known as workforce planning. The aim should be to achieve a staffing establishment and skill mix in the department that suit the size, complexity and clinical activity of the hospital and the demands and workloads placed on the pharmacy service; benchmarking information is a useful tool to support this.

Local intelligence must be used when reviewing all benchmarking data, as it is important to ensure similar services are being compared. Ideally, benchmarks should be sufficiently sensitive to demonstrate whether gaps in service provision may lead to less effective medicines management and increased risk for patients, but often quantitative data will not on their own be able to provide this level of sophistication. For example, the quantitative data may show that one service runs with half of the staffing costs of its neighbouring hospital but it may be that the more expensive trust provides services under service level agreements to other organisations or that the lack of trained, experienced clinical pharmacists in the 'more efficient' organisation may reduce the quality of prescription intervention monitoring, provide insufficient prescribing support for the junior doctors and reduce the ability to implement the formulary and thus contain medicine expenditure. Similarly, within the pharmacy department, an inadequate staffing establishment required to manage dispensing workloads may cause increased error rates. It is important to remember when interpreting benchmarking information that the natural position for any staff member to take is that the information provided is inaccurate or inappropriate and to defend the existing staffing or service position. However, chief pharmacists and other pharmacy team leaders must look at information gathered and review comparisons with an open mind to ensure efficiency opportunities are not overlooked. Involving team members in the data collection can help to support the robustness and acceptability of data used to provide benchmarking information.

Staff management

This is where leadership and management are the most closely entwined. Developing the staff and aligning them with the business needs of the organisation is probably the single most difficult and least predictable aspect of management, being the most challenging, the most frustrating and the most rewarding all at once. It is also the aspect of management that has historically received the least attention, frequently regarded as common sense and not requiring special training. Whereas other aspects of managers' jobs are thought to require qualifications and training, the human aspect, competence in handling and getting the best out of people, was all too frequently regarded as something that develops automatically without help: this can be a serious and potentially costly error. The ability of a manager, at any level, to lead a group of staff, create a vision, sell that vision, engage staff in how the vision will be delivered and then manage the implementation plan needs a level of self and team awareness that can be developed with training and feedback. Leading and managing a team effectively can be difficult and can make a manager feel isolated at times if decisions have to be made which are right for patients and service development but are unpopular with staff. Leadership is the subject of much narrative and broad reading with self-reflection as well as formal training and the support of a good manager can help leadership skills develop. The NHS leadership qualities framework provides a structured approach to the elements of leadership, although identifying the elements and performing as a good leader are not the same.[6]

Selection strategy

The starting point for the management of others is the selection of the right person for each job advertised.

Every pharmacist with responsibility for recruitment from preregistration onwards needs to be skilled in staff selection. Pharmacists will have access to expert advice and assistance on policies and procedures from human resource colleagues, but they will not take over the responsibilities of the employing manager. The pharmacy team's performance remains the ultimate responsibility of the chief pharmacist, but at all management levels an individual's performance will only be as good as the performance of the team – so getting the right people in the team is crucial to success.

The ability to choose the right person for the right job with the skills to complement the rest of the team is essential. A review of the ability of the pharmacy team to deliver its objectives must be undertaken before a post is advertised. The following questions should be considered before the recruitment process begins, so that the manager has considered whether the post in its current format is needed or whether a different post or professional could fulfil the current requirements:

- What kind of team does the pharmacy department currently have?
- What roles does the department need individuals within the team to fulfil?
- What skills are needed to meet the departmental objectives?
- What skills are currently present in the team members and what are the gaps?
- What type of professional is needed to fill the gap role and so what changes in team composition are required?
- What personal dynamics does the group entail?

Often, an important source of information about the purpose and function of the pharmacy team comes from the pharmacy business plan and trust objectives. Other issues to be considered include service developments on the horizon, potential workload volume changes, structural changes in the health service, professional developments and political changes. A chief pharmacist or pharmacy team manager must have a clear vision of both service and team development if he or she is to create a team with the ability to meet its objectives. Once the role and skills needed are decided the next step is producing the right job description.

Job analysis, job description and personnel specification

Before placing a job advertisement, the job description and person specification should be reviewed to ensure they describe the role accurately – new staff members will quickly become disillusioned if the post for which they have applied does not undertake the role as described in practice. Table 19.2 illustrates the criteria used to analyse a job and award its pay banding in the national *Agenda for Change* pay scales using a points system. The job description should describe the role to be undertaken and state the job-holder's responsibilities and authority level. Usually the accountability (who manages the post) is stated. There is no standard format for job descriptions in the NHS, although local templates are usually developed in departments or trusts. Additional sheets can be added to the back of these forms by applicants for extra supporting information. When a job advertisement generates a large

Table 19.2 *Agenda for Change* role criteria and relevant job information

Factor	Relevant job information
Communication and relationship skills	Details the provision and receipt of information and how complex it is, what barriers need to be overcome by the post-holder and how much agreement/cooperation may be required
Knowledge, training and experience	What are the qualifications, theoretical and practical knowledge and experience needed for the role?
Analytical and judgement skills	What level of complexity of facts requires comparison and interpretation by the post-holder?
Planning and organisational skills	Is there a range of planning required in the role? Over short- or long-term timescales and with what level of adjustment?
Physical skills	What physical skills obtained through practice are needed in the role? For example, are keyboard skills used, or is there manipulation of pharmaceuticals?
Responsibility for patient care	What is the level of clinical care provided and is there accountability for services?
Responsibility for policy/service development	Is there responsibility in the role for policy development or simply the implementation of policy developed by others?
Responsibility for financial and physical resources	What is the range of financial responsibilities, including budgetary responsibilities?
Responsibility for human resources	Does the post-holder manage or supervise staff?
Responsibility for information resources	Is the post-holder responsible for the provision of information, and what type?
Responsibility for research and development	Does the role involve research or audit?
Freedom to act	What discretion does the post-holder have to work alone?
Physical effort	What level of effort is required – mainly sitting, walking, moving objects or people?
Mental effort	How much concentration is required and what are the levels of interruptions?
Emotional effort	How distressing is the role? Is the post-holder dealing with emotional circumstances regularly?
Working conditions	How often is the post-holder exposed to unpleasant conditions, e.g. body fluids, cytotoxics?

response rate it is easier for the shortlisting team to find all of the information pertaining to an applicant in one place rather than certain elements on an application form and the remainder on an accompanying curriculum vitae which repeats much of the information on the form.

A person specification will also be provided for any role advertised and this will identify the characteristics of the future post-holder. This includes the skills, knowledge, experience, qualifications and attributes needed, but also the personal characteristics that are required in the successful candidate. A person specification will describe the essential minimum standards for the post as well as the desirable qualities that the best candidates may have. The essential criteria for the post will, with the job description, have resulted in the *Agenda for Change* pay scale of the post and so, to be appointed, a candidate must possess all of the descriptors in the essential criteria. These criteria are often separated into two categories in the person specification: (1) A, to be demonstrated in the application form; and (2) I, to be demonstrated at interview. It is important for applicants to ensure that they provide supporting information to indicate that they meet any criteria described as 'application form essential' in order to secure an interview. If a number of applicants meet the essential criteria and the recruiters wish to restrict the numbers of candidates interviewed, they may eliminate candidates based on the criteria that are classified desirable that are requested at the application form stage.

It is also useful to remember that a person specification will often cite written communication skills as a criterion to be demonstrated at the application stage and for this reason application forms containing typographical errors and those not coherently structured may be cast aside. In addition a form should not simply regurgitate the criteria in the specification. Many applicants will state that they are self-motivated, enthusiastic and have good organisational or team skills without providing examples of past experience to demonstrate this. It is for this reason that an application for any job needs to be well prepared and it is advisable for applicants to ask someone to review the form before it is submitted. This can be a review by a friend to check for typos and understanding or it may be particularly useful to find someone who is regularly involved in recruitment to give advice and guidance.

Advertising

The aim of an advertisement is to ensure a good range of applicants at a reasonable cost. The choice of advertising medium is important: the *Pharmaceutical Journal* is the obvious choice for pharmacist posts but local papers and in-house hospital magazines can be better for other staff groups. Expense may prohibit this in many organisations and the NHS jobs website is now commonly used to advertise a range of pharmacy posts. Candidates looking for specific roles or jobs in specific areas can sign up for alerts from the website to their work or home e-mail. The content of the advertisement should encourage suitable people to apply and discourage those who are not suitable. The information needs to be informative and yet remain clear and concise. A telephone number is normally given through which further information can be obtained.

It is advisable that a potential applicant calls to make enquiries regarding a job. This will familiarise the employer with the name of an applicant and a little bit about them, which is a useful ice-breaker during an interview if an applicant is called for one. If applying for a senior position, it is advisable to visit the department and get a feel for the job and the team dynamics. While it is important that the department wants the candidate to be part of that team, it is essential that the applicant feels comfortable with the line manager, the team and the strategic direction of the department. For an appointment to be successful it needs to be 'best fit' for both the applicant and the employer.

When the interview stage arrives, candidates should be clear that they would accept the post if the terms and conditions are suitable and they are offered it. It is frustrating for an interview panel to offer a post to a candidate who has decided he or she does not want the job but cannot offer a reasonable explanation for this decision.

Methods of selection

Most candidates for pharmacy posts will be chosen following an interview. It is often difficult to relax at interview but it is important that the candidate is open and honest so that the panel can assess accurately the personality of the individual and previous experience. An experienced interview panel should help put a candidate at ease and will describe the framework for the interview before it starts. If candidates have questions that they wish to ask there is usually time allocated at the end. It is advisable that a candidate makes a list before arriving at the interview as these questions may be forgotten in the pressure of the moment. When preparing for interview there are some standard questions that are often asked and can be anticipated by the candidate. Answers should not simply be regurgitated but some preparation should help the interviewee relax while providing some easy wins. Common themes include:

- summarising career and achievements to date
- why does the candidate have a particular interest in the job advertised?
- what will the candidate bring to the post?

In addition, the person specification can provide hints towards the other questions that may be asked. Criteria in the person specification that are recorded as 'I for interview' should be assessed by questioning or via a presentation during the interview. It is important to listen carefully to the questions posed to ensure that the answers are appropriate, concise, honest and do not meander. It is acceptable to pause before answering a question to think of the best response or consider the most appropriate example when replying to a question, rather than rushing in to provide an answer and then being less coherent with the final reply.

It is now common practice to ask candidates to give a presentation, usually at the beginning of the interview. This will help identify the candidate's communication, presentation and influencing skills. It is important that the candidate keeps to the allotted time and remembers mainly to discuss the pharmaceutical aspects of the subject rather than providing lots of background information, as this will be what will interest the panel.

Prioritisation exercises present candidates with a selection of situations that they are required to place in order of priority. It is usual to be able to ask for points of clarification or explanation in these exercises to aid prioritisation, to show that impulsive decisions are not being made before all the facts are known.

Sometimes candidates may be invited to meet informally with departmental or other trust staff prior to the interview during what is often described as 'trial by buffet'. This is usually reserved for more senior appointments. For the successful candidate it is the first step towards building relationships with new colleagues and so it is important to circulate during the session and speak to as many of the staff as possible.

Psychometric testing is sometimes used in senior management appointments in a hospital, although the costs and availability of trained personnel needed to administer and analyse the tests limit their use.

Recruitment and retention

The national shortage of pharmacists has left every branch of the profession with vacancies. The hospital sector has had to compete with higher rates of pay for junior pharmacists in the community sectors of the profession and attractive locum rates of pay. Furthermore, the establishment of prescribing adviser roles in primary care trusts has provided some of the clinical opportunities seen within the hospital sector without the unsociable hours required to meet the 7-day nature of busy acute trusts. There are also issues with the recruitment and retention of technicians resulting from their expanding roles and the creation of new posts during the past decade.

Much work has been undertaken by managers across the hospital sector to improve recruitment and retention. Senior hospital pharmacist and technician posts at more senior levels of *Agenda for Change* scales are more attractive if juniors take a longer-term view of their career pathway. Other local enhancements are offered in some organisations to attract the juniors for future progression. A greater emphasis has been placed on providing vacation work for undergraduates. For some time the extensive undergraduate programme developed by Boots has successfully resulted in the attraction of newly qualified pharmacists into their employment. In many hospitals a training package for vacation students has been established to offer experience in many aspects of the services provided by hospital pharmacy departments.

Rotational training programmes have been established by managers to encourage applicants and to improve retention within the hospital sector, and many organisations will offer a guaranteed postgraduate clinical diploma place as part of their recruitment strategy. The myth that it is difficult to transfer to the hospital sector once a community or industrial career has been started is being dispelled now and the skills offered by many pharmacists from other branches of the profession are welcomed within UK hospitals. Work is being undertaken by many hospital managers to develop accelerated clinical induction packages which will develop the clinical knowledge required for a role in hospital pharmacy while recognising other well-developed and valuable skills on offer from a colleague who has previously only practised outside the hospital sector.

One of the major attractions of a career in hospital pharmacy is the well-developed roles of support staff. Skill mix management has progressed over recent years, with technical staff taking on more and more of the non-clinical roles previously held by pharmacists. This is a positive direction as it leads to retention of good technical staff and releases pharmacists' time to deal with more in-depth clinical issues at a ward level. Dispensaries in some hospitals are run as 'pharmacist-free' zones. Pharmacists are becoming more involved in multidisciplinary team working at a ward level, attending ward rounds, giving prescribing advice to medical staff or practising as independent prescribers themselves, providing administration advice to nursing staff and getting involved in aspects of discharge planning such as preparing discharge prescriptions on behalf of the multidisciplinary team.

Flexible working arrangements are a common feature of hospital pharmacies: job-sharing, part-time hours, modified start and finish times, career breaks and so on. There is also a growing need to meet the needs of patients and other clinical staff better by providing services beyond conventional working hours.

As well as attracting staff, retaining them is an important part of a manager's role. One aspect of this is to provide a comprehensive induction programme for new appointees. The length and nature of the induction programme will depend on the appointee's experience and post. Typical features will be an introduction to colleagues, an overview of the departmental and trust structures, information about trust and pharmacy policies, procedures and guidelines, essential health and safety information and training at a ward and dispensary level.

Staff appraisal

Under the *Agenda for Change* pay system all staff are required to demonstrate that they have core and role-specific competencies (the knowledge and skills framework) and have met their objectives to pass through what is described, under the system, as the foundation gateway and receive their incremental pay award at the end of the first year. As a result an initial induction should be followed up by regular reviews during the first year as the manager must support the individual to pass through this gateway by agreeing clear objectives with the new staff member and ensuring he or she has a personal development plan which enables him or her to achieve the necessary criteria. An annual appraisal is essential thereafter to review performance, celebrate successes, agree objectives or targets and identify training needs to support the employee's achievement for the coming year.

Management of misconduct

Ensuring the best staff are appointed, retained and developed are all important roles for the pharmacy manager but occasionally things go wrong. Trusts have disciplinary procedures to deal with misconduct and personnel departments provide help and advice to managers. The first step for minor problems (for example, lateness) will be to counsel the staff member; this is not considered part of the formal process, but does give an opportunity for improvement. Discussion is confidential, based on evidence and will give the member of staff an opportunity to explain his or her viewpoint. Clear timescales, expected standards and review dates have to be specified and agreed with the staff member. If improvement is not achieved or if a more serious matter occurs, the formal steps of the disciplinary policy will be followed. Usually the steps are: verbal warning, written warning, final warning, dismissal. However, for theft, assault or other very serious acts (usually called gross misconduct), dismissal may follow the first event. Those undertaking performance management or addressing misconduct are well advised to ensure written records are kept – even if counselling or a verbal warning is given it is important to confirm this to the member of staff involved.

Sickness

On appointment, staff will be reviewed by occupational health staff to check suitability for employment. Inevitably, staff have periods of sickness from time to time. Their manager should be aware of these episodes and ensure appropriate certificates are completed and records made upon the employee's return to work. The aim of any trust sickness absence (sometimes called attendance capability) policy is to support staff to attend work and achieve their maximum potential whilst they are there. Support from the hospital's occupational health department can be provided if needed and should be proactively advocated to support staff and prevent sickness absence rather than being seen as the place where staff are 'sent' when their attendance is poor. Work itself can cause sickness – stress or physical problems – so such causes need to be identified and addressed. When underlying disease or disability is identified as the cause, efforts should be made to adapt the job to retain the employee – an aspect of encouraging diversity in the workplace. Repeated incidents of sickness absence and therefore the ability of the employee to fulfil the role for which he or she was employed may result in the formal stages of the procedure being implemented and can result in dismissal.

Conclusion

The need for good leadership within pharmacy is vital for the success of the pharmacy service. The responsibility for leading a complex pharmacy service in a changing environment is challenging, but seeing success, providing good care and developing people and practice can be extremely rewarding. Under *Agenda for Change*, the pay scales allow for senior advancement in purely clinical roles and many pharmacists may not find the senior management positions, with the pressures that go with the associated responsibility, as a less attractive option than in previous years. It is important to recognise, however, that even solely clinical posts will require leadership and management skills for the post-holder to be successful and so whatever route an individual takes, these skills must be developed. The Audit Commission emphasised the importance of the role of the chief pharmacist and succession planning is essential if chief and deputy posts are to continue to be filled with those who are enthusiastic to advance pharmacy services and protect the reputation of the profession.[7] The growth in spending on medicines and the risks associated with their use add to the need for high-quality managers. The satisfaction of knowing that you have improved care for large numbers of patients through changes in service provision or developed large numbers of staff should always make these roles an option when planning a career pathway.

References

1. Department of Health. *Agenda for Change, Modernising the NHS Pay System*. London: The Stationery Office, 1999.
2. Care Quality Commission. *Essential Standards of Quality and Safety*. London: Care Quality Commission, 2010.
3. Department of Health. *Improving Working Lives for the Pharmacy Team*. London: Department of Health, 2001.
4. Campbell D, Fowler A. Benchmarking: concepts and frameworks. *Pharm Manage* 2001; 17: 52–55.
5. Campbell D, Fowler A. Benchmarking: project planning and implementation. *Pharm Manage* 2001; 17: 56–59.
6. The NHS leadership qualities framework. Available online at: http://www.nhsleadershipqualities.nhs.uk/ (accessed 18 August 2010).
7. Audit Commission. *A Spoonful of Sugar – Medicines in NHS Hospitals*. London: Audit Commission, 2001.

Further reading

Blanchard K, Johnson S. *One Minute Manager*. New York: Harper Collins, 2000.

Covey S. *Principle Centred Leadership*. London: Simon & Schuster, 1999.

Department of Health National Leadership Council. Available online at: http://www.dh.gov.uk/ en/Aboutus/HowDHworks/BoardsandCommittees/NationalLeadershipCouncil/index.htm (accessed 27 August 2010).

Gareth L. *Mentoring Manager*. London: Institute of Management, 2000.

Iles V. *Really Managing Healthcare*. Buckingham: Open University Press, 2001.

Pedlar M, Burgoyne J, Boydell TA. *A Manager's Guide to Leadership*. Berkshire: McGraw-Hill Professional, 2004.

Smith B. Using the Lean approach to transform pharmacy services in an acute trust. *Pharm J* 2009; 282: 457–461.

Further reading

Index